Ding-Geng (Din) Chen and Karl E. Peace

Applied Meta-Analysis with R and Stata, Second Edition

Chapman & Hall/CRC Biostatistics Series

Series Editors:
Shein-Chung Chow
Duke University School of Medicine, USA

Byron Jones
Novartis Pharma AG, Switzerland

Jen-pei Liu
National Taiwan University, Taiwan

Karl E. Peace
Georgia Southern University, USA

Bruce W. Turnbull
Cornell University, USA

Bayesian Methods in Pharmaceutical Research
Emmanuel Lesaffre, Gianluca Baio, Bruno Boulanger

Biomarker Analysis in Clinical Trials with R
Nusrat Rabbee

Interface between Regulation and Statistics in Drug Development
Demissie Alemayehu, Birol Emir, Michael Gaffney

Innovative Methods for Rare Disease Drug Development
Shein-Chung Chow

Medical Risk Prediction Models: With Ties to Machine Learning
Thomas A Gerds, Michael W. Kattan

VReal-World Evidence in Drug Development and Evaluation
Harry Yang, Binbing Yu

Cure Models: Methods, Applications, and Implementation
Yingwei Peng, Binbing Yu

Bayesian Analysis of Infectious Diseases
COVID-19 and Beyond
Lyle D. Broemeling

Applied Meta-Analysis with R and Stata, Second Edition
Ding-Geng (Din) Chen and Karl E. Peace

For more information about this series, please visit: https://www.routledge.com/
Chapman–Hall-CRC-Biostatistics-Series/book-series/CHBIOSTATIS

Applied Meta-Analysis with R and Stata, Second Edition

Ding-Geng (Din) Chen and Karl E. Peace

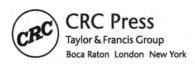

CRC Press
Taylor & Francis Group
Boca Raton London New York

CRC Press is an imprint of the
Taylor & Francis Group, an **informa** business

A CHAPMAN & HALL BOOK

First edition published 2021
by CRC Press
6000 Broken Sound Parkway NW, Suite 300, Boca Raton, FL 33487-2742

and by CRC Press
2 Park Square, Milton Park, Abingdon, Oxon, OX14 4RN

ISBN: 978-0-367-18383-7 (hbk)
ISBN: 978-0-367-70934-1 (pbk)
ISBN: 978-0-429-06124-0 (ebk)

Typeset in Palatino
by codeMantra

To my parents and parents-in-law, who value higher education and hardwork, and to my wife, Ke, my son, John D. Chen, and my daughter, Jenny K. Chen, for their love and support.

Ding-Geng (Din) Chen

To the memory of my late mother, Elsie Mae Cloud Peace, my late wife, Jiann-Ping Hsu, and to my son, Christopher K. Peace, daughter-in-law, Ashley Hopkins Peace, and grandchildren, Camden and Henry.

Karl E. Peace

Contents

Preface for the Second Edition

Since the publication of the first edition (Chen and Peace, 2013), we have received extensive compliments on how well it was structured for use by meta-analysts in analyzing their own meta-data following the detailed step-by-step illustrations using R and R packages. We are also aware of excellent reviews from a variety of social media sources and professionals.

For example, all "Editorial Reviews," from the Journal of the American Statistical Association (December 2014), Journal of Applied Statistics (2014), Biometrics (September 2015), Psychometrika (Vol. 80, June 2015), Journal of Biopharmaceutical Statistics (2015), and ISCB News (59, June 2015): ... a well-written book suitable for graduate students and practitioners in the fields of medicine and health. This book should equally serve as a valuable reference regarding self-study and as a learning tool for related practitioners and biostatisticians, particularly those with little or no experience in using R to provide ...detailed, step-by-step explanations that make this book a nice reference. Larry Hedges, who perhaps more so than anyone stimulated greater use of and research in meta-analysis with his book published in the mid-1980s said about our first edition: "A useful book on meta-analysis in R is Chen and Peace (2013) although all the examples are all from medicine."

Dr. Oscar A. Linares, director of the Mathematical Medicine & Biostatistics Unit, at Plymouth Pharmacokinetic Modeling Study Group wrote:

I highly recommend this book to anyone doing meta-analysis in general, and meta-analysis with R, in particular. The book brings you up to speed quickly and the examples are relevant to actual research. Using R for meta-analysis in this book is like "standing on the shoulders of giants" as one does their work on meta-analysis (2014).

We have also received suggestions and comments for further improvement, among which is to add Stata to the new edition. Therefore, a feature of this second edition is to also illustrate data analyses using the Stata system. Thus, in this second edition, we have incorporated all suggestions and comments from enthusiastic readers and corrected all errors and typos in addition to including Stata programs for meta-analysis. The Stata programs appear in the last section as an appendix of each chapter corresponding to the subsections where analyses using R were performed.

Another major update is to change the way data are loaded into R. In the first edition, we used R package gdata to read the data set from an Excel book (named as dat4Meta.xls) where all data are stored. Many readers communicated to us that they had some difficulties in using gdata due to its dependence on Perl. Therefore, in this edition, we use R package readxl, a standalone package, to read the data from this Excel book using its function read_excel. The Excel book dat4Meta.xls is in the Microsoft version 97-2003 worksheet and we include a newer version (2007 and newer) dat4Meta.xlsx in this edition. Readers can also use read_excel to read both data into R for practice of the contents in this book as well as for their own meta-analysis in their future research.

We have updated the chapters. In Chapter 1, we combined Sections 1.1, 1.2, and 1.3 in the first edition into Section 1.1 now specifically for R, and included Section 1.2 to introduce Stata for meta-analysis. The simple simulation on multi-center studies is then changed from Section 1.4 in the first edition to Section 1.3 in this edition.

In Chapter 2, we deleted accesses to some databases that were no longer supported and updated the references to the Cochrane Collaborative using the most current links. Finally, we added a link to RISmed, a package that is very helpful in searching for and identifying articles for potential inclusion in meta-analyses.

In Chapter 3, we split the Section 3.3 (Data Analysis in R) into two sections in this edition. The new Section 3.3 is now "Meta-Analysis for Data from Cochrane Collaboration Logo" and the new Section 3.4 is "Meta-Analysis of Amlodipinne Trial Data." In Section 3.4, we updated the meta-analysis from R meta only to include meta-analysis using the metafor package as a comparison. We further updated the Sections 3.5 and 3.6 and included the Stata programs as an appendix for meta-analyses in this chapter.

In Chapter 4, we updated all the meta-analyses with the metafor package with additional Sections 4.2.1.5, 4.2.2.4, and 4.2.3.4. We included the Stata programs as an appendix for meta-analyses in this chapter.

In Chapter 5, we updated Section 5.2.3 and created a new section, i.e., Section 5.3 "Meta-Analysis of the Impact of Intervention." In this section, we included meta-analysis with the R package metafor to compare with the results from meta and the step-by-step calculation. With this new section, we updated the "Meta-Analysis of Tubeless vs Standard Percutaneous Nephrolithotomy" in Section 5.4 and in Section 5.5 "Discussion" we included the Stata programs as an appendix for meta-analyses in this chapter.

In Chapter 6, we split Section 6.3 (Step-by-Step Implementation in R) into two sections. The new Section 6.3 is now "Illustration with Cochrane Collaboration Logo Data - Binomial Data" and the new Section 6.4 is "Illustration with PCNL Meta-Data - Continuous Data." In both sections, we updated the meta-analysis from R meta and the step-by-step implementation in R to include meta-analysis using the metafor package as a comparison. We further updated Section 6.5 and included the Stata programs as an appendix for meta-analyses in this chapter.

We updated Chapter 7 on meta-regression with a different section structure: Section 7.1 "Data" describes the three meta-data sets; Section 7.2 "The Methods in Meta-Regression" holds the discussions of methods for meta-regression, which was Section 7.2.1 in the first edition; Section 7.3 "Meta-Analysis of BCG Data" is produced from Sections 7.2.2 and 7.2.3 in the first edition; Section 7.4 "Meta-Analysis of IHD Data" is updated from Section 7.3.1; Section 7.5 "Meta-Analysis of ADHD Data" is updated from Section 7.3.2 in the first edition. We updated Section 7.6 for discussion on meta-regression and included the Stata programs as an appendix for meta-analyses in this chapter.

Chapter 8 "Multivariate Meta-Analysis" is a new chapter, which is updated from Section 10.3 in the first edition. In this chapter, Section 8.1 described the models for the multivariate meta-analysis and the associated R package mvmeta. In Section 8.2, we introduced the bivariate meta-data from five clinical trials on periodontal disease, followed by meta-analyses with R package mvmeta in Section 8.3 and metafor in Section 8.4. We updated the discussions for multivariate meta-analysis in Section 8.5 and included the Stata programs as an appendix for meta-analyses in this chapter.

Chapters 9 to 12 are new chapters contributed from our colleagues: Dr. Hani Samawi, Haresh Rochani, Jingjing Yin, Lili Yu, and Abby Zhang. We invited Dr. Hani Samawi to contribute Chapter 9 on "Publication Bias in Meta-Analysis"; Dr. Haresh Rochani and Mario Keko to contribute Chapter 10 on "Strategies to Handle Missing Data in Meta-Analysis"; Dr. Jingjing Yin and Jing Kersey to contribute Chapter 11 on "Meta-Analysis for Evaluating Diagnostic Accuracy"; and Drs. Lili Yu and Abby Zhang to contribute Chapter 12 on "Network Meta-Analysis".

Dr. Hani Samawi is Acting Chair and Professor, and Drs. Lili Yu, JingJing Yin, and Haresh Rochani are Associate Professors in the Department of Biostatistics at the Jiann-Ping College of Public Health (JPHCOPH) at Georgia Southern University, Statesboro, GA 30460. Abby Zhang was assistant professor of Biostatistics in JPHCOPH at the time of writing and is now assistant professor of Biostatistics at Kennesaw State University. Jing Kersey (who subsequently received the DrPH in Biostatistics) and Mario Keko are doctorate students in biostatistics at JPHCOPH.

With these new chapters, the chapter on "Meta-Analysis for Rare Events" is now Chapter 13 and "Meta-Analyses with Individual Patient-Level Data versus Summary Statistics" is Chapter 14. We updated both chapters accordingly.

Chapter 15 is updated from "Other R Packages for Meta-Analysis" to "Other R/Stata Packages for Meta-Analysis" to include Stata. Specifically, we give a brief summary and comparison of the three R packages in Section 15.1. We further present methods to combine p-values from studies in Section 15.2. In Section 15.3, we introduce several R packages for meta-analysis of correlation coefficients and illustrate their applications to a real data set on land-use intensity across 18 gradients from nine countries. We complete this book with Section 15.4 in which we discuss additional R packages and Section 15.5 to discuss additional Stata packages for meta-analysis.

All R and Stata programs and data sets used in this book can be requested from Professor Ding-Geng (Din) Chen at DrDG.Chen@gmail.com. Readers can follow the R and Stata programs in each chapter to load the specific data from the Excel databook for practice. Also, readers may use and modify the R and Stata programs for their own applications. To facilitate the understanding of implementation in R, we annotated all the computing programs with comments and explanations starting with # (i.e., the R command for "comment") so that the readers can understand exactly the meaning of the corresponding R programs. Note that some of the R outputs are reformatted and modified to fit the pages and figures in finalizing the entire LaTeX document.

We would like to express our gratitude to many individuals. First, thanks to David Grubbs from Taylor & Francis for his encouragement in this new edition. Also, thanks to Fabio Valeri from the Institute of Primary Care, University of Zurich and University Hospital Zurich, Switzerland, who points out the errors we made in equations (3.9) and (3.10), which are now corrected. Huge thanks go to Manyun Liu, BASS Fellow in the Jiann-Ping Hsu College of Public Health, for her dedicated and valuable assistance in Stata.

Special thanks are due to Professors Robert Gentleman and Ross Ihaka, who created the R language with visionary open source code, as well as to the developers and contributing authors in the R community, for their endless efforts and contributed packages. We welcome any comments and suggestions on typos, errors, and future improvements about this book. Please contact Professor Ding-Geng (Din) Chen at email: DrDG.Chen@gmail.com.

Chapel Hill, NC, Ding-Geng (Din) Chen
Statesboro, GA, Karl E. Peace
September 09, 2020

Preface for the First Edition

In Chapter 8 of our previous book (Chen and Peace, 2010), we briefly introduced meta-analysis using R. Since then, we have been encouraged to develop an entire book on meta-analyses using R that would include a wide variety of applications – which is the theme of this book.

In this book we provide a thorough presentation of meta-analysis with detailed step-by-step illustrations on their implementation using R. In each chapter, examples of real studies compiled from the literature and scientific publications are presented. After presenting the data and sufficient background to permit understanding of the application, various meta-analysis methods appropriate for analyzing data are identified. Then analysis code is developed using appropriate R packages and functions to meta-analyze the data. Analysis code development and results are presented in a stepwise fashion. This stepwise approach should enable readers to follow the logic and gain an understanding of the analysis methods and the R implementation so that they may use R and the steps in this book to analyze their own meta-data.

Based on their experience in biostatistical research and teaching biostatistical meta-analysis, the authors understand that there are gaps between developed statistical methods and applications of statistical methods by students and practitioners. This book is intended to fill this gap by illustrating the implementation of statistical meta-analysis methods using R applied to real data following a step-by-step presentation style.

With this style, the book is suitable as a text for a course in meta-data analysis at the graduate level (Master's or Doctorate's), particularly for students seeking degrees in statistics or biostatistics. In addition, the book should be a valuable reference for self-study and a learning tool for practitioners and biostatisticians in public health, medical research universities, governmental agencies, and the pharmaceutical industry, particularly those with little or no experience in using R.

R has become widely used in statistical modeling and computing since its creation in the mid-1990s and it is now an integrated and essential software for statistical analyses. Becoming familiar with R is then imperative for the next generation of statistical data analysts. In Chapter 1, we present a basic introduction to the R system, where to get R, how to install R, and how to upgrade R packages. Readers who are already familiar with R may skip this chapter and go directly to any of the remaining chapters.

In Chapter 2, we provide an overview of the research protocols for meta-analysis. In Chapter 3, we provide an overall introduction to meta-analysis for both fixed-effects and random-effects models in meta-analysis. Two real data sets are introduced along with two commonly used R packages of meta and rmeta.

In Chapters 4 and 5, we present meta-analysis for specific data types. In Chapter 4, we consider meta-analysis with binary data. We begin this chapter with two real data sets. The first is a meta-analysis of "Statin Clinical Trials" to compare intensive statin therapy to moderate statin therapy in the reduction of cardiovascular outcomes. The second is a meta-analysis of five studies on Lamotrigine for the treatment of bipolar depression. In Chapter 5, we consider meta-analysis for continuous data. Similarly to Chapter 4, we introduce two published data sets. The first data set uses 6 studies on the impact of intervention. The second data set is of studies from the literature comparing tubeless to standard percutaneous nephrolithotomy.

Chapter 6 is on the development of measures to quantify heterogeneity as well as to test the significance of heterogeneity among studies in a meta-analysis. Continuing from Chapter 6 to explain heterogeneity in meta-analysis, Chapter 7 is to introduce meta-regression to explain extra heterogeneity (or the residual heterogeneity) using study-level moderators or study-level independent predictors. Three data sets are used in this chapter to illustrate the application of meta-regression with fixed-effects and random-effects meta-regressions. The first data set contains summary information from 13 studies on the effectiveness of BCG vaccine against tuberculosis. The second data set contains summary information from 28 studies on ischemic heart disease (IHD) to assess the association between IHD risk reduction and reduction in serum cholesterol. Both data sets are widely used in meta-regression as examples. We recompiled a third data set to assess whether the ability to inhibit motor responses is impaired for adolescents with attention-deficit hyperactivity disorder. The R library metafor is introduced in this chapter for both meta-analysis and meta-regression.

There are extensive discussions between individual-patient data (IPD) analysis and meta-analysis (MA) in the situations where IPD are accessible. Some favor IPD and others favor MA. So in Chapter 8, we make use of actual individual-level patient data on lamotrigine (obtained from the manufacturer) to treat bipolar depression to illustrate the pros and cons of IPD and MA. Simulations are conducted in this chapter to compare IPD with MA on efficiency. All demonstrated that both models yielded very comparable results. This chapter thus serves to further promote meta-analysis using study-level summary statistics. Without much loss in relative efficiency for testing treatment effect, MA is recommended since it is usually difficult to obtain original individual-level data and is costlier and more time-consuming.

All the methods presented to Chapter 8 are based on the theory of large sample approximations. For rare events, these methods usually break down. The typical remedies are to remove the studies with zero events from the meta-analysis, or add a small value as continuity correction, say 0.5, to the rare events which usually lead to biased statistical inferences. In Chapter 9, we use the well-known Rosiglitazone meta-analysis data to illustrate the bias and then introduce a novel confidence distributions approach for meta-analysis where two methods are implemented for meta-analysis of rare events. We conclude the book with Chapter 10 to review other specific R packages for meta-analysis.

All R programs and data sets used in this book can be requested from Professor Ding-Geng (Din) Chen at DrDG.Chen@gmail.com. Readers can refer to Section 1.3 to load the specific data from the Excel databook into R. Also readers may use and modify the R programs for their own applications. To facilitate the understanding of implementation in R, we annotated all the R programs with comments and explanations starting with # (i.e., the R command for "comment") so that the readers can understand exactly the meaning of the corresponding R programs. Note that some of the R outputs are reformatted and modified to fit the pages and figures in finalizing the entire LaTeX document.

We would like to express our gratitude to many individuals. First, thanks to David Grubbs from Taylor & Francis for his interest in the book and to Shashi Kumar for assistance in LaTeX. Also thanks to Dr. Gary Evoniuk (GlaxoSmithKline, NC), Ms. Suzanne Edwards (GlaxoSmithKline, NC), and Dr. Dungang Liu (Yale University, CT) for their suggestions and comments to Chapter 8, and to Professor Minge Xie (Rutgers University, NJ), Drs. Dungang Liu (Yale University, CT) and Guang Yang (Rutgers University, NJ) for their suggestions and comments to Chapter 9 as well as their wonderful job to produce the R package gmeta.

Special thanks are due to Professors Robert Gentleman and Ross Ihaka who created the R language with visionary open source, as well as to the developers and contributing authors in the R community for their endless efforts and contributed packages.

Finally, thanks go to Xinyan(Abby) Yan, our graduate assistant, for her dedicated and valuable assistance in compiling data sets, and to Dr. Nicole Trabold (University of Rochester, NY) for her careful reading of the book.

We welcome any comments and suggestions on typos, errors, and future improvements about this book. Please contact Professor Ding-Geng (Din) Chen at email: DrDG.Chen@gmail.com.

Rochester, NY, Ding-Geng (Din) Chen
Statesboro, GA, Karl E. Peace
December 12, 2012

Authors

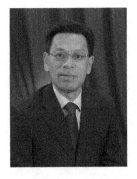

Ding-Geng (Din) Chen is a fellow of American Statistical Association and currently the Wallace H. Kuralt Distinguished Professor at the University of North Carolina-Chapel Hill, USA. Formerly, he was a Professor of Biostatistics at the University of Rochester, New York, USA, the Karl E. Peace Endowed Eminent Scholar Chair and professor in Biostatistics in the Jiann-Ping Hsu College of Public Health at Georgia Southern University, USA, and a professor of statistics at South Dakota State University, USA. Dr. Chen's research interests include clinical trial biostatistical methodological development in Bayesian models, survival analysis, multi-level modeling and longitudinal data analysis, and statistical meta-analysis. He has published more than 200 refereed papers and co-authored/co-edited 30 books in statistics.

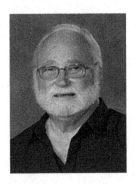

Karl E. Peace is the Georgia Cancer Coalition Distinguished Cancer Scholar, Founding Director of the Center for Biostatistics, Professor of Biostatistics, and Senior Research Scientist in the Jiann-Ping Hsu College of Public Health at Georgia Southern University (GSU). Dr. Peace has made pivotal contributions in the development and approval of drugs to treat numerous diseases and disorders. A fellow of the ASA, he has been a recipient of many honors, including the Drug Information Association Outstanding Service Award, the American Public Health Association Statistics Section Award, the first recipient of the President's Medal for outstanding contributions to GSU, and recognition by the Georgia and US Houses of Representatives, and the Virginia House of Delegates, for his contributions to drug development, biostatistics, and public health education. He has published over 150 papers and 15 books.

List of Figures

List of Tables

1

Introduction to R and Stata for Meta-Analysis

In this chapter, we begin with a basic introduction to the R and Stata for meta-analysis. We focus this introduction on R since R will be the main software in this book and the Stata program will be included at the end of each chapter for Stata users to practise the meta-analysis in each chapter.

We assume that readers have no experience in R. So this introduction to R will be from the very basic R system on where to get R and how to install R and upgrade R packages. We then proceed to show how easy it is to use R for data management as well as to simulate and analyze data from multi-center studies with a brief introduction to meta-analysis. We conclude the chapter with a brief summary and some recommendations for further reading and references.

The main goal for this chapter is to introduce R to readers. For readers who already know and have familiarity with R, you can skip this chapter and go directly to any of the remaining chapters.

1.1 Introduction to R for Meta-Analysis

1.1.1 What is R?

R was initially created by Ihaka and Gentleman (1996) from University of Auckland, New Zealand. Since its creation in the middle of 1990s, R has quickly become a popular programming language and an environment for statistical computing. The continuing development of R is carried out by a core team from different institutions around the world.

To obtain an introduction to R, go to the official home page of the R project at http://www.R-project.org and click "What is R?":

R is a language and environment for statistical computing and graphics. It is a GNU project which is similar to the S language and environment which was developed at Bell Laboratories (formerly AT&T, now Lucent Technologies) by John

Chambers and colleagues. R can be considered as a different implementation of S. There are some important differences, but much code written for S runs unaltered under R.

R provides a wide variety of statistical (linear and nonlinear modeling, classical statistical tests, time-series analysis, classification, clustering, ...) and graphical techniques, and is highly extensible. The S language is often the vehicle of choice for research in statistical methodology and R provides an Open Source route to participation in that activity.

One of R's strengths is the ease with which well-designed publication-quality plots can be produced, including mathematical symbols and formulae wherever needed. Great care has been taken over the defaults for the minor design choices in graphics, but the user retains full control.

R is available as Free Software under the terms of the Free Software Foundation's GNU General Public License in source code form. It compiles and runs on a wide variety of UNIX platforms and similar systems (including FreeBSD and Linux), Windows, and MacOS.

To some users, "free" software may be a "negative" word for software that is difficult to use, has lower quality, or utilizes procedures that have not been validated or verified, etc. However to other users, "free" software means software from an open source that not only allows use of the software but also permits modifications to handle a variety of applications. This latter description is the fundamental principle for R system.

We now proceed to the steps for installing and using R.

1.1.2   Steps on Installing **R** and Updating **R** Packages

In general, the R system consists of two parts. One is the so-called R *base system* for the core R language and associated fundamental libraries. The other consists of user contributed *packages* that are more specialized applications. Both the *base system* and the *packages* may be obtained from the Comprehensive R Archive Network (CRAN) from the weblink:

$$\text{http://CRAN.r-project.org}$$

Installation of R system is described in the following sections.

1.1.2.1   First Step: Install **R** *Base System*

The *base system* can be downloaded from

$$\text{http://CRAN.r-project.org}$$

for different platforms of "Linux," "MacOS X," and "Windows." In this book, we illustrate the use of R for "Windows." "Windows" users can download the latest version of R using the link:

http://CRAN.r-project.org/bin/windows/base/release.htm

(At the writing of this book, version *R 4.0.0* is available.). To download and install R to your computer simply follow the instructions from the installer to install R to the "Program Files" subdirectory in your C. You are ready to use R for statistical computing and data analysis.

Note to LATEX and *R/Sweave* users (in fact, this book is written using R/Sweave): LATEX will complain about the extra space in the path as in "Program Files." Therefore if you want to use R along with LATEX, you need to make a subdirectory *without* space in the path to install R.

You should now have an icon with shortcut to R. Simply click the icon to start R. You should see some introductory information about R and a command prompt '>':

To illustrate R computation, suppose we wish to calculate the sum of 2013 (i.e., the year we published the first edition of this book) and 8 (i.e., the years lagged from the publication of the first edition of this book to this second edition). The first line of R computation is:

```
> # The year of publication of the second edition
> year2nd = 2013+8
```

The computed value may be printed using:

```
> print(year2nd)
```

```
[1] 2021
```

You should get "2021," the year of the publication of this second edition!

1.1.2.2 Second Step: Installing and Updating R Packages

The R *base system* contains a variety of standard statistical functions, descriptive and inferential statistical analysis methods, and graphics which are appropriate for many statistical computing and data analysis requirements.

However, the *packages* are more specialized applications that are contributed by advanced R users who are expert in their field. From our view, *packages* in R is the most important component in R development and upgrading. At the time of writing this book, there are more than 16000 packages in the R system spanning almost all fields of statistical computing and methodology which can be downloaded from http://cran.r-project.org/web/packages/. For reassurance, *we can say that you can find anything you need in R.*

You may install any *packages* from the R prompt by clicking `install.packages` from the R menu *Packages*.

For example, for researchers and practitioners who are interested in meta-analysis, there are several R packages for this purpose, such as the *meta*, *rmeta*, *metafor* which can be installed from this pull-down manual. All the functionalities of this package are then available by loading it to R as:

```
> # Load the `meta' package
> library(meta)
> # Load `rmeta" package
> library(rmeta)
> # Load `metafor' package
> library(metafor)
```

For first-time users for this package, information about its use may be obtained by invoking the 'help' manual, such as:

```
> library(help=metafor)
```

A help page is then available which explains all the functionality of this package. For readers who desire a comprehensive list of available packages, go to

http://CRAN.R-project.org/src/contrib/PACKAGES.html

1.1.2.3   Steps to Get Help and Documentation

A striking feature of R is the easy access of its "Help and Documentation" which may distinguish it from other software systems. There are several ways to access "Help and Documentation."

A general help for R can be obtained by typing `help.start` where you can find help on

1. `Manuals` on

   - An Introduction to R
   - The R Language Definition
   - Writing R Extensions
   - R Installation and Administration
   - R Data Import/Export
   - R Internals

2. `Reference` on

   - Packages
   - Search Engine & Keywords

3. `Miscellaneous Material` about

   - R

- Authors
- Resources
- License
- Frequently Asked Questions
- Thanks
- NEWS
- User Manuals
- Technical papers

4. `Material specific to the Windows port`

- CHANGES
- Windows FAQ

A general reference may be obtained from *RGui* in R. When R is started, click "Help" to access R help items on "FAQ on R," "FAQ on R on Windows," "Manuals (in PDF)," etc. We recommend that readers print the online PDF manual "Introduction to R" for future reference.

Additional "Help and Documentation" may be obtained from the R Homepage. Documentations and online discussion about R are available from the R homepage http://www.r-project.org/. The online "Documentation" section consists of almost all the manuals, FAQs, R Journal, books, and other related information. We recommend readers spend some time in reviewing the online documents to gain familiarity with R.

The most convenient way to access "Help" is from the R command prompt. You can always obtain specific help information from the R command prompt by using "help()." For example, if you want help on "Calculate Effect Size and Outcome Measures" in the library *metafor*, type:

```
> help(escalc)
```

This will load an information page on "Calculate Effect Size and Outcome Measures" containing relevant information. This includes the description of the function, detailed usage for the function and some examples on how to use this function.

1.1.3 Database Management and Data Manipulations

1.1.3.1 Data Management with RMySQL

There are several packages in R for database management and data manipulations. One of the most popular databases used with R is MySQL which is freely available at http://mysql.com for a variety of platforms and is relatively easy to configure and operate. Corresponding to MySQL, there is a R package RMYSQL which is maintained by Jeffrey Horner and available at http://cran.r-project.org/web/packages/RMySQL/. For readers who are familiar with MySQL and relational databases, we highly recommend this R package to create tables and store data into MySQL.

1.1.3.2 Data Management with Microsoft Excel and R Package gdata

Microsoft Excel is the most commonly and easiest to use in data management for most of the readers. In writing this book, we make use of the familiar Microsoft Excel spreadsheet structures and have created excel datasheets in an excel book (named *dat4Meta.xls* for Microsoft Excel 2003 and earlier, and *dat4Meta.xlsx* for Microsoft Excel 2007 and later) for each data set used in each chapter. So we will introduce R functionalities to read Excel data.

There are several ways to access excel databook. In writing the book Chen and Peace (2010), we used R package RODBC (i.e. R for Open DataBase Connectivity) to read data from excel databook to R with the odbcConnectExcel and odbcConnectExcel2007 since at that time, our computer system is 32-bit. This package is available at http://cran.r-project.org/web/packages/RODBC/.

Since 64-bit computers have more or less replaced those 32-bit computers, in this first edition of this book we introduced gdata, another more general R package to read the data from Excel databook. This package is available at http://cran.r-project.org/web/packages/gdata/.

As an alternative to the functions in the RODBC package, the function of read.xls in gdata can be used to read an excel datasheet into R. Since this function is linked to a module from perl language (http://perl.org), you are required to install perl first into your computer. This can be easily done from http://perl.org since perl is free, for example, we install perl at path "c:/myprograms/perl64." With installed perl, read.xls translates the excel spreadsheet into a comma-separated values (CSV) file and then calls another R function read.csv to read the .csv file.

For example, to read the data in Statin Clinical Trials to be used in Section 4.1.1, the R code chunk is as follows:

```
> # Load the library
> require(gdata)
> # Get the data path from your Excel data book "data4Meta.xls"
> datfile = "file path to  the data 'dat4Meta.xls'"
> # Call "read.xls" to read the Excel data at specific data sheet
> dat  = read.xls(datfile, sheet="Data_Statin2006",
        perl="c:/myprograms/perl64/perl/bin/perl.exe")
> # Print the data
> print(dat)
```

```
     Study nhigh evhigh nstd evstd  ntot evtot
1 Prove It  2099    147 2063   172  4162   319
```

```
2   A-to-Z  2265    205 2232   235  4497   440
3     TNT   4995    334 5006   418  10001  752
4    IDEAL  4439    411 4449   463  8888   874
```

We used this structure in the first edition of this book to read the data from the Excel databook we created in writing this book and will continue using this package to read the excel files into R in this second edition. We recommend readers gain familiarity with this format if you have *perl* installed in your computer. Note that you will need to specify your file path at your computer where you store the excel databook.

1.1.3.3 Data Management with Microsoft Excel and R Package xlsx

Another R package xlsx, which is a java-based package and dependent on *Java*, can be used to read excel files into R. To use this package, you will need to install *Java* first based on your computer system, which can be freely downloaded from www.java.com.

Then you will need to install R package rJava and xlsx. There are two main functions in xlsx package for reading both *xls* and *xlsx* Excel files: read.xlsx and read.xlsx2 (faster on big files compared to read.xlsx function).

1.1.3.4 Data Management with Microsoft Excel and R Package readxl

Different from the existing packages (e.g. *gdata* and *xlsx*), the readxl package, developed by Hadley Wickham and his colleagues, has no external dependencies to other packages. Therefore, it is easy to install and use on all operating systems to work with *tabular* data from Excel (i.e., xls or xlsx). Detailed description can be found from https://readxl.tidyverse.org.

To illustrate this package, let us first install and load the readxl package as follows:

```
> # Install the package if not done
> install.packages("readxl")
> # Load the package to R session
> library("readxl")
> # To help with this package
> library(help="readxl")
```

With the loaded package, we can now follow the steps below to read .xls or .xlsx files into R:

```
> # 1. Read xls file format
> # File path to xls
> datfilexls = " file path to the data 'dat4Meta.xls'"
> # Call function "read_excel"
```

```
> datxls = read_excel(datfilexls, sheet="Data_Statin2006")
> # Print the file
> datxls

# A tibble: 4 x 7
   Study   nhigh evhigh  nstd evstd  ntot evtot
   <chr>    <dbl>  <dbl> <dbl> <dbl> <dbl> <dbl>
1 Prove It  2099    147  2063   172  4162   319
2 A-to-Z    2265    205  2232   235  4497   440
3 TNT       4995    334  5006   418 10001   752
4 IDEAL     4439    411  4449   463  8888   874

> # 2. Read xlsx file format:
> # File path to xlsx
> datfilexlsx= "file path to the data 'dat4Meta.xlsx'"
> # Call "read_excel" to read the xlsx file
> datxlsx = read_excel(datfilexlsx, sheet="Data_Statin2006")
> # Print the file
> datxlsx

# A tibble: 4 x 7
   Study   nhigh evhigh  nstd evstd  ntot evtot
   <chr>    <dbl>  <dbl> <dbl> <dbl> <dbl> <dbl>
1 Prove It  2099    147  2063   172  4162   319
2 A-to-Z    2265    205  2232   235  4497   440
3 TNT       4995    334  5006   418 10001   752
4 IDEAL     4439    411  4449   463  8888   874
```

We can see that both "datxls" and "datxlsx" are the same.

1.1.3.5   Other Methods to Read Data into R

If you have Microsoft Excel in your computer, the easiest way to access the data is to export the data into a tab-delimited or comma-separated form, and use `read.table` or `read.csv` to import the data into R.

The `read.table` function is a generic and flexible function used to read data into R in the form of a dataframe. To get familiar with its full functionality, use "help" as follows:

```
> help(read.table)
```

You will see the description and detailed usage. Examples are given on how to use this function. Some of the functionalities are re-iterated here for easy reference:

- `header=TRUE`: If the first line in the data is the variable names, the `header=TRUE` argument is used in `read.table` to use these names to identify the columns of the output dataframe. Otherwise `read.table` would just name the variables using a `V` followed by the column number. In this case, we can use `col.names=` argument in `read.table` to specify a name vector for the dataframe.

- `row.names=`: The `row.names` argument is used to name the rows in the dataframe from `read.table`. Without `row.names` or with `row.names=NULL`, the rows in the dataframe will be listed as the observations numbers.

- `Missing Values`: As its default, `read.table` automatically treats the symbol `NA` to represent a missing value for any data type. For numeric data, `NaN`, `Inf`, and `-Inf` will be treated as missing. If other structure is used for missing values, the `na.strings` argument should be used to refer to that structure to represent missing values.

- `skip=`: The `skip=` argument is used to control the number of lines to skip at the beginning of the file to be read, which is useful in situations where the data have embedded explanation at the beginning. For a very large datafile, we can specify `nrows=` argument to limit the maximum number of rows to read and increase the speed of data processing.

As wrappers for `read.table`, there are three functions of `read.csv`, `read.csv2`, and `read.delim` used specifically for comma-, semicolon-, or tab-delimited data, respectively.

1.1.3.6   R Package `foreign`

For other data formats, the R core team created a package called `foreign`, to read and write data from other statistical packages, such as Minitab, S, SAS, SPSS, Stata, Systat, and dBase. This package is available at http://cran.r-project.org/web/packages/foreign/ with a detailed manual at http://cran.r-project.org/web/packages/foreign/foreign.pdf to describe its functionalities.

1.2   A Simple Simulation on Multicenter Studies for Meta-Analysis

To demonstrate basic application of R and its functionality for data analysis as well as meta-analysis, we simulate a simple multi-center study to compare a new anti-hypertensive drug (denoted by `Drug`) to a conventional control drug (denoted by `CTRL`) on reducing diastolic blood pressure in hypertensive adult men.

    Let us assume an appropriate power analysis indicated that the sample size required to detect a specified treatment difference is $N = 1,000$. Since it is difficult to recruit 1,000 participants at one location during the specified time frame, the research team decided to conduct a multi-center study to recruit these participants from 5 centers, which led to a 5-center study with 200 participants from each center. For these N participants, we record their age and measure baseline diastolic blood pressure just before randomization since *age* is an important risk factor linked to blood pressure.

The new and the control drugs are administered and blood pressure is measured and recorded periodically thereafter, including at the end of the study. Then the change in blood pressure between the endpoint and baseline may be calculated and used to evaluate the anti-hypertensive efficacy of the new drug.

We illustrate the simulation of the data, data manipulation, and analysis with appropriate statistical graphics. Since this is the very first introduction to R, we intentionally use the basic R command so that readers can follow the logic without difficulty.

1.2.1   Data Simulation

1.2.1.1   R Functions

R has a wide range of functions to handle probability distributions and data simulation. For example, for the commonly used normal distribution, the values of its *density, cumulative distribution function, quantile function* and *random generation* with mean equal to *mean* and standard deviation equal to *sd* can be generated using the following R functions:

```
dnorm(x, mean = 0, sd = 1, log = FALSE)
pnorm(q, mean = 0, sd = 1, lower.tail = TRUE, log.p = FALSE)
qnorm(p, mean = 0, sd = 1, lower.tail = TRUE, log.p = FALSE)
rnorm(n, mean = 0, sd = 1)
```

where

x, q	*is*	vector of quantiles
p	*is*	vector of probabilities
n	*is*	number of observations
mean	*is*	vector of means
sd	*is*	vector of standard deviations.

The above specification can be found using the *Help* function as follows:

```
> help(rnorm)
```

There are similar sets of *d, p, q, r* functions for *Poisson, binomial, t, F, hypergeometric, χ^2, Beta*, etc. Also there is a *sample* function for sampling from a vector *replicate* for repeating computations.

1.2.1.2   Data Generation and Manipulation

With this introduction, we can now simulate data center-by-center. For example in center 1, assuming that the baseline diastolic blood pressures for these 200 ($n = 100$ for each treatment) recruited participants are normally distributed with mean (mu) = 100 (mmHg) and standard deviation $sd = 20$ (mmHg). The *age* for these 200 middle-age men is assumed to be normally distributed with mean age $age.mu = 50$ (year old) and standard deviation $age.sd = 10$ (year). In addition, we assume the new drug will decrease diastolic blood pressure by $mu.d = 20$(mmHg).

These input values at center 1 for this simulation can be specified in R as follows:

```
> # Number of participants each arm
> n      = 100
> # Mean blood pressure at baseline
> mu     = 100
> # Standard deviations for blood pressure
> sd     = 20
> # Mean changes for blood pressure
> mu.d   = 10
> # Mean age for participants
> age.mu = 50
> # sd of age for participants
> age.sd = 10
```

We first simulate data for the *n* *CTRL* participants with *age*, baseline blood pressure (denoted by *bp.base*), endpoint blood pressure (denoted by *bp.end*), and change in blood pressure from baseline to endpoint (denoted by *bp.diff=bp.end-bp.base*) with following R code chunk:

```
> # Fix the seed for random number generation
> set.seed(123)
> # Use "rnorm" to generate random normal
> age        = rnorm(n, age.mu, age.sd)
> bp.base    = rnorm(n,mu,sd)
> bp.end     = rnorm(n,mu,sd)
> # Take the difference between endpoint and baseline
> bp.diff    = bp.end-bp.base
> # put the data together using "cbind" to column-bind
> dat4CTRL   = round(cbind(age,bp.base,bp.end,bp.diff))
```

Note that the simulation seed is set at 123 so that simulation can be reproduced, which is done by set.seed(123). Otherwise, results can be different from each simulation.

We can manipulate the data using column bind (R command cbind) to combine all the simulated data together and round the data into the nearest whole number (R command **round**) to produce a data set and give the data matrix a name: *dat4CTRL*. The first few observations may be viewed using following R code:

```
> # Print the first 6 observations
> head(dat4CTRL)

    age bp.base bp.end bp.diff
[1,] 44      86    144      58
[2,] 48     105    126      21
[3,] 66      95     95       0
[4,] 51      93    111      18
[5,] 51      81     92      11
[6,] 67      99     90      -9
```

Similarly, we can simulate data for the new drug *Drug*. We use the same variable names here, but give a different name to the final data set: *dat4drug*. Note that the *mean* for the *bp.end* is now *mu-mu.d* to simulate the decrease in mean value:

```
> # Simulate `age'
> age      = rnorm(n, age.mu, age.sd)
> # Simulate `baseline' blood pressure
> bp.base  = rnorm(n,mu,sd)
> # Simulate `endpoint' blood pressure
> bp.end   = rnorm(n,mu-mu.d,sd)
> # The changes in blood pressure
> bp.diff  = bp.end-bp.base
> # Make the data matrix
> dat4drug = round(cbind(age,bp.base,bp.end,bp.diff))
```

We do not print the observations at this time. To further manipulate the data, we stack the two data sets from *CTRL* and *Drug* using R command **rbind** to produce a data frame using R command **data.frame**. We also create a column *TRT* with two factors of *CTRL* and *Drug* to indicate there are two treatments in this data set and another column *Center* to represent the data is from which center. Finally, we name this data as *dat1*:

```
> # Make a dataframe to hold all data
> dat1     = data.frame(rbind(dat4CTRL,dat4drug))
> # Make "TRT" as a factor for treatment.
> dat1$TRT    = as.factor(rep(c("CTRL", "Drug"), each=n))
> # Make a "Center" to represent the center number
> dat1$Center = 1
```

With these manipulations, the data frame *dat1* should have 200 observations with 100 from *CTRL* and 100 from *Drug*. Also this dataframe should have 6 variables like *age, bp.base, bp.end, bp.diff, TRT, Center* as its columns. We can check it using the following R code chunk:

```
> # check the data dimension
> dim(dat1)

[1] 200   6

> # print the first 6 observations to see the variable names
> head(dat1)

  age bp.base bp.end bp.diff  TRT Center
1  44      86    144      58 CTRL      1
2  48     105    126      21 CTRL      1
3  66      95     95       0 CTRL      1
4  51      93    111      18 CTRL      1
5  51      81     92      11 CTRL      1
6  67      99     90      -9 CTRL      1
```

We can then write this process of data generation into a function so that we can call this function to simulate data for other centers. We name this function as *data.generator* as follows:

```
> data.generator = function(n,age.mu,age.sd,mu,mu.d,sd, center){
# Data from CTRL
age      = rnorm(n, age.mu, age.sd)
bp.base  = rnorm(n,mu,sd)
bp.end   = rnorm(n,mu,sd)
bp.diff  = bp.end-bp.base
dat4CTRL = round(cbind(age,bp.base,bp.end,bp.diff))
# Data from Drug
age      = rnorm(n, age.mu, age.sd)
bp.base  = rnorm(n,mu,sd)
bp.end   = rnorm(n,mu-mu.d,sd)
bp.diff  = bp.end-bp.base
dat4drug = round(cbind(age,bp.base,bp.end,bp.diff))
# Put both data matrice\tilde{}s together
dat      = data.frame(rbind(dat4CTRL,dat4drug))
# Make "TRT" as a factor for treatment.
dat$TRT  = as.factor(rep(c("CTRL", "Drug"), each=n))
# Make a "Center" to represent the center number
dat$Center = center
# Return the simulated data
dat
} # end of function
```

With this new function of `data.generator`, we can regenerate the data from center 1 as follows:

```
> d1 = data.generator(n,age.mu,age.sd,mu,mu.d,sd, 1)
```

To generate data from other centers, we suppose mean and standard deviation for baseline blood pressure and age are similar for all centers, but the new drug has different effectiveness for each center with mu.d2 = 13 for center 2, mu.d3 = 15 for center 3, mu.d4 = 8 for center 4 and mu.d5 = 10 for center 5, respectively. Then we can generate data from each center as follows:

```
> # Data from Center 2
> mu.d2 = 13
> d2     = data.generator(n,age.mu,age.sd,mu,mu.d2,sd,2)
> # Data from Center 3
> mu.d3 = 15
> d3     = data.generator(n,age.mu,age.sd,mu,mu.d3,sd,3)
> # Data from Center 4
> mu.d4 = 8
> d4     = data.generator(n,age.mu,age.sd,mu,mu.d4,sd,4)
> # Data from Center 5
> mu.d5 = 10
> d5     = data.generator(n,age.mu,age.sd,mu,mu.d5,sd,5)
```

Putting these data from 5 centers together, we create one final data set for this study which is named as dat as follows:

```
> dat = data.frame(rbind(d1,d2,d3,d4,d5))
> # Change `Center' from numeric to factor
> dat$Center = as.factor(dat$Center)
```

This data should have 1000 observations from 5 centers each having 100 from *CTRL* and 100 from *Drug*. Also this dataframe should have 6 variables like *age*, *bp.base*, *bp.end*, *bp.diff*, *TRT*, *Center* as its columns.

1.2.1.3   Basic R Graphics

R is well-known for its graphics capabilities. We can display the distributions for the data just generated to view whether they appear to be normally distributed using the R command boxplot for the first center as follows:

```
> # Call boxplot
> boxplot(dat4CTRL, las=1, main="Control Drug")
```

Notice in the boxplot, we used las=1 which is to change the orientation of the tick mark labels from the default parallel to the axis (the default, las = 0) to horizontal (i.e., las = 1).

This will generate Figure 1.1 from which one can see that the data appear to be normally distributed except for one outlier from the baseline data.

Similarly we can produce the distribution for *Drug* using the following R code chunk:

```
> boxplot(dat4drug, las=1, main="New Drug")
```

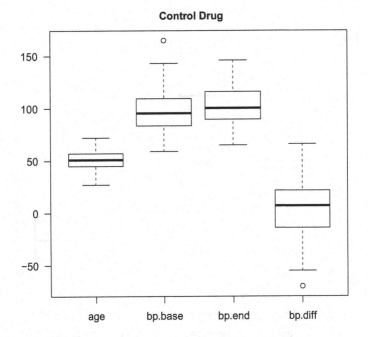

FIGURE 1.1
Distributions for data generated for "Control Drug".

This will produce Figure 1.2 to show that the data are in fact normally distributed. The boxplot for endpoint is 10 mmHG lower than the baseline blood pressure.

Before performing any statistical analysis, we recommend exploring the data using appropriate plots to assess whether distributional or other relevant assumptions required for the validity of the analysis methods hold for the data. There is another suite of advanced R graphics to use for this purpose, i.e. the package *lattice* with implementation of Trellis Graphics .

This package is maintained by Deepayan Sarkar (2008) and can be downloaded from

http://r-forge.r-project.org/projects/lattice/

or simply from RGUI. We first load the package into R by `library(lattice)` and display the relationship between the blood pressure difference as a function of *age* for each treatment to assess whether there exists a statistically significant relationship in addition to a treatment difference. This can be done with the following R code chunk:

```
> #load the lattice library
> library(lattice)
> # call xyplot function and print it
```

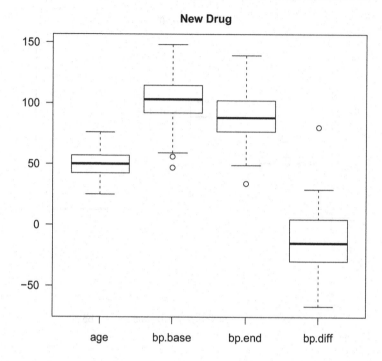

FIGURE 1.2
Distributions for data generated for "New Drug".

```
> print(xyplot(bp.diff~age|Center*TRT, data=dat,xlab="Age",
  strip=strip.custom(bg="yellow"),
  ylab="Blood Pressure Difference",lwd=3,cex=1.3,pch=20,
  type=c("p", "r")))
```

This produces Figure 1.3. From this figure, we can see graphically that the relationship between the blood pressure decreases and age is not significant, but that the new drug did reduce blood pressure.

To illustrate the treatment effect by center, we can make use of the `bwplot` in this `lattice` library to produce Figure 1.4 as follows.

```
> # Call bwplot
> print(bwplot(bp.diff~TRT|Center, data=dat,xlab="TRT",
  strip=strip.custom(bg="yellow"),
  ylab="Blood Pressure Difference",lwd=3,cex=1.3,pch=20,
  type=c("p", "r")))
```

Another way to illustrate the treatment effect is to group the treatment by center which can be produced in Figure 1.5 with following R code chunk. We can see there are some variations within centers which is exactly what we simulated with different `mu.d`.

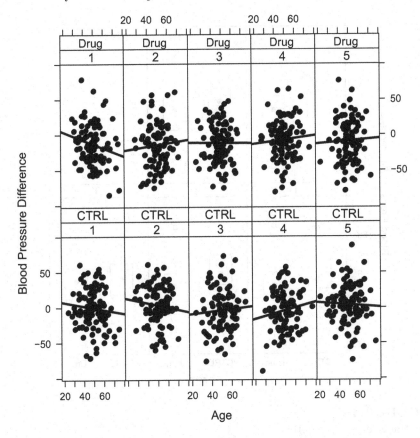

FIGURE 1.3
Data with regression line for each treatment and center.

```
> # Call bwplot
> print(bwplot(bp.diff~Center|TRT, data=dat,xlab="Center",
  strip=strip.custom(bg="yellow"),
  ylab="Blood Pressure Difference",lwd=3,cex=1.3,pch=20,
  type=c("p", "r")))
```

1.2.2   Data Analysis

With these preliminary graphical illustrations, we now comfortably proceed to data analysis. We will compare the treatment effect with results using data from each center as well as the results from pooled data from 5 centers. We will then briefly introduce the concept of meta-analysis with this simulated data.

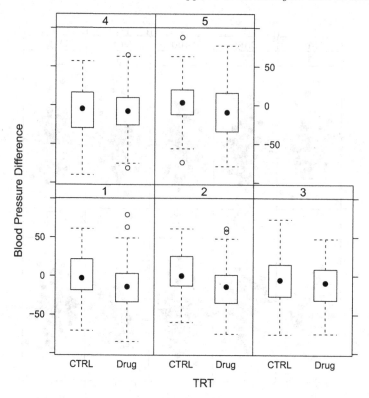

FIGURE 1.4
Treatment effect by center.

1.2.2.1 Data Analysis from Each Center

Before we pool the data together for analysis, let us start to look into the treatment effect from each individual center first, which we would expect a less statistical powerful results.

We subset the data from each center to perform an analysis of variance using following R code chunk:

```
> # Model for Center 1
> m.c1 = aov(bp.diff~TRT, data=dat[dat$Center==1,])
> # Print the summary
> summary(m.c1)

            Df Sum Sq Mean Sq F value Pr(>F)
TRT          1   7963    7963    9.56 0.0023 **
Residuals  198 164958     833
---
```

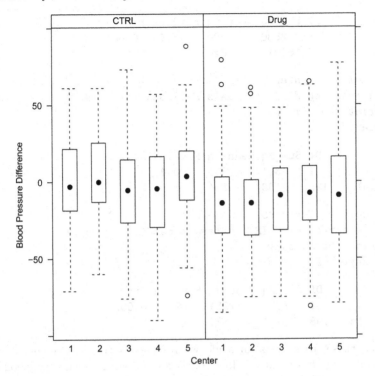

FIGURE 1.5
Treatment effect grouped by center.

```
Signif. codes:
0 *** 0.001 ** 0.01 * 0.05 . 0.1


> # Model for Center 2
> m.c2 = aov(bp.diff~TRT, data=dat[dat$Center==2,])
> # Print the summary
> summary(m.c2)


            Df Sum Sq Mean Sq F value  Pr(>F)
TRT          1  14775   14775    17.7 3.9e-05 ***
Residuals  198 165407     835


> # Model for Center 3
> m.c3 = aov(bp.diff~TRT, data=dat[dat$Center==3,])
> # Print the summary
> summary(m.c3)
```

```
              Df Sum Sq Mean Sq F value Pr(>F)
TRT            1    2880    2880    3.48  0.064 .
Residuals    198 164018     828
```

```
> # Model for Center 4
> m.c4 = aov(bp.diff~TRT, data=dat[dat$Center==4,])
> # Print the summary
> summary(m.c4)
```

```
              Df Sum Sq Mean Sq F value Pr(>F)
TRT            1     341     341    0.42   0.52
Residuals    198 159168     804
```

```
> # Model for Center 5
> m.c5 = aov(bp.diff~TRT, data=dat[dat$Center==5,])
> # Print the summary
> summary(m.c5)
```

```
              Df Sum Sq Mean Sq F value Pr(>F)
TRT            1    7951    7951    9.14 0.0028 **
Residuals    198 172241     870
```

From these fittings, as an aside we notice that the treatment effect is statistically significant (at p-value <0.05) for centers 1 (p-value $= 0.0023$), 2 (p-value $= 3.9e\text{-}05$) and 5(p-value $= 0.0028$) , but not for centers 3 (p-value $= 0.064$) and 4 (p-value $= 0.52$).

1.2.2.2   Data Analysis with Pooled Data from Five Centers

To pool all the data from the 5 centers, we start to fit a full model with 3-way interactions among treatment, center, and covariate as follows:

$$
\begin{aligned}
y = {}& \beta_0 + \beta_1 TRT + \beta_2 Center + \beta_3 age \\
& + \beta_4 TRT \times Center + \beta_5 TRT \times age + \beta_6 Center \times age \\
& + \beta_7 TRT \times Center \times age + \epsilon
\end{aligned}
\tag{1.1}
$$

where y denotes the change in blood pressure and β's are the parameters. ϵ is the error term which is assumed to be independently identically distributed (*i.i.d.*) with normal distribution with standard deviation σ.

The fitting of this linear model (1.1) is accomplished in one line of R code using aov as:

```
> # Call 'aov' to fit the 3-way model
> lm1 = aov(bp.diff~TRT*Center*age, data=dat)
> summary(lm1)
```

```
              Df Sum Sq Mean Sq F value  Pr(>F)
TRT            1  27689   27689   33.17 1.1e-08 ***
```

Center	4	2978	745	0.89	0.47
age	1	71	71	0.08	0.77
TRT:Center	4	6194	1548	1.85	0.12
TRT:age	1	9	9	0.01	0.92
Center:age	4	5391	1348	1.61	0.17
TRT:Center:age	4	2261	565	0.68	0.61
Residuals	980	818088	835		

```
---
Signif. codes:
0 *** 0.001 ** 0.01 * 0.05 . 0.1
```

The `summary` prints a summary of the model fitting including the analysis of variance (ANOVA) table and we can see that there is no statistically significant 3-way and 2-way interactions. So we drop the `age` covariate and refit a reduced model with `Center` as block to pool the data from 5 centers. This model can be expressed as

$$y = \beta_0 + \beta_1 TRT + \beta_2 Center + \epsilon \qquad (1.2)$$

And the R implementation can be done as follows:

```
> # Call 'aov' to fit the reduced model
> lm2 = aov(bp.diff~TRT+Center, data=dat)
> summary(lm2)
```

	Df	Sum Sq	Mean Sq	F value	Pr(>F)	
TRT	1	27689	27689	33.08	1.2e-08	***
Center	4	2978	745	0.89	0.47	
Residuals	994	832014	837			

It can be seen from the output that there is a statistically significant treatment effect with data pooled from 5 centers which confirmed with the illustration from Figure 1.5 that the new drug statistically significantly reduced blood pressure.

1.2.2.3 A Brief Introduction to Meta-Analysis

As an alternative to the pooled multi-center analysis in the previous section, we will briefly introduce the concept of meta-analysis. We will make use of the R library `metafor` which will be illustrated in later chapters.

In order to carry out a meta-analysis, we first need to `aggregate` the individual data by study for their sample size, means, and standard deviations which can be done with following R code chunk:

```
> # Get the study sample size
> ndat = aggregate(dat$bp.diff,
      list(Center=dat$Center,TRT = dat$TRT), length)
```

```
> # Print the study specific sample size
> ndat

   Center  TRT   x
1       1 CTRL 100
2       2 CTRL 100
3       3 CTRL 100
4       4 CTRL 100
5       5 CTRL 100
6       1 Drug 100
7       2 Drug 100
8       3 Drug 100
9       4 Drug 100
10      5 Drug 100

> # Calcuate the means by study
> mdat = aggregate(dat$bp.diff,
     list(Center=dat$Center,TRT = dat$TRT), mean)
> # Print the means
> mdat

   Center  TRT       x
1       1 CTRL   -0.24
2       2 CTRL    3.05
3       3 CTRL   -3.84
4       4 CTRL   -4.43
5       5 CTRL    3.84
6       1 Drug  -12.86
7       2 Drug  -14.14
8       3 Drug  -11.43
9       4 Drug   -7.04
10      5 Drug   -8.77

> # Calculate the standard deviations
> sddat = aggregate(dat$bp.diff,
     list(Center=dat$Center,TRT = dat$TRT), sd)
> # Print the SDs
> sddat

   Center  TRT    x
1       1 CTRL 29.2
2       2 CTRL 27.4
3       3 CTRL 30.0
4       4 CTRL 28.3
5       5 CTRL 28.3
6       1 Drug 28.5
```

7	2 Drug 30.3
8	3 Drug 27.5
9	4 Drug 28.4
10	5 Drug 30.6

To carry out the meta-analysis, we load the **metafor** library and calculate the effect-size (ES) using mean-difference as follows:

```
> # Call the library
> library(metafor)
> # Calculate the ESs
> esdat = escalc(measure="MD",
          n1i= ndat$x[ndat$TRT=="Drug"],
          n2i= ndat$x[ndat$TRT=="CTRL"],
          m1i= mdat$x[mdat$TRT=="Drug"],
          m2i= mdat$x[mdat$TRT=="CTRL"],
          sd1i= sddat$x[sddat$TRT=="Drug"],
          sd2i= sddat$x[sddat$TRT=="CTRL"], append=T)
> rownames(esdat) = ndat$Study[ndat$TRT=="TRT"]
> # Print the ES dataframe
> esdat

         yi       vi
1 -12.6200  16.6625
2 -17.1900  16.7078
3  -7.5900  16.5675
4  -2.6100  16.0776
5 -12.6100  17.3981
```

With this calculated ES as mean-difference, we can then calculate the study-specific p-values as follows:

```
> # Calculate the z-values for each study
> z = esdat$yi/sqrt(esdat$vi)
> # Calculate the p-values for each study
> pval.studywise = 2*(1-pnorm(abs(z)))
> # Print the p-values
> pval.studywise

[1] 1.99e-03 2.61e-05 6.22e-02 5.15e-01 2.50e-03
attr(,"ni")
[1] 200 200 200 200 200
attr(,"measure")
[1] "MD"
```

This results are similar to the results from the ANOVAs in Section 1.2.2.1 which concludes that the treatment effect is statistically significant (at p-value <0.05) for centers 1, 2, and 5, but not for centers 3 and 4.

For meta-analysis, we use a random-effects meta-model with DerSimonian-Laird estimator which will be explained in the later chapter using the following R code chunk:

```
> # Random-effects meta-analysis with DL
> meta.MD.DL = rma(yi,vi,measure="MD",method="DL", data=esdat)
> # Print the result
> meta.MD.DL

Random-Effects Model (k = 5; tau^2 estimator: DL)

tau^2 (estimated amount of total heterogeneity): 14.9509
                                                 (SE = 22.3638)
tau (square root of estimated tau^2 value):       3.8666
I^2 (total heterogeneity / total variability):   47.27%
H^2 (total variability / sampling variability):   1.90

Test for Heterogeneity:
Q(df = 4) = 7.5865, p-val = 0.1080

Model Results:

estimate      se     zval    pval    ci.lb    ci.ub
-10.4810   2.5151   -4.1673  <.0001  -15.4104  -5.5515  ***


---
Signif. codes:
0 *** 0.001 ** 0.01 * 0.05 . 0.1
```

It can be seen that the treatment effect from the meta-estimate of -10.4810 is statistically significant with p-value < 0.0001 which indicated that the new drug significantly reduced blood pressure if we meta-analyze the data from 5 centers together. This coincides with the pooled multi-center analysis in Section 1.2.2.2.

1.3   Introduction of Stata for Meta-Analysis

As introduced in Section 1.1, the R packages of meta, rmeta, and metafor will be used in this book for meta-analysis using R. For Stata, we will use metan in this book.

Stata has a long history of building methods for meta-analyses. The suite of meta and metan offers a comprehensive compilation of commands to perform meta-analyses, which is very broad, but also very easy to use, with similar functionalities as in R packages of meta, rmeta and metafor.

If `Stata` users have an earlier version than Stata 16, install `meta` with the following code:

```
net from http://www.stata.com
net cd stb
net cd stb43
net describe sbe16_2
net install sbe16_2
```

To use `metan`, `Stata` users need to install this meta-analysis suite with the following command:

```
ssc install metan.
```

An easy to follow "Quick Workflow" and the summary of all features in four tables for meta-analysis in `Stata` can be found in the link https://www.stata.com/new-in-stata/meta-analysis/#four-tables. More resources about `Stata` for meta-analysis can be found in https://www.stata.com/support/faqs/statistics/meta-analysis/ and https://journals.sagepub.com/doi/pdf/10.1177/1536867X0800800102.

1.4 Summary and Recommendations for Further Reading about Using R

In this chapter, we introduced the reader to the R system, its installation, and its related packages. We illustrated the use of R for data simulation and manipulation, statistical graphics, and statistical modeling by simulating data from a simple multi-center study.

For further reading to gain more familiar with the R system, we recommend:

- **R fundamentals to *S* languages**: Two books from John Chambers (1998, 2008) are excellent references to understand the R language and its programming structures.

- **R graphics:** Besides Sarkar's book (Sarkar, 2008) on *lattice*, we also recommend Paul Murrell's book (Murrell, 2005).

- **Statistical data analysis using R:** we recommend Faraway's two books published in 2004 (Faraway, 2004) and 2006 (Faraway, 2006) which are two excellent books using R for statistical modeling. Everitt and Hothorn's book (Everitt and Hothorn, 2006) on statistical data analysis using R is another excellent book we used in the classroom which interested students. For biostatistics using R, interested readers can read our books with the first edition of

the "Clinical Trial Data Analysis Using R" (Chen and Peace, 2010)
and the second edition of the "Clinical Trial Data Analysis Using R
and SAS" (Chen, Peace, and Zhang, 2017).

- **Statistical computing:** Maria Rizzo's book on "Statistical Computing with R (Rizzo, 2008) is an excellent book.

- **Meta-Analysis Using R:** After the publication of our first edition
  in 2013 of "Applied Meta-analysis with R" (Chen and Peace, 2013),
  there was another excellent book "Meta-Analysis with R" published
  in 2015 by Schwarzer, Carpenter, and Rucker (2015). We like to
  make aware to interested readers so that they can read both books.

- **Books for light-reading:**. There are a series of books in the bookstores which are written in very nonstatistical fashion for readers to
  get familiar with R. We recommend Kabacoff (2011) which is a R
  language tutorial with focus on step-by-step practical problem solving, Gardener (2012) which is written for users and data analysts
  with/without R knowledge, Adler (2012) which covers every aspects
  of R and it is an excellent reference book for R.

- **R online documentations:** we emphasize again that there are
  many free online books, manuals, journals, and others to be
  downloaded from R homepage at "Documentation".

2

Research Protocol for Meta-Analyses

2.1 Introduction

In this book, we present numerous examples of detailed meta-analysis in many areas of application using features of R and Stata. In doing so, with the exception of having access to patient-level data in one chapter, we used summary data for a set of studies to be combined already meta-analyzed and reported in the literature. In presenting statistical details and results of our meta-analyses, we identified the research questions to which the meta-analyses appearing in the literature were directed. So we did not start by specifying a research question of interest, then perform searches of databases such as PUBMED, MEDLINE and identify the totality of studies that could provide summary information relative to the question, obtain publications of the studies, and then abstract the summary data to be synthesized.

In actual practice, if one were to have a question that a meta-analysis could possibly answer, the first and most important step is to write a protocol under which the totality of the meta-analysis inquiry as a scientific research effort would be conducted. The purpose of this chapter is to inform the reader of this most important exercise, briefly outline the steps involved in writing a meta-analysis protocol, and point the reader to publications that provide much detail and guidance in writing the protocol for a meta-analysis.

2.2 Defining the Research Objective

In developing a protocol for a clinical trial of a new drug, the first step is to formulate the objective or question that the trial seeks to answer as seen in Chapter 6 of Peace and Chen (2010). Beginning with a well-defined question as the first step in developing a protocol for a meta-analysis is of no less importance than beginning development of a protocol for a new drug with a well-defined question or objective. Some would argue that it may be more important as the opportunity for injecting bias may be greater.

As an example, suppose we were interested in performing a meta-analysis based upon published studies of the following objective:

Objective: To assess the overall evidence of the effectiveness of calcium-channel blockers in the treatment of mild-to-moderate hypertension.

There are elements of the objective statement that are well defined; i.e., the drug class and the disease. However, searching the literature for mild-to-moderate hypertension may lead to publications that vary according to what is considered mild-to-moderate. So there is a need to specify

1. what is meant by mild-to-moderate. What is considered as normal blood pressure has changed over the years. So searching the literature for mild-to-moderate hypertension may identify older published studies where mild-to-moderate hypertension has a range of blood pressure that is shifted to the right of that in more recent studies. In addition, no mention is made of:

2. the effectiveness measure or outcome (and how assessed),

3. the type of control group,

4. study characteristics such as (1) type of design (parallel, crossover), (2) method of assignment (e.g., balanced random assignment) of patients to drug and control groups, (3) other measures to guard against bias (e.g., double-blinded),

5. type of patient (e.g., age range, race or ethnicity, gender, concomitant disease, etc.), or perhaps

6. length of study.

These six items along with specifying what is meant by mild-to-moderate essentially define parameters that govern the search for studies to be included in the meta-analysis to address the question or objective. Their importance relative to the objective statement is discussed in the following section of the protocol.

2.3 Criteria for Identifying Studies to Include in the Meta-Analysis

2.3.1 Clarifying the Disease under Study (What Is Meant by Mild-to-Moderate?)

What is considered as normal blood pressure has changed over the years (and thus so has what is considered as mild-to-moderate hypertension). For many years, the American Heart Association considered normal blood pressure for adults to be systolic blood pressure less than 140 mmHG and diastolic blood pressure (DBP) less than 90 mmHG. More recently, the National Heart, Lung, and Blood Institute (NHLBI) in Bethesda, Maryland, released new clinical guidelines for normal blood pressure in adults. They considered normal blood pressure in adults to be systolic less than 120 and diastolic to be less than 80. Over about a 20 year period, the definition of normal tension dropped by 20 mmHG supine and 10 mmHG DBPs. Hypertensive patients who entered trials per the AHA definition of normal blood pressure are likely to have blood pressure at baseline greater than that of patients who entered trials per the NHLBI.

After reviewing the references obtained, the meta-analysis researcher may wish to revise the objective, search for studies of hypertension and not restrict the search to mild-to-moderate hypertension.

2.3.2 The Effectiveness Measure or Outcome

In clinical trials of hypertension, the primary endpoint or effectiveness measure is change in DBP, where change in DBP is DBP after beginning treatment minus DBP just before beginning treatment (baseline). Systolic blood pressure (SBP) is measured and analyzed but is not considered primary. Since blood pressure varies with the position (sitting, standing, or supine) of the patient and with the method of assessment (digital recorder or sphygmomanometer), this information should be included as search parameters. Some trials may also report the proportion of patients in each treatment group who became normotensive. Older publications may include reports of change in mean arterial pressure, which is a weighted average of DBP and SBP. The point is that to synthesize results across trials, the same effectiveness measure must be determinable from each trial.

2.3.3 The Type of Control Group

Efficacy of a drug from a clinical trial is assessed relative to a control group. If the control is a matching placebo (negative control) then efficacy is viewed as direct efficacy. If the comparison of drug to placebo is statistically significant at some prespecified small false positive rate, then direct evidence of efficacy would have been demonstrated. If the control is another drug (positive control), then the comparison of drug to the positive control provides a measure of the extent to which the drug is efficacious relative to the positive control. If positive control was already regulatory approved as efficacious, the difference between the drug and the positive control being small enough to conclude that drug was equivalent to the positive control supports indirect efficacy of the drug. There are other issues here relative to the comparability of the trial population to the population in which the efficacy of the positive control was established. But it should be clear that in identifying a group of studies for meta-analysis of a specific drug, studies included should contain both the drug group and the same control group.

2.3.4 Study Characteristics

Study characteristics are important in searching for studies that may be synthesized to address the objective of the meta-analysis. These include the (1) type of experimental design, such as whether it is crossover (each patient serves as his/ her own control) or parallel; (2) whether patients are randomly assigned to the treatment and control groups in balanced (equal numbers of patients to each group) or imbalanced (such as twice as many patients randomly assigned to the treatment group as to the control group) fashion or whether randomization is in blocks to ensure balance across time of entry; (3) whether patients are stratified on prognostic factors prior to randomization; and (4) measures taken to eliminate or minimize bias (such as double-blinded: both investigational site personnel and patients are blinded as to identification of the intervention groups) or preserving blinding and preservation of the Type I error if group sequential analyses are performed in the study.

2.3.5 Type of Patient

Patient characteristics such as age, race or ethnicity, gender, whether patients in the studies are in or out of hospital during the treatment period, the existence of concurrent disease other than the one being treated by the new drug, and whether patients are permitted to take concomitant medications for the concurrent diseases all help to identify the type of patient in the inferenced population from the individual studies. Synthesizing studies that share common patient characteristics ensure that inference from the meta-analysis is to the same inferenced population. It is advisable for the researcher to abstract summary measures (e.g., mean, St.Dev., etc.) by treatment group for subgroups induced by the patient characteristics. The researcher could then address the extent to which inference to the general population extended to subgroups.

2.3.6 Length of Study

The length of the treatment period of the study is important in the study of hypertension (as well as in the study of many other diseases). Change in blood pressure from a study of say 1 month of treatment is different than blood pressure from a study of 6 months duration.

2.4 Searching for and Collecting the Studies

There are many databases that may be searched for a particular meta-analysis. More popular ones are PubMed (MEDLINE), Embase, Web of Science (Science Citation Index), ClinicalTrials.gov, and the Cochrane Central

Register of Controlled Trials. PubMed contains more than 30 million citations for biomedical literature from MEDLINE (www.ncbi.nlm.nih.gov/pubmed). MEDLINE is the largest component of PubMed as pointed in Katcher (2006).

Embase contains more than 31 million indexed records and over 8,500 currently indexed peer-reviewed journals. Embase is a highly versatile, multi-purpose, and up-to-date database covering the most important international biomedical literature from 1947 to the present day (http://www.embase.com/info/what-embase).

The Web of Science core collection indexes more than 21,294 journals, books, and conference proceedings. The Web of Science Platform contains more than 34,502 journals, books, proceedings, patents, and data sets (https://clarivate.libguides.com/webofscienceplatform/coverage).

ClinicalTrials.gov lists 340,643 research studies with locations in all 50 states and in 214 countries (http://www.clinicaltrials.gov/). Using the search function located on the home page, we found 136 studies when searching for mild-to-moderate hypertension and 7,955 studies were found when dropping mild-to-moderate and searching for hypertension.

The Cochrane Collaboration is an international network of over 11,000 members and over 68,000 supporters from more than 130 countries. They work together to help healthcare providers, policy-makers, patients, their advocates and care givers, make well-informed decisions about health care, by preparing, updating, and promoting the accessibility of Cochrane Reviews – numbering over 7,500 and published online in the Cochrane Database of Systematic Reviews, part of The Cochrane Library. They also prepare the largest collection of records of randomized controlled trials in the world, called CENTRAL, which is published as part of The Cochrane Library. Their work is recognized internationally as the benchmark for high-quality information about the effectiveness of healthcare (http://www.cochrane.org/about-us).

The Cochrane Handbook consists of four Parts: About Cochrane Reviews, Core Methods, Specific Perspectives in Reviews, and Other Topics. Chapters 3 and 4, of Part II, are particularly helpful in outlining and explaining the search and selection of studies (https://training.cochrane.org/handbook/current/chapter-04). The criteria for Identifying studies to include in the meta-analysis are synonymous to the Inclusion/Exclusion Criteria of a clinical trial protocol. Inclusion means the researcher decides which studies to keep for the meta-analysis. Exclusion means the researcher decides which studies not to keep. For a clinical trial protocol, inclusion/exclusion criteria apply at the patient level. Inclusion/exclusion criteria for meta-analysis apply at the study level.

Chapter 2 of Part II of the Cochrane Handbook (https://training.cochrane.org/handbook/current/chapter-02) is particularly helpful in determining the scope of the meta-analysis investigation and defining the question or objective of the investigation.

Many other databases are available for searching. In addition to those noted above, GIDEON, CINAHL, Micromedex, and Dynamed

(https://databases.hollis.harvard.edu/primo-explore/search?query=lsr39,
exact,Medicine%20and%20Public%20Health&tab=databases&search_scope=
default_scope&vid=HVD_DB&lang=en_US&offset=0&sortby=lso03)   are
accessible via Countway Library at Harvard (https://countway.harvard.edu/).
These are of particular importance in the fields of Medicine and Public Health.

The databases listed represent a start for researchers in the areas identified. Researchers in other areas of meta-analysis application may identify
other databases by searching the WWW and/or making use of university
libraries.

A package that is very helpful in searching for and identifying articles
for potential inclusion in meta-analyses is "RISmed." This package describes
a set of tools to extract bibliographic content from the National Center for
Biotechnology Information (NCBI) databases, including `PubMed`. The name
`RISmed` is a portmanteau of RIS (for Research Information Systems, a common
tag format for bibliographic data) and `PubMed`. `RISmed` may be accessed using
the link: https://cran.r-project.org/web/packages/RISmed/RISmed.pdf.

2.5   Data Abstraction and Extraction

The researcher should design a data extraction form (DAF) that is clear and
unambiguous. It will be used to extract and record the data from studies that
will be synthesized to address the objective of the meta-analysis. Chapter
5, Collecting Data, of Part II of the Cochrane Handbook is helpful in facil-
itating the design of a Data Collection Form which is needed in extracting
data from studies to be used in the researchers' meta-analysis investigation.
(https://training.cochrane.org/handbook/current/chapter-05).

Synthesis of the individual study findings proceeds easier from the DAF
than working directly from the publication to analysis file creation. The DAF
with extracted data creates a documentation record that can be used in a quality assurance process or used by future researchers who may wish to update
meta-analysis findings as more studies become available.

Reports of studies may vary in terms of the summary measures (e.g., means
versus medians, standard deviations versus standard errors, etc.) reported and
the level of study detail. Meta-analysis researchers may need to contact the
authors of the studies for any additional study details. In addition, researchers
may find more than one report of the same study. Data from all reports should
be abstracted and referenced on the DAF, but the researcher must determine
which report is most accurate with respect to the numbers of patients and
summary statistics. Again, the researcher may need to contact the authors to
determine which report provides the appropriate summary measures to use
for their meta-analysis.

It is a good practice for researchers to pilot the DAF on a small group of studies to ensure that it captures all information required for their meta-analysis. If multiple reviewers and data extractors differ, every effort should be made to explain any differences among extractors and arrive at a consensus.

What to include on the DAF is guided primarily by the criteria for identifying studies to include in the meta-analysis. That is, the disease under study; the effectiveness measures or outcomes; the type of control group; study characteristics; type of patient and length of study.

As noted previously, the researcher will find Chapter 4 Part II of the Cochrane Handbook helpful in selecting studies (https://training.cochrane.org/handbook/current/chapter-04).

2.6   Meta-Analysis Methods

The meta-analysis methods section of the protocol will be guided by the objective, the type of data to be synthesized, and the statistical methods appropriate for the data collected and the design of the study. This section should be written before undertaking searches for appropriate studies. It is important to address how heterogeneity of summary measures across studies will be addressed.

As is the case in writing the data analysis section of a protocol, the meta-analysis methods section may need to be modified based upon peculiarities found among studies identified in the search and data abstracted therefrom.

Chapter 10 of Part II of the Cochrane Handbook: Analysing data and undertaking meta-analyses (https://training.cochrane.org/handbook/current/chapter-10) is helpful to researchers in developing the meta-analysis methods section.

Of course meta-analysis methods (using R) is primarily the subject of this book. The researcher is encouraged to review Chapters 3–9 for help in identifying methods appropriate for various summary data.

2.7   Results

We recommend that researchers produce stand-alone reports of their meta-analysis research efforts. The outline of such a report would follow the protocol contents outline but may include appendices to make the report standalone. The report would include an Abstract or Executive Summary,

Objectives, Study Population, Locating (Searching for) Studies, Screening and Evaluation Methods (which includes Inclusion/ Exclusion Criteria, Study Characteristics), Data abstraction and Extraction, Meta-Analysis Methods, Results, Summary and Discussion, Conclusions, and Appendices.

Readers should view the results from the numerous meta-analyses in Chapters 3–9 of this book for specificity of output (results) including graphical displays of effect sizes, assessment of heterogeneity, and bias. The meta-analysis report plays the same role for the meta-analysis protocol as the clinical study report for a clinical trial protocol.

The meta-analysis report becomes the single best source of documentation of the meta-analysis research as a process. Once the report is developed, articles for publication may be developed.

2.8   Summary and Discussion

This chapter called attention to the importance of writing a protocol as the first step in a meta-analysis investigation. After an initial introduction, we noted that a meta-analysis protocol (i.e. plan of study) would contain sections with content related to **Defining the Research Objective, Criteria for Identifying Studies to include in the Meta-analysis, Searching for and Collecting the Studies, Data Abstraction, Meta-analysis Methods** and **Results**.

The section on Criteria for Identifying Studies to include in the Meta-analysis had six subsections for further clarity. These are Clarifying the Disease under Study, the effectiveness measure or outcome, the type of control group, study characteristics, type of patient, and length of study.

Berman and Parker (2002) acknowledge that the totality of a meta-analysis resembles a conventional study, requiring a written protocol. They provide a structure for creating a meta-analysis protocol and list some guidelines for measuring the quality of papers that may provide summary information to be synthesized.

In addition, Part II of the Cochrane Handbook is helpful to researchers in developing a meta-analysis protocol and for using methods appropriate for the objective and analysis of data.

The report authored by West et al. (2002) for the Agency for Healthcare Research and Quality entitled "Systems to Rate the Strength of Scientific Evidence" is a must read. It recognizes the importance of developing a well-designed protocol to guide the totality of the meta-analysis inquiry as a scientific research effort. "Thus, **before** a research team conducts a systematic review, it develops a well-designed protocol that lists: (1) a focused study question, (2) a specific search strategy, including the databases to be searched, and how studies will be identified and selected for the review according to inclusion and exclusion criteria, (3) the types of data to be abstracted from each article, and (4) how the data will be synthesized, either as a text summary or as some type of quantitative aggregation or meta-analysis. These steps are taken to protect the work against various forms of unintended bias in the identification, selection, and use of published work in these reviews."

Further, the main sections of this chapter and subsections of Section 2.3 pertain largely to medical questions or questions based on clinical trials. Section and subsection topics are applicable regardless of the application with few modifications. For example, Subsection 2.3.1 Clarifying the Disease under Study in general would be Clarifying the Area of Application; Section 2.3.5 Type of Patients would be Specifying the Experimental, Sampling, or Analysis Unit.

Regardless of the application, the researcher must first write a scientifically defensible protocol that will guide the totality of the meta-analysis inquiry as a scientific research effort. The protocol should include the sections: Defining the Research Objective, Criteria for Identifying Studies to include in the Meta-analysis, Searching for and Collecting the Studies, Data Abstraction, Meta-analysis Methods, and Results. After writing the protocol, identifying data sources, abstracting the data, the data may be meta-analyzed by methods that are largely independent of the application.

3

Fixed Effects and Random Effects in Meta-Analysis

To any analyst performing a meta-analysis, the first terminology is probably fixed-effects versus random-effects models. Therefore to give readers an introductory and broad view of meta-analysis, we begin by presenting these models with limited details in this chapter along with the commonly used R packages of `rmeta` , `meta` , and `metafor` using two data sets described in Section 3.1. Detailed descriptions of these models and their applications will be learned in future chapters.

The first data set is the classical and famous data from Cochrane Collaboration logo that resulted from systematic reviews of the entire, pre-1980 clinical study literature of corticosteroid therapy in premature labor and its effect on neonatal death. The meta-analysis figure is part of the logo of the Cochrane Collaboration (http://www.cochrane.org). We present meta-analyses of this data set using the R system. The response measure in this data set is binary (death or alive).

The second data set contains estimates of treatment effect from eight randomized controlled trials of the effectiveness of amlodipine as compared to placebo in improving work capacity in patients with angina. The response measure in this data set is "work capacity" which is continuous.

In Section 3.2, we introduce fixed-effects and random-effects models used in meta-analysis where fixed-effects is the weighted mean method and random effects is the DerSimonian-Laird random-effects model implemented in R libraries `rmeta` (Author: Thomas Lumley from the Department of Biostatistics at the University of Washington, USA), `meta` (Author: Guido Schwarzer from the Institute for Medical Biometry and Medical Informatics at the University Hospital Freiburg, Germany), and `metafor` (Author: Wolfgang Viechtbauer, Viechtbauer (2010)).

In this chapter, we demonstrate how to use R and the R functionalities from the three libraries to analyze the two data sets. Specifically, we will use the library `rmete` in Section 3.3 to meta-analyze the data from Cochrane Collaboration Logo, which is binary, whereas the libraries `meta` and `metafor` are used in Section 3.4 to meta-analyze the continuous primary endpoint from clinical trial studies on amlodipine. In Section 3.5, we give some guidelines on which models, i.e., fixed-effects or random-effects, should be used. Discussion and recommendations appear in Section 3.6.

Note: to run the R programs in this chapter, readers should first install the following R packages: readxl to read the data, rmeta, meta, and metafor to perform meta-analysis.

3.1 Two Data Sets from Clinical Studies

3.1.1 Data for Cochrane Collaboration Logo: Binary Data

Data from 7 randomized controlled trials conducted prior to 1980 of corticosteroid therapy in premature labor and its effect on neonatal death were meta-analyzed. These data are included in R meta-analysis library rmeta and are reproduced in Table 3.1 for easy reference. This dataframe contains five columns. Column 1 contains the "name" as an identifier for the study. Column 2 contains the number ("ev.trt") of deaths among patients in the treated group. Column 3 contains the total number of patients ("n.trt") in the treated group. Column 4 contains the number of deaths ("ev.ctrl") in the control group. Column 5 contains the total number of patients ("n.ctrl") in the control group.

3.1.2 Clinical Studies on Amlodipine: Continuous Data

Eight randomized controlled trials of the effectiveness of the calcium channel blocker amlodipine as compared to placebo in improving work capacity in patients with angina are summarized in Table 3.2. These data are used in Li et al. (1994) to illustrate potential bias in meta-analysis. The data are reproduced further in Hartung et al. (2008). The change in work capacity is defined as the ratio of exercise time after the patient receives the intervention (i.e., drug or placebo) to the exercise time at baseline (before receiving the intervention). It is assumed that the logarithms of these ratios are normally distributed. Table 3.2 lists the observed sample size, mean, and variance for

TABLE 3.1

Data for Cochrane Collaboration Logo

Name	ev.trt	n.trt	ev.ctrl	n.ctrl
Auckland	36	532	60	538
Block	1	69	5	61
Doran	4	81	11	63
Gamsu	14	131	20	137
Morrison	3	67	7	59
Papageorgiou	1	71	7	75
Tauesch	8	56	10	71

TABLE 3.2

Angina Study Data

Protocol	nE	meanE	varE	nC	meanC	varC
154	46	0.2316	0.2254	48	−0.0027	0.0007
156	30	0.2811	0.1441	26	0.0270	0.1139
157	75	0.1894	0.1981	72	0.0443	0.4972
162	12	0.0930	0.1389	12	0.2277	0.0488
163	32	0.1622	0.0961	34	0.0056	0.0955
166	31	0.1837	0.1246	31	0.0943	0.1734
303	27	0.6612	0.7060	27	−0.0057	0.9891
306	46	0.1366	0.1211	47	−0.0057	0.1291

both treatment and placebo groups. We meta-analyze these data to illustrate application of (meta-analysis) methods for continuous data.

3.2 Fixed-Effects and Random-Effects Models in Meta-Analysis

As described in Wikipedia, "In statistics, a meta-analysis combines the results of several studies that address a set of related research hypotheses. This is normally done by identification of a common measure of *effect size*, which is modeled using a form of meta-regression. Resulting overall averages when controlling for study characteristics can be considered meta-effect sizes, which are more powerful estimates of the true effect size than those derived in a single study under a given single set of assumptions and conditions." We thus begin introducing this *effect size* (ES) in Section 3.2.1.

3.2.1 Hypotheses and Effect Size

The fundamental objective for conducting a clinical study of the efficacy of a new drug (D) in the treatment of some disease is to demonstrate that the new drug is effective in treating the disease. Translating into the statistical hypothesis framework, the objective becomes the alternative hypothesis in contrast to the null hypothesis of inefficacy given by:

H_0 : Effect of D is no different from that of control (placebo = P)

H_a : Effect of D is better than that of P

Treatment effect size is a comparative function of the efficacy response measure among patients in the drug groups to that among patients in the control group. The comparative function may be the difference in means if response is continuous, or the difference in proportions if response is dichotomous or binary. Other comparative functions of effect size for binary data are the log-odds ratio or relative risk. It is noted that the comparative function specifies an arithmetical order of the interventions; e.g., drug-control or drug/control. The treatment effect size is denoted by δ to be compatible with the notations used in Peace and Chen (2010), Chen and Peace (2013), and Chen et al. (2017). Then H_0 and H_a above become:

$$H_0 : \delta = 0$$
$$H_a : \delta > 0$$

For multiple randomized, controlled, efficacy studies of a drug, H_0 and H_a are the same for each study. Randomization of patients to treatment groups within studies and conducting the study in a blinded and quality manner ensures valid, unbiased estimates of treatment effect within studies.

Fundamentally a design-based analysis strategy is no different than a meta-analysis of the treatment effect estimates across the centers. That is, first compute the estimates of treatment effect $\hat{\delta}_i$ and the within variance $\hat{\sigma}_i^2$ of treatment effect at each study or center $i (i = 1, \cdots, K)$, and then meta-analyze the $\hat{\delta}_i$ across studies or centers.

To obtain an estimate of the overall efficacy of the drug across all studies and to provide an inference as to the statistical significance of the overall effect, the individual study estimates are meta-analyzed. There are typically two meta-analysis approaches in this direction with one as *fixed-effects* and the other as *random-effects*.

In fixed-effects meta-analysis, we assume that we have an estimate of *treatment effect* $\hat{\delta}_i$ and its (within) variability estimate $\hat{\sigma}_i^2$ from each clinical study i. Each $\hat{\delta}_i$ is an estimate of the underlying global overall effect of δ across all studies. To meta-analyze this set of $\hat{\delta}_i$ means that we combine them using some weighting scheme.

However for the random-effects meta-analysis model, we assume that each $\hat{\delta}_i$ is an estimate of its own underlying true effect δ_i which is one realization from the overall global effect δ. Therefore, the random-effects meta-analysis model can incorporate both within-study variability and between-study variability – which may be an important source of heterogeneity in multiple studies.

3.2.2   Fixed-Effects Meta-Analysis Model: The Weighted-Average

3.2.2.1   Fixed-Effects Model

The underlying assumption for the fixed-effects model is that all studies in the meta-analysis share a common (true) overall effect size δ with same impacts from all other risk factors. With that assumption, the true effect size is the same (and therefore the name of *fixed-effects*) in all the studies.

In this fixed-effects model, each observed effect size $\hat{\delta}_i$ could vary among studies because of the random errors from each study and is assumed to be an estimate of the underlying global overall effect δ.

Under the fixed-effects model, we assume that all factors that could influence the effect size are the same in all the studies and that

$$\hat{\delta}_i = \delta + \epsilon_i \tag{3.1}$$

where ϵ_i is assumed to be normally distributed by $N(0, \hat{\sigma}_i^2)$. That is

$$\hat{\delta}_i \sim N(\delta, \hat{\sigma}_i^2) \tag{3.2}$$

The global δ is then estimated by combining the individual estimates by some weighting scheme in order to obtain the most precise estimate of the global effect. That is, we weight $\hat{\delta}_i$ for each study i with an appropriate weight w_i, then compute the weighted mean or pooled estimate $\hat{\delta}$ of treatment effect as well as its variance $\hat{\sigma}^2$, where

$$\hat{\delta} = \sum_{i=1}^{K} w_i \hat{\delta}_i \tag{3.3}$$

$$\hat{\sigma}^2 = Var(\hat{\delta}) = \sum_{i=1}^{K} w_i^2 \hat{\sigma}_i^2 \text{(under independence of the K studies)} \tag{3.4}$$

Using the weighted mean in equation (3.3) and its variance in equation (3.4), an approximate 95% confidence interval (CI) for δ is:

$$\hat{\delta} \pm 1.96 \times \sqrt{\hat{\sigma}^2} \tag{3.5}$$

In addition, we may formulate a t-type of test as:

$$T = \frac{\hat{\delta} - \delta}{\sqrt{\hat{\sigma}^2}} \tag{3.6}$$

to be used to test $H_0 : \delta = 0$. Based on the test statistic in equation (3.6), we construct confidence intervals on the overall global effect of δ in the usual manner.

3.2.2.2 The Weighting Schemes

The weighted mean in equation (3.3) requires $\sum_{i=1}^{K} w_i = 1$. Typical choices of w_i are:

1. Weighting by the number of studies.

    In this scheme, the weights are fixed to a constant for all studies as

$$w_i = \frac{1}{K} \tag{3.7}$$

    where K is the number of studies(fixed);

2. Weighting by the number of patients in each study.

In this scheme, the weights are defined as the proportion between the number of patients in each study and the total number of patients from all K studies as:

$$w_i = \frac{N_i}{N} \tag{3.8}$$

where N_i is the number of patients in study i and N is the total number of patients as $N = \sum_{i=1}^{K} N_i$;

3. Weighting by the number of patients from each study and each treatment.

In this scheme, we first calculate the initial weight for each study as $w_i' = \frac{N_{iD} N_{iP}}{N_{iD} + N_{iP}}$ and the total weight $w = \sum_{i=1}^{K} w_i'$. We then rescale w_i' by the total weight w to define the weighting as follows:

$$w_i = \frac{w_i'}{w} \tag{3.9}$$

where N_{iD} and N_{iP} are the numbers of patients in the new drug treatment (D) and Placebo (P) groups, respectively, at study i;

4. Weighting by the inverse variance.

In this scheme, we first calculate the initial weight for each study as $w_i' = \frac{1}{\hat{\sigma}_i^2}$ and the total weight $w = \sum_{i=1}^{K} w_i'$. We then rescale w_i' by the total weight w to define the weighting as follows:

$$w_i = \frac{w_i'}{w}. \tag{3.10}$$

The weighting scheme 1 in equation (3.7) yields the unweighted mean or arithmetic average of the estimates of treatment effect across studies.

The weighting scheme 2 in equation (3.8) yields the average of the estimates of treatment effect across studies weighted according to the number of patients in each study. Note that the weighting scheme 2 in equation (3.8) reduces to weight scheme 1 in equation (3.7) if there is balance across studies.

The weighting scheme 3 in equation (3.9) yields the average of the estimates of treatment effect across studies weighted to allow treatment group imbalance in each study. Note that scheme 3 in equation (3.9) reduces to scheme 2 in equation (3.8) if treatment groups are balanced across studies.

The weighting scheme 4 in equation (3.10) yields the average of the estimates of treatment effect across studies weighting the estimates inversely to their variance which is used in almost all fixed-effects models and we will use this weighting hereafter. Note that scheme 4 in equation (3.10) reduces to scheme 1 in equation (3.7) if the $\hat{\sigma}_i^2$ are the same (true homogeneity) across studies.

It should be noted that for dichotomous response data, the data at each study may be summarized by a two-by-two table with responders versus non-responders as columns and treatment groups as rows. Let O_i denote the number of responders in the pivotal cell of the two-by-two table at each study, and $E(O_i)$ and $Var(O_i)$ denote the expected value and variance of O_i, respectively, computed from the hypergeometric distribution. The square of equation (3.6) becomes the Mantel-Haenszel statistic (unadjusted for lack of continuity) proposed by Mantel and Haenszel (1959) for addressing association between treatment and response across studies. For this reason, the weighted mean estimate in (3.3) with its variance in (3.4) using weighting scheme 4 is implemented in R library `rmeta` as function `meta.MH` for "*Fixed effects (Mantel-Haenszel) meta-analysis.*" This R library is created by Professor Thomas Lumley at the University of Washington with functions for simple fixed- and random-effects meta-analysis for two-sample comparisons and cumulative meta-analyses as well as drawing standard summary plots, funnel plots, and computing summaries and tests for association and heterogeneity.

3.2.3   Random-Effects Meta-Analysis Model: DerSimonian-Laird

3.2.3.1   Random-Effects Model

When meta-analyzing effect sizes from different studies (such as separate clinical trials), the fundamental assumption in the fixed-effects model that the true effect size is the same for all studies may be impractical. When we attempt to synthesize a group of studies with a meta-analysis, we expect that these studies have enough in common to combine the information for statistical inference, but it may be impractical to require that these studies have identical true effect size.

The random-effects meta-analysis model assumes the treatment effect $\hat{\delta}_{iR}$ from each study i is an estimate of its own underlying true treatment effect δ_{iR} with an estimated within-study sampling variance $\hat{\sigma}_i^2$ (so assumed known) and further that the δ_{iR} from all the K studies follow some overall global distribution denoted by $N(\delta, \tau^2)$. This random-effects meta model can be written as:

$$\hat{\delta}_{iR} \sim N(\delta_{iR}, \hat{\sigma}_i^2)$$
$$\delta_{iR} \sim N(\delta, \tau^2) \qquad (3.11)$$

This random-effects model can be described as an extension of the fixed-effects model in equation (3.1) as:

$$\hat{\delta}_{iR} = \delta + \nu_i + \epsilon_i \qquad (3.12)$$

where $\nu_i \sim N(0, \tau^2)$ describes the between-center (or between-study) variation.

We make the assumption that ν_i and ϵ_i are independent, and therefore, the random-effects model in equation (3.11) can be rewritten as:

$$\hat{\delta}_{iR} \sim N(\delta, \hat{\sigma}_i^2 + \tau^2) \tag{3.13}$$

In this formulation, the extra parameter τ^2 represents the between-study variability around the underlying global treatment effect δ. It is easy to show in this formulation that the global δ is also estimated by the weighted mean similar to the fixed-effects meta-model as given in equation (3.3) as:

$$\hat{\delta}_R = \frac{\sum_{i=1}^{K} w_{iR} \hat{\delta}_{iR}}{\sum_{i=1}^{K} w_{iR}} \tag{3.14}$$

with standard error estimated as:

$$se\left(\hat{\delta}_R\right) = \sqrt{\frac{1}{\sum_{i=1}^{K} w_{iR}}} \tag{3.15}$$

where the weights now are given by:

$$\hat{w}_{iR} = \frac{1}{\hat{\sigma}_i^2 + \hat{\tau}^2} \tag{3.16}$$

$$se\left(\hat{\delta}_R\right) = \sqrt{\frac{1}{\sum_{i=1}^{K} w_{iR}}} \tag{3.17}$$

Therefore, a 95% CI may be formulated to provide statistical inference similar to the fixed-effects model.

There are several methods to estimate the $\hat{\tau}^2$. The most commonly used estimate is from DerSimonian and Laird (1986) and is derived using the method of moments (which does not involve iterative search algorithms as do likelihood-based ones). Parenthetically, we note that the Dersimonian-Laird procedure is commonly referred to as the Cochran-Dersimonian-Laird procedure due to the work Cochran did in the mid-1950s on combining data from a series of experiments. This estimate is given as:

$$\hat{\tau}^2 = \frac{Q - (K - 1)}{U} \tag{3.18}$$

if $Q > K - 1$, otherwise, $\hat{\tau}^2 = 0$ where

$$Q = \sum_{i=1}^{K} w_i(\hat{\delta}_i - \hat{\delta})^2 \tag{3.19}$$

$$U = \sum_{i=1}^{K} w_i - \frac{\sum_{i=1}^{K} w_i^2}{\sum_{i=1}^{K} w_i} \tag{3.20}$$

Note that the statistic Q is used for testing the statistical significance of heterogeneity across studies. This random-effects meta-model is implemented in the R library `rmeta` as function `meta.DSL` for "*Random effects (DerSimonian-Laird) meta-analysis.*" It is implemented as `metabin` and `meta-cont` in library `meta`. It is also implemented as `method = "DL"` in the function `rma` in R package `metafor`.

Therefore, the random-effects meta-analysis model can incorporate both within-study and between-study variability which may be an important source of heterogeneity for meta-analysis. In this sense, the random-effects meta-analysis model is more conservative since $w_{iR} \leq w_i$ which leads to

$$se(\hat{\delta}_R) = \sqrt{\frac{1}{\sum_{i=1}^{K} w_{iR}}} \geq \sqrt{\frac{1}{\sum_{i=1}^{K} w_i}} = se(\hat{\delta}). \tag{3.21}$$

3.2.3.2 Derivation of DerSimonian-Laird Estimator of τ^2

The derivation of DerSimonian-Laird estimator of τ^2 in equation (3.18) is based on the method of moments by equating the sample statistic of Q to the corresponding expected value.

To emphasize here again that the only difference between the fixed-effects and the random-effects is the weighting factors in the weighted-average where in the random-effects $\hat{w}_{iR} = \frac{1}{\hat{\sigma}_i^2 + \hat{\tau}^2}$ and in the fixed-effects $\hat{w}_i = \frac{1}{\hat{\sigma}_i^2}$. Corresponding to these weighting factors, the meta-estimators are $\hat{\delta}_R = \frac{\sum_{i=1}^{K} w_{iR}\hat{\delta}_{iR}}{\sum_{i=1}^{K} w_{iR}}$ for random-effects and $\hat{\delta} = \frac{\sum_{i=1}^{K} w_i\hat{\delta}_i}{\sum_{i=1}^{K} w_i}$ for fixed-effects.

It can be shown that both estimators of $\hat{\delta}_R$ and $\hat{\delta}$ are unbiased with expected value of δ. The variances are

$$var\left(\hat{\delta}\right) = \frac{1}{\sum_{i=1}^{K} w_i} \tag{3.22}$$

$$var\left(\hat{\delta}_R\right) = \frac{1}{\sum_{i=1}^{K} w_{iR}} \tag{3.23}$$

With these facts, we can now derive the DerSimonian-Laird estimator. Let us first decompose the Q as

$$Q = \sum_{i=1}^{K} w_i(\hat{\delta}_i - \hat{\delta})^2 = \sum_{i=1}^{K} w_i \left[(\hat{\delta}_i - \delta) - (\hat{\delta} - \delta)\right]^2$$

$$= \sum_{i=1}^{K} w_i(\hat{\delta}_i - \delta)^2 - 2\sum_{i=1}^{K} w_i(\hat{\delta}_i - \delta)(\hat{\delta} - \delta) + \sum_{i=1}^{K} w_i(\hat{\delta} - \delta)^2 \tag{3.24}$$

Therefore, the expected values of Q under random-effects model in equation (3.11) can be shown as follows:

$$E(Q) = \sum_{i=1}^{K} w_i E(\hat{\delta}_i - \delta)^2 - \left(\sum_{i=1}^{K} w_i \right) E(\hat{\delta} - \delta)^2$$

$$= \sum_{i=1}^{K} w_i var(\hat{\delta}_i) - \left(\sum_{i=1}^{K} w_i \right) var(\hat{\delta})$$

$$= \sum_{i=1}^{K} w_i var(\hat{\delta}_i) - \left(\sum_{i=1}^{K} w_i \right) var\left[\frac{\sum_{i=1}^{K} w_i \hat{\delta}_i}{\sum_{i=1}^{K} w_i} \right]$$

$$= \sum_{i=1}^{K} w_i var(\hat{\delta}_i) - \left(\sum_{i=1}^{K} w_i \right) \frac{\sum_{i=1}^{K} w_i^2 var\left(\hat{\delta}_i \right)}{\left(\sum_{i=1}^{K} w_i \right)^2}$$

$$= \sum_{i=1}^{K} w_i (w_i^{-1} + \tau^2) - \left(\sum_{i=1}^{K} w_i \right) \frac{\sum_{i=1}^{K} w_i^2 (w_i^{-1} + \tau^2)}{\left(\sum_{i=1}^{K} w_i \right)^2}$$

$$= \sum_{i=1}^{K} w_i (w_i^{-1} + \tau^2) - \left(\sum_{i=1}^{K} w_i \right) \left[\frac{1}{\sum_{i=1}^{K} w_i} + \frac{\tau^2 \sum_{i=1}^{K} w_i^2}{\left(\sum_{i=1}^{K} w_i \right)^2} \right]$$

$$= (K-1) + \tau^2 \left[\sum_{i=1}^{K} w_i - \frac{\sum_{i=1}^{K} w_i^2}{\sum_{i=1}^{K} w_i} \right] \tag{3.25}$$

For the method of moments, let $E(Q) \approx Q$ to estimate the τ^2 as

$$\hat{\tau}^2 = \frac{Q - (K-1)}{\sum_{i=1}^{K} w_i - \frac{\sum_{i=1}^{K} w_i^2}{\sum_{i=1}^{K} w_i}} \tag{3.26}$$

which is the well-known DerSimonian-Laird method of moments for τ^2 in equation (3.18). Notice that the estimated variance $\hat{\tau}^2$ can be less than zero even though the true variance of τ^2 can never be. This happens when $Q < df = K - 1$ and when this happens, the estimated $\hat{\tau}^2$ is set to zero.

3.2.4 Publication Bias

Publication bias is sometimes referred to as selection bias. In meta-analysis, the studies selected to be included are vital to the inferential conclusion. Publication bias could arise when only positive studies (those that demonstrate statistical significance or if not statistically significant do not reflect qualitative interaction) of a drug are published. Therefore even though all published studies of a drug for the treatment of some disease may be selected for a meta-analysis, the resulting inferential results may be biased (may overestimate the efficacy of the drug). The bias may be particularly significant when meta-analyses are conducted or are sponsored by a group with a vested interest in the results.

In meta-analysis, Begg's *funnel plot* or Egger's plot is used to graphically display the existence of publication bias. Statistical tests for publication bias are usually based on the fact that clinical studies with small sample sizes (and therefore large variances) may be more prone to publication bias in contrast to large clinical studies. Therefore, when estimates from all studies are plotted against their variances (sample size), a symmetrical funnel should be seen when there is no publication bias, while a skewed asymmetrical funnel is a signal of potential publication bias.

We will briefly illustrate this funnel plot along with the data analysis using the R system in this chapter. Chapter 9 will have more extensive discussions and illustrations about publication bias. Readers may review Chapter 9 for a broader discussion and presentation of Publication Bias.

3.3   Meta-Analysis for Data from Cochrane Collaboration Logo

3.3.1   The Data

We illustrate meta-analysis using R package **rmeta**. First we access the "Cochrane" data and load it into R as:

```
> # Load the data
> data(cochrane)
> # print it
> cochrane
```

	name	ev.trt	n.trt	ev.ctrl	n.ctrl
1	Auckland	36	532	60	538
2	Block	1	69	5	61
3	Doran	4	81	11	63
4	Gamsu	14	131	20	137
5	Morrison	3	67	7	59
6	Papageorgiou	1	71	7	75
7	Tauesch	8	56	10	71

This gives the data in Table 3.1.

3.3.2   Fitting the Fixed-Effects Model

With this dataframe, we first fit the fixed-effects model as described in Section 3.2.2 using the R function **meta.MH** to compute the individual odds ratios or relative risks, the Mantel-Haenszel weighted mean estimate, and Woolf's test for heterogeneity. The R implementation is illustrated by the following R code chunk:

```
> # Fit the fixed-effects model
> steroid = meta.MH(n.trt, n.ctrl, ev.trt, ev.ctrl,
                        names=name, data=cochrane)
> # Print the model fit
> summary(steroid)

Fixed effects ( Mantel-Haenszel ) meta-analysis
Call: meta.MH(ntrt = n.trt, nctrl = n.ctrl, ptrt = ev.trt,
        pctrl = ev.ctrl, names = name, data = cochrane)
------------------------------------
                OR (lower  95% upper)
Auckland       0.58    0.38      0.89
Block          0.16    0.02      1.45
Doran          0.25    0.07      0.81
Gamsu          0.70    0.34      1.45
Morrison       0.35    0.09      1.41
Papageorgiou   0.14    0.02      1.16
Tauesch        1.02    0.37      2.77
------------------------------------

Mantel-Haenszel OR =0.53 95% CI ( 0.39,0.73 )
Test for heterogeneity: X^2( 6 ) = 6.9 ( p-value 0.3303 )
```

It is observed from the model fit that the overall OR is 0.53 with 95% CI of (0.39, 0.73), indicating significant overall effect for steroid treatment in reducing neonatal death. However, if analyzed individually, in only two ("Auckland" and "Doran") of the 7 studies, the steroid treatment was statistically significant. In addition, the χ^2 test for heterogeneity yielded a p-value of 0.3303 indicating nonstatistically significant heterogeneity.

We could call the default function `plot` to plot the meta-analysis, but we can produce a more comprehensive figure for this analysis by calling the `forestplot` using the following R code chunk which gives Figure 3.1.

This is the so-called "forest plot" in meta-analysis; i.e., a plot of the estimates and their associated 95% CIs for each study, as well as the global (summary or combined) estimate. The 95%CI intervals are the lines; the squares in the middle of the lines represent the point estimates. The global estimate or "Summary" is the diamond whose width is the associated 95% CI.

```
> # Create the ``tabletext" to include all the outputs
> tabletext = cbind(c("","Study",steroid$names,NA,"Summary"),
                c("Deaths","(Steroid)",cochrane$ev.trt,NA,NA),
                c("Deaths","(Placebo)",cochrane$ev.ctrl, NA,NA),
                c("","OR",format(exp(steroid$logOR),digits=2),
                    NA,format(exp(steroid$logMH),digits=2)))
> # Generate the CI
> mean    = c(NA,NA,steroid$logOR,NA,steroid$logMH)
> stderr  = c(NA,NA,steroid$selogOR,NA,steroid$selogMH)
```

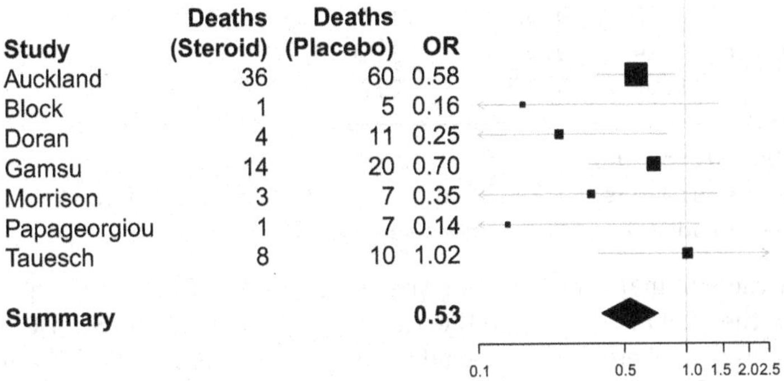

Study	Deaths (Steroid)	Deaths (Placebo)	OR
Auckland	36	60	0.58
Block	1	5	0.16
Doran	4	11	0.25
Gamsu	14	20	0.70
Morrison	3	7	0.35
Papageorgiou	1	7	0.14
Tauesch	8	10	1.02
Summary			**0.53**

FIGURE 3.1
Forestplot for Cochrane data.

```
> l       = mean-1.96*stderr
> u       = mean+1.96*stderr
> # Call forestplot
> forestplot(tabletext,mean,l,u,zero=0,
         is.summary=c(TRUE,TRUE,rep(FALSE,8),TRUE),
            clip=c(log(0.1),log(2.5)), xlog=TRUE)
```

3.3.3 Fitting the Random-Effects Model

Similarly, the random-effects model as described in Section 3.2.3 can be implemented using R function meta.DSL to compute the individual odds ratios or relative risks, the Mantel-Haenszel weighted mean estimate and Woolf's test for heterogeneity along with the estimate of the random-effects variance. The R implementation is illustrated by the following R code chunk:

```
> # Call the meta.DSL for calculations
> steroidDSL  = meta.DSL(n.trt,n.ctrl,ev.trt,ev.ctrl,
         names=name, data=cochrane)
> # Print the summary from meta.DSL
> summary(steroidDSL)

Random effects ( DerSimonian-Laird ) meta-analysis
Call: meta.DSL(ntrt = n.trt, nctrl = n.ctrl, ptrt = ev.trt,
         pctrl = ev.ctrl, names = name, data = cochrane)
------------------------------------
              OR (lower  95% upper)
Auckland    0.58    0.38       0.89
Block       0.16    0.02       1.45
Doran       0.25    0.07       0.81
Gamsu       0.70    0.34       1.45
```

```
Morrison     0.35      0.09       1.41
Papageorgiou 0.14      0.02       1.16
Tauesch      1.02      0.37       2.77
-----------------------------------------
SummaryOR= 0.53  95% CI ( 0.37,0.78 )
Test for heterogeneity: X^2( 6 ) = 6.86 ( p-value 0.334 )
Estimated random effects variance: 0.03
```

From the summary, we see that the estimated between-study variance = 0.03 and the global OR = 0.53 with 95% CI of (0.37, 0.78). Because of the estimated nonzero between-study variance, the 95% CIs from individual studies and the one based on the global estimate are slightly wider than those from the fixed-effects meta-analysis – which is consistent with the theory described in Section 3.2.3. Both fixed-effects and random-effects models indicate a significant overall effect for steroid treatment in reducing neonatal death.

Similarly, the random-effects meta-analysis can be easily shown graphically in Figure 3.2 with the default `plot` setting. We encourage readers to use `forestplot` to reproduce this figure with different settings.

```
> plot(steroidDSL)
```

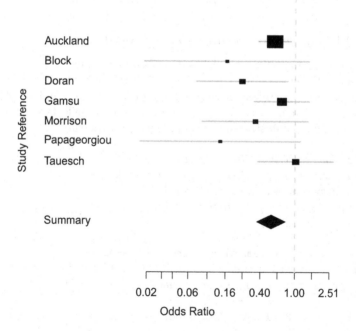

FIGURE 3.2
Forest plot for the Cochran trial with 95% CIs from random-effects meta-analysis.

3.4 Meta-Analysis of Amlodipine Trial Data

For this data, we illustrate the application of the R libraries `meta` and `metafor` for their functionalities in meta-analysis.

3.4.1 The Data

We load the data in Table 3.2 into R using R library `readxl` as follows:

```
> # Load the library "readxl"
> require(readxl)
> # Get the data path
> datfile = " Your data file path  to 'dat4Meta.xls'"
> # Call "read_excel" to read the Excel data in specific data
      sheet
> angina  = read_excel(datfile, sheet="Data_Angina")
> # Print the data
> angina
```

```
# A tibble: 8 x 7
  Protocol    nE meanE   varE    nC  meanC    varC
     <dbl> <dbl> <dbl>  <dbl> <dbl>  <dbl>   <dbl>
1      154    46 0.232  0.225    48 -0.0027 0.0007
2      156    30 0.281  0.144    26  0.027  0.114
3      157    75 0.189  0.198    72  0.0443 0.497
4      162    12 0.093  0.139    12  0.228  0.0488
5      163    32 0.162  0.0961   34  0.0056 0.0955
6      166    31 0.184  0.125    31  0.0943 0.173
7      303    27 0.661  0.706    27 -0.0057 0.989
8      306    46 0.137  0.121    47 -0.0057 0.129
```

We see that there are eight protocols or studies, each with the number of observations, mean, and variance for treatment and control groups.

Also note that in above R code chunk, we define the `datfile` to where you store the Excel file, i.e., `datfile = your datafile path/dat4Meta.xls`, and so you need to change your `datafile path` to where you actually store this excel databook (i.e., `dat4Meta.xls`) in your computer.

3.4.2 Meta-Analysis with `meta` Package

To illustrate the application of the R library `meta` for its functionalities in meta-analysis, we load the library as:

```
> library(meta)
```

The functions associated with this library may be seen using:

```
> library(help=meta)
```

As seen, this library may be used also for fixed- and random-effects meta-analysis. In addition, there are functions that can be used for tests of bias, and for producing forest and funnel plots.

3.4.2.1 Fit the Fixed-Effects Model

This is a data set with continuous response data and we use the `metacont` to model the data with the following R chunk:

```
> # Fit fixed-effects model
> fixed.angina = metacont(nE, meanE, sqrt(varE),nC,meanC,sqrt(varC),
        data=angina,studlab=Protocol,comb.random=FALSE)
> # Print the fitted model
> fixed.angina
```

```
           MD              95%-CI %W(fixed)
154    0.2343 [ 0.0969;  0.3717]      21.2
156    0.2541 [ 0.0663;  0.4419]      11.4
157    0.1451 [-0.0464;  0.3366]      10.9
162   -0.1347 [-0.3798;  0.1104]       6.7
163    0.1566 [ 0.0072;  0.3060]      17.9
166    0.0894 [-0.1028;  0.2816]      10.8
303    0.6669 [ 0.1758;  1.1580]       1.7
306    0.1423 [-0.0015;  0.2861]      19.4

Number of studies combined: k = 8


                         MD             95%-CI    z    p-value
Fixed effect model 0.1619 [0.0986;  0.2252] 5.01    < 0.0001

Quantifying heterogeneity:
 tau^2 = 0.0066 [0.0000; 0.1028]; tau = 0.0812 [0.0000; 0.3207];
 I^2 = 43.2% [0.0%; 74.9%]; H = 1.33 [1.00; 2.00]

Test of heterogeneity:
     Q d.f. p-value
 12.33    7  0.0902

Details on meta-analytical method:
- Inverse variance method
- DerSimonian-Laird estimator for tau^2
- Jackson method for confidence interval of tau^2 and tau
```

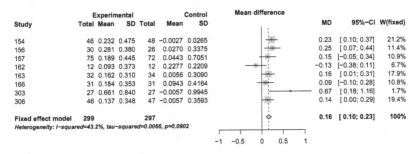

FIGURE 3.3

A detailed forest plot for the Angina trial with 95% CIs.

From this fixed-effects model fitting, we note from the 95% CIs that amlodipine treatment is not statistically significant in four of the eight protocols. However, the overall effect of amlodipine from the fixed-effects model is 0.1619 with corresponding 95% CI of [0.0986; 0.2252] and p-value < 0.001 – indicating a statistically significant treatment effect. The test of heterogeneity gave a p-value of 0.09 from $Q = 12.33$ with 7 degrees of freedom indicating that there is no strong evidence against homogeneity.

A typical forest plot can be generated by calling the `forest.meta` as follows to produce Figure 3.3.

```
> # Call forest.meta to make the forest plot
> forest.meta(fixed.angina)
```

To assess potential publication bias informally, we generate the funnel plot and visually assess whether it is symmetric. This funnel plot can be generated using the following R code chunk which produces Figure 3.4:

```
> # Call funnel to make funnel plot
> funnel(fixed.angina)
```

From this figure, we note that protocol 303 has the largest mean difference of 0.6669 on the right and protocol 162 has the smallest mean difference of −0.1347 on the left. The remaining are quite symmetric. A statistical significance test can be performed using `metabias`. This test is based on the rank correlation between standardized treatment estimates and variance estimates of estimated treatment effects where Kendall's tau is used as the correlation measure (see from Begg and Mazumdar, 1994) to test the null hypothesis that there is no publication bias. Other tests may be performed and may be seen in the library `meta`.

By calling `metabias` for this model fitting as follows:

```
> # Call metabias for statistical test
> metabias(fixed.angina, k.min=5)
```

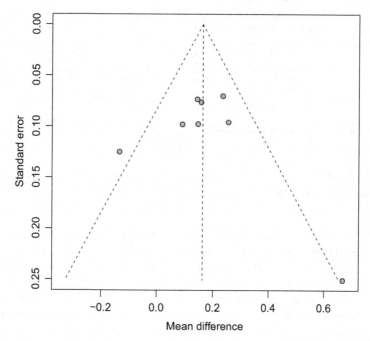

FIGURE 3.4
Funnel plot for the Angina trial.

```
          Linear regression test of funnel plot asymmetry

data:  fixed.angina
t = 0.33779, df = 6, p-value = 0.747
alternative hypothesis: asymmetry in funnel plot
sample estimates:
bias    se.bias      slope
0.5885126 1.7422260 0.1104225
```

we see the *p*-value associated with this test is 0.747 indicating symmetry of
the funnel plot.

3.4.2.2   Fit the Random-Effects Model

Similar to the fixed-effects model in Section 3.4.2.1, we can fit the random-
effects model as follows:

```
> # fit random-effects model
> random.angina = metacont(nE, meanE, sqrt(varE),nC,meanC,
  sqrt(varC),
          data=angina,studlab=Protocol,comb.random=T)
```

```
> # print the summary fit
> random.angina
```

	MD	95%-CI	%W(fixed)	%W(random)
154	0.2343	[0.0969; 0.3717]	21.2	17.5
156	0.2541	[0.0663; 0.4419]	11.4	12.7
157	0.1451	[-0.0464; 0.3366]	10.9	12.5
162	-0.1347	[-0.3798; 0.1104]	6.7	9.0
163	0.1566	[0.0072; 0.3060]	17.9	16.2
166	0.0894	[-0.1028; 0.2816]	10.8	12.4
303	0.6669	[0.1758; 1.1580]	1.7	2.9
306	0.1423	[-0.0015; 0.2861]	19.4	16.8

```
Number of studies combined: k = 8
```

	MD	95%-CI	z	p-value
Fixed effect model	0.1619	[0.0986; 0.2252]	5.01	< 0.0001
Random effects model	0.1589	[0.0710; 0.2467]	3.54	0.0004

```
Quantifying heterogeneity:
 tau^2 = 0.0066 [0.0000; 0.1028]; tau = 0.0812 [0.0000; 0.3207];
 I^2 = 43.2% [0.0%; 74.9%]; H = 1.33 [1.00; 2.00]
```

```
Test of heterogeneity:
     Q d.f. p-value
 12.33    7  0.0902
```

```
Details on meta-analytical method:
- Inverse variance method
- DerSimonian-Laird estimator for tau^2
- Jackson method for confidence interval of tau^2 and tau
```

This gives the model fitting for random-effects as well as for fixed-effects. We note from the output that the estimated between-protocol variance $\hat{\tau}^2 = 0.0066$ and that the mean difference is estimated as 0.159 from the random-effects model as compared to 0.162 from the fixed-effects model. The 95% CI from the random-effects model is $(0.071, 0.247)$ as compared to $(0.098, 0.225)$ from fixed-effects model. Again the 95% CI from the random-effects model is wider than that for the fixed-effects model. We leave generating the forest plot as an exercise for interested readers.

3.4.3 Meta-Analysis with the metafor Package

This package is considered as the most general R package for all meta-analyses. Interested readers can use any of these packages for meta-analysis since they all give the same results.

In this section, we briefly illustrate the application of the `metafor` for its functionalities in meta-analysis to familiarize interested readers for this package. We load the library as:

```
> # Load the package
> library(metafor)
```

The functions associated with this library may be seen using:

```
> library(help=metafor)
```

As seen, this library can be also used for fixed- and random-effects meta-analysis. As a comprehensive collection of functions for conducting meta-analyses in R, this package includes many other functions for meta-analysis, such as meta-regression analyses, multivariate/multilevel meta-analysis, network meta-analyses, etc., as discussed in Viechtbauer (2010).

3.4.3.1 Calculate the Effect Size

The first step in using `metafor` for meta-analysis is to calculate the effect-size (ES) for each study to obtain a set of effect size estimates along with their corresponding within-study sampling variances. With these calculated ESs, the meta-analysis is then to combine these ESs.

This calculation is done by calling the function `escalc` as illustrated as follows:

```
> # Call escalc to calculate effect sizes
> ES.MD = escalc(measure="MD", n1i=nE, n2i=nC,
                 m1i=meanE, m2i=meanC,
                 sd1i=sqrt(varE), sd2i=sqrt(varC), data=angina)
> # Print the ES
> ES.MD
```

	Protocol	nE	meanE	varE	nC	meanC	varC	yi	vi
1	154	46	0.232	0.2254	48	-0.0027	0.0007	0.2343	0.0049
2	156	30	0.281	0.1441	26	0.0270	0.1139	0.2541	0.0092
3	157	75	0.189	0.1981	72	0.0443	0.4972	0.1451	0.0095
4	162	12	0.093	0.1389	12	0.2277	0.0488	-0.1347	0.0156
5	163	32	0.162	0.0961	34	0.0056	0.0955	0.1566	0.0058
6	166	31	0.184	0.1246	31	0.0943	0.1734	0.0894	0.0096
7	303	27	0.661	0.7060	27	-0.0057	0.9891	0.6669	0.0628
8	306	46	0.137	0.1211	47	-0.0057	0.1291	0.1423	0.0054

As seen from above code chunk, we use `n1i=nE`, `n2i=nC`, `m1i=meanE`, `m2i=meanC`, `sd1i=sqrt(varE)`, `sd2i=sqrt(varC)` from the data `data=angina` to calculate the ESs. The ESs are calculated with `measure="MD"` which is to calculate the mean difference (MD) between the treatment of amlodipine and control.

As seen further from the output, two extra columns are added to the data ES.MD along with the original data. Specifically, the column yi is the calculated ES, i.e., the MD and the column vi are the associated sample variances for each ES from that study.

With these two columns of data, we can easily apply the model equations described in Section 3.2 for fixed-effects and random-effects meta-analysis using the weighted-average schemes.

3.4.3.2 Fit the Fixed-Effects Model

For fixed-effects meta-analysis, we call function rma with the method="FE" as follows:

```
> # Fit the fixed-effects model
> FE.angina = rma(yi, vi, data=ES.MD, method="FE")
> # Print the Summary of model fit
> FE.angina

Fixed-Effects Model (k = 8)

I^2 (total heterogeneity / total variability):    43.23%
H^2 (total variability / sampling variability):   1.76

Test for Heterogeneity:
Q(df = 7) = 12.3311, p-val = 0.0902


Model Results:

estimate      se    zval    pval   ci.lb   ci.ub
  0.1619  0.0323  5.0134  <.0001  0.0986  0.2252  ***


---
Signif. codes: 0 *** 0.001 ** 0.01 * 0.05 . 0.1
```

We have the same conclusion as in the output of fixed.angina. The estimated overall treatment MD is 0.1619 with SE = 0.0323, z-value = 5.0134, and p-value < 0.0001. The 95% confidence interval is (0.0986, 0.2252).

3.4.3.3 Fit the Random-Effects Model

Similarly, for random-effects meta-analysis to reproduce the results in random.angina, we call function rma with the method="DL" as follows:

```
> # Fit the DL random-effects model
> RE.angina = rma(yi, vi, data=ES.MD, method="DL")
```

```
> # Print the summary of model fit
> RE.angina


Random-Effects Model (k = 8; tau^2 estimator: DL)

tau^2 (estimated amount of total heterogeneity): 0.0066
                                               (SE = 0.0083)
tau (square root of estimated tau^2 value):      0.0812
I^2 (total heterogeneity / total variability):   43.23%
H^2 (total variability / sampling variability):  1.76

Test for Heterogeneity:
Q(df = 7) = 12.3311, $p$-val = 0.0902

Model Results:

estimate     se     zval     pval    ci.lb    ci.ub
  0.1589  0.0448   3.5443   0.0004   0.0710   0.2467  ***


---
Signif. codes: 0 *** 0.001 ** 0.01 * 0.05 . 0.1
```

Again, we have reproduced the same conclusion as in the output of `random.angina`. The estimated overall treatment MD is 0.1589 with SE = 0.0448, z-value = 3.5443, and p-value = 0.0004. The 95% CI is (0.0710, 0.2467).

3.5   Which Model Should We Use? Fixed Effects or Random Effects?

Whether a fixed-effects model or a random-effects model should be used to synthesize treatment effects across studies in a meta-analysis should not be entirely based upon a test for heterogeneity of treatment effects among the studies. Rather model selection should be based on whether the studies share a common effect size and on the goals in performing the meta-analysis. This requires the analyst to review the studies to be included in the meta-analysis in detail. In fact for the results of a meta-analysis to accrue the highest level of scientific credibility, a protocol (see Chapter 2) should be written to guide all aspects of the meta-analysis as a process: defining the question(s), defining the endpoint(s), or response variable(s), specifying criteria for study inclusion/exclusion, retrieval of study reports, abstracting information from the studies, statistical methods, etc.

3.5.1 Fixed Effects

In reviewing the studies to be included in a fixed-effects meta-analysis, attention should be given to whether it is reasonable to believe "a priori" that each study would provide an estimate of the same (or common) treatment effect. If so, then a fixed-effects model may be used.

As an example consider a Phase III, multi-center, randomized, double-blind, controlled clinical trial of a dose of a new drug. Such trials are conducted to confirm efficacy (as compared to control) of the new drug. Patients are randomized to drug or control at each center and all centers follow a common protocol. All patients entered have the same disease and have similar characteristics – as defined by the inclusion/exclusion criteria. Further, investigator meetings which are attended by the investigator and research nurse (at a minimum) are conducted prior to entering any patients. The purpose of this meeting is to thoroughly familiarize center personnel with the protocol and data collection requirements so as to minimize heterogeneity among sites. Although such a trial is usually analyzed using a linear model blocking on center, the trial could be analyzed using a meta-analysis model considering each center as a separate study. Since each center (study) is expected to provide an independent estimate of the same or common treatment effect, a fixed-effects meta-analysis model is reasonable.

3.5.2 Random Effects

If in reviewing the studies to be included in a meta-analysis, it is unreasonable to believe "a priori" that each study would provide an estimate of the same (or common) treatment effect, then a random-effects model should be used.

As an example, suppose a pharmaceutical company conducts several randomized, controlled clinical trials of the efficacy of a drug at a given dose in different populations; e.g., six trials in the young- ($18 \leq$ age <45), middle- ($45 \leq$ age < 65), and old- ($65 \leq$ age) age groups of either sex (male, female). It is reasonable to expect that efficacy of the drug will differ across these six populations. Thus a random-effects model would be appropriate to synthesize the estimates of the treatment effect (drug versus control) across the six populations. Note that separate meta-analyses using a random-effects model across age groups could be conducted to obtain the estimate of treatment effect by sex.

3.5.3 Performing Both a Fixed-Effects and a Random-Effects Meta-Analysis

In practice, many analysts perform both a fixed-effects and a random-effects meta-analysis of the same set of studies – even if there is an "a priori" basis for believing the fixed-effects model is appropriate. If inference is provided via a confidence interval, generally the confidence interval from the random-effects model analysis will be wider (providing a more conservative inference) than the one from the fixed-effects model analysis. The confidence intervals would be identical only in the case when the interstudy variability (the extent of heterogeneity) is 0. The text book by Borenstein et al Borenstein et al. (2009) as well as The Cochrane Collaborative (http://www.cochrane-net.org/openlearning/HTML/mod13-4.htm) and the presentation by Michael Brannick (http://luna.cas.usf.edu/ mbrannic/files/meta/FixedvRandom.doc) provide excellent discussion contrasting the fixed-effects versus random-effects cases.

3.6 Summary and Conclusions

In this chapter, we introduced meta-analysis methods for synthesizing studies using publicly available data sets with both fixed-effects and random-effects models. Woolf's test was used to test for lack of homogeneity. Note that this chapter was expanded from Chapter 8 in Chen and Peace (2010) with greater detail and better presentation. Also notice that in this second edition, we included the illustration of the `metafor` package which was not in the first edition as seen in Chen and Peace (2013).

Readers of this chapter may use the models and associated R code contained herein to perform their own meta-analyses of studies by synthesizing treatment effects across studies. For further reading, we recommend Hedges and Olkin (1985), Whitehead (2003), Hartung et al. (2008), and Borenstein et al. (2009). For R application, we recommend the reader become more familiar with the `rmeta`, `meta`, and `metafor` libraries. Chapter 12 (Meta-Analysis) in Everitt and Hothorn (2006) is again an excellent reference on the subject. The commercial software of `Comprehensive Meta-Analysis` associated with the book of Borenstein et al. (2009) is also a must-read in this arena.

Appendix: Stata Programs for Fixed-Effects and Random-Effects in Meta-Analysis by Manyun Liu

The `Stata` program below corresponds to the R program in the chapter.

```
/*### Reproduce R results in Subsection 3.3.1 ###*/
/* Note: Because the "cochrane" data is in R "rmeta" package,
         we created a new Excel sheet "Data_cochrane"
         in "dat4Meta.xls" to provide the data. */
```

```
/*  Load the data:
Stata can directly load the excel files by clicking
"File-Import-Excel Spreadsheet", then input the Excel
file path and choose "Import first row as variable names
Or you can use the following command to
load the excel file */

/*Changes the Working Directory*/
cd "your "dat4Meta.xls" path"
    import excel using dat4Meta.xls, sheet("Data_cochrane")
cellrange(A1:E8) firstrow clear

/*  Present the data */
browse

/*  Or we can use list command to present the data */
list

/*### Reproduce R results in Subsection 3.3.2 ###*/
/* Generate two new variables,
 which are the survival of patients of each group */
generate strt = ntrt-evtrt
generate sctrl = nctrl-evctrl

/* Fit the fixed-effects model, print the results and
also automatically produces the forest plot */
metan evtrt strt evctrl sctrl, or fixed label(namevar=name)

/*### Reproduce R results in Subsection 3.3.3 ###*/
/* Fit the random-effects model, print the results
and also automatically produces the forest plot */
metan evtrt strt evctrl sctrl, or random label(namevar=name)

/*### Reproduce R results in Subsection 3.4.1 ###*/
/* Load the excel file */
import excel using dat4Meta.xls, sheet("Data_Angina")
cellrange(A1:G9) firstrow clear

/*  Present the data */
browse

/*### Reproduce R results in Subsection 3.4.2 ###*/
ssc install metan
```

```
/*### Reproduce R results in Subsection 3.4.2 ###*/
help metan

/*### Reproduce R results in Subsection 3.4.2.1 ###*/
/* Generate two new variables,
which are the standard deviation of each group */
generate sdE = sqrt(varE)
generate sdC = sqrt(varC)

/*  R metacont implemented weighted mean difference,
therefore we utilize weighted mean difference in Stata as well.
Fit the fix-effects model, print the results and also
automatically produces the forest plot */

metan nE meanE sdE nC meanC sdC, nostandard fixed
  label(namevar=Protocol)

/*### Reproduce R results in Subsection 3.4.2.1 ###*/
/* Call funnel to make funnel plot */
ssc install metafunnel

metafunnel _ES _seES

/*### Reproduce R Results in Subsection 3.4.2.1 ###*/
/*  Call metabias for statistical test */
ssc install metabias

metabias _ES _seES, begg

/*### Reproduce R Results in Subsection 3.4.2.2 ###*/
/* Fit the random-effects model, print the results and
also automatically produces the forest plot */

metan nE meanE sdE nC meanC sdC, nostandard random
label(namevar=Protocol)

/*  The two R codes are unique to R,
    and we still use metan in Stata */

/*### Reproduce R Results in Subsection 3.4.3.1 ###*/
/*  For the fix-effects model, still use the previous Stata code,

which also provides effect sizes _ES and standard error _seES */
```

```
metan nE meanE sdE nC meanC sdC, nostandard fixed
label(namevar=Protocol)
generate _varES = _seES^2

/*  view the data */
browse
```

4

Meta-Analysis with Binary Data

With the conceptual introduction in Chapter 3, we now come to a more detailed discussion on meta-analysis for a specific data type.

The first and probably most commonly seen meta-analysis is of binary or binomial data where the number of successes is considered in a sequence of independent studies each of which has success with probability p.

We begin this chapter with two real data sets in Section 4.1 and then describe the meta-analysis models associated with this type of data in Section 4.2 with step-by-step R implementation using the first data set so interested readers can follow these steps to understand the principles and theoretical background of meta-analysis. Following this step-by-step illustration in this section, we further use R packages `meta` and `metafor` to show how to analyze this data with their built-in functions so to enhance the understanding of meta-analysis and to improve the learning for interested readers.

The second data set will be used in Section 4.3 to illustrate the application of R package `meta` corresponding to the meta-analysis methods detailed in Section 4.2 with discussion in Section 4.4.

Note to the readers: you need to install R packages `readxl` to read in the excel data file, R packages `meta`, and `metafor` for meta-analysis.

4.1 Data from Real Life Studies

4.1.1 Statin Clinical Trials

This study is about meta-analysis of cardiovascular clinical trials designed to compare intensive statin therapy to moderate statin therapy in the reduction of cardiovascular outcomes. The data are from Cannon et al. (2006). Recent clinical trials have demonstrated that high-dose statins (also referred to as intensive statin therapy) appear to be more effective than standard-dose statins in reducing cardiovascular events, as seen in (1) the PROVE IT-TIMI-22 (Pravastatin or Atorvastatin Evaluation and Infection Therapy-Thrombolysis In Myocardial Infarction-22) and (2) the TNT (Treating to New Targets) trials. However, two trials, (3) the A-to-Z (Aggrastat to Zocor) and (4) the IDEAL (Incremental Decrease in End Points Through Aggressive

Lipid Lowering), had nonstatistically significant trends toward benefit of intensive statin therapy for their pre-specified primary endpoint, raising questions regarding the reliability of this observation. In order to determine more accurately the clinical utility of intensive statin therapy, we performed a meta-analysis of these four trials, which represent more than 100,000 patient-years of observation directly comparing high-dose versus standard dose statin therapy. The data set is shown in Table 4.1.

Note that in this table, nhigh is the total number of patients randomized to high dose, evhigh is the number of patients with event (defined as the combined incidence of coronary death or nonfatal myocardial infarction (MI)) in the high dose group, nstd is the total number of patients randomized to standard dose, evstd is the number of patients with event in the standard dose group, ntot is the total number of patients in both treatment groups, and evtot is the total number of patients with events in both treatment groups.

Figure 4.1 summarizes the results of a meta-analysis that shows the relative risk of high dose versus standard dose of statins in preventing death and nonfatal MI from both fixed-effects and random-effects models described in Chapter 3. This analysis is detailed in Section 4.2.1 with the R package meta, and we encourage interested readers to read Cannon et al. (2006) which was published in the Journal of the American College of Cardiology.

In this figure, the first four rows specify the four individual studies. For each, the study name is shown on the left, followed by detailed information of the studies as:

TABLE 4.1

Data for Coronary Death or MI of Statin Use

Study	nhigh	evhigh	nstd	evstd	ntot	evtot
Prove It	2099	147	2063	172	4162	319
A-to-Z	2265	205	2232	235	4497	440
TNT	4995	334	5006	418	10001	752
IDEAL	4439	411	4449	463	8888	874

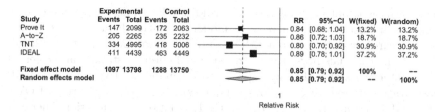

FIGURE 4.1

Meta-analysis with risk-ratio (RR).

- the observed number of events and total number of patients from both experimental and control groups;

- a forest plot summarizes all the statistics,

- effect size (ES) of relative ratios,

- the 95% confidence intervals (CIs),

- the relative weight assigned to the study from both fixed- and random-effects models

Also, the last two rows represent the summary information from both fixed- and random-effects models.

In this chapter, we will use this data set to illustrate both the detailed steps in implementing the meta-analysis methods and the application of R packages `meta` and `metafor` to analyze these data to reproduce the results.

4.1.2 Five Studies on Lamotrigine for Treatment of Bipolar Depression

Bipolar disorder is a psychiatric condition historically known as manic-depressive disorder. Bipolar disorder is among the top causes of worldwide disability and is characterized by both depressive and manic episodes as described in Geddes et al. (2009). Bipolar disorder is a lifelong recurrent illness and there is no known cure. Patients usually require long-term treatment with psychotherapy drugs to control symptoms. Lamotrigine is one of several drugs used in the treatment of bipolar disorder. It is an anticonvulsant and has been approved by the US FDA as an adjunctive treatment for epilepsy and for maintenance treatment for Bipolar I disorder. Lamotrigine is marketed in the USA and in some European countries as "Lamictal" by GlaxoSmithKline.

Although there is evidence of long-term efficacy of lamotrigine as maintenance treatment for Bipolar I disorder, five placebo-controlled clinical trials of lamotrigine in acute phase therapy have been reported as individually neutral and there was no statistically significant benefit from this medication as reported in Calabrese et al. (2008). To further investigate the efficacy of lamotrigine in acute bipolar depression, Geddes et al. (2009) conducted a meta-analysis of these five trials (see Table 1 in Geddes) using patient-level data. The authors also conducted an extensive database search on MEDLINE, EMBASE, CINAHL, PsyINFO, and CENTRAL and found two more studies which reported substantially statistically significant benefits with lamotrigine. However, these two studies were not used because of substantial differences in protocols. In this chapter, we will illustrate meta-analyses of binary response variables by performing a meta-analysis on two binary response efficacy variables defined in the paper using summary information (count data) from the five placebo-controlled trials.

A patient was considered a responder if he/she experienced at least a 50% reduction from baseline in terms of the Hamilton rating scale for depression (HRSD) or in terms of the Montgomery-Asberg depression rating scale (MADRS). In addition to meta-analyzing these two binary response variables, we also meta-analyze the MADRS response variable according to whether the patient suffered severe depression (HRSD $\geq$ 24) or mild-to-moderate depression (HRSD $<$ 24) at baseline.

Summary count data on the above four binary response variables from Geddes et al. (2009) were re-typed into the excel datafile "dat4Meta." The file can be loaded into R as follows:

```
> # Load the library "readxl"
> require(readxl)
> # Get the data path
> datfile = " File path to data 'dat4Meta.xls'"
> # Call "read_excel" to read the Excel data in specific data
        sheet
> Lamo  = read_excel(datfile, sheet="Data_Lamo")
```

The data can be seen from Table 4.2 where `Trial` is the name for the clinical trials, `Events` is the number of patients who responded to "lamotrigine" or "Placebo" as seen in `Group`, and `Total` is the total number of patients in the corresponding group. `Response Category` is a variable created to correspond to the four analyses summarized in Figures 1 and 2 of the Geddes et al where 1 is for $>$ 50% reduction in HRSD, 2 for $>$ 50% reduction on MADRS, 3 MADRS response for baseline Hamilton rating scale for depression $<$ 24, 4 MADRS response for baseline HRSD $\geq$ 24.

This data set will be used to illustrate meta-analyses using the R `meta` package. We will first reproduce the results from the paper using the RR as the treatment effect, followed by meta-analyses using the risk-difference and odds-ratio (OR) as treatment effects.

4.2   Meta-Analysis Methods

A goal of meta-analysis is to combine estimates of treatment effect or ESs across similar studies. If estimates of treatment effect or ES are not provided, but the number of patients responding out of the total number studied on treatment and control are, we have to calculate the ES for each study and then combine the ESs to assess the consistency of the effect across studies and to compute a summary effect.

Commonly used ESs for binomial data are the RR, the risk-difference, and the OR. We will discuss these ESs in meta-analyses conducted.

TABLE 4.2

Data for Five Lamotrigine Clinical Trials

Trial	Events	Total	Group	Category
SCA100223	59	111	Lamotrigine	1
SCA30924	47	131	Lamotrigine	1
SCA40910	51	133	Lamotrigine	1
SCAA2010	51	103	Lamotrigine	1
SCAB2001	32	63	Lamotrigine	1
SCA100223	44	109	Placebo	1
SCA30924	37	128	Placebo	1
SCA40910	39	124	Placebo	1
SCAA2010	45	103	Placebo	1
SCAB2001	21	66	Placebo	1
SCA100223	59	111	Lamotrigine	2
SCA30924	56	131	Lamotrigine	2
SCA40910	55	133	Lamotrigine	2
SCAA2010	51	103	Lamotrigine	2
SCAB2001	31	63	Lamotrigine	2
SCA100223	44	109	Placebo	2
SCA30924	44	128	Placebo	2
SCA40910	47	124	Placebo	2
SCAA2010	46	103	Placebo	2
SCAB2001	19	66	Placebo	2
SCA100223	25	57	Lamotrigine	3
SCA30924	32	65	Lamotrigine	3
SCA40910	34	86	Lamotrigine	3
SCAA2010	31	56	Lamotrigine	3
SCAB2001	20	35	Lamotrigine	3
SCA100223	29	65	Placebo	3
SCA30924	26	62	Placebo	3
SCA40910	31	76	Placebo	3
SCAA2010	31	60	Placebo	3
SCAB2001	14	31	Placebo	3
SCA100223	34	54	Lamotrigine	4
SCA30924	24	66	Lamotrigine	4
SCA40910	21	47	Lamotrigine	4
SCAA2010	20	47	Lamotrigine	4
SCAB2001	11	28	Lamotrigine	4
SCA100223	17	44	Placebo	4
SCA30924	18	66	Placebo	4
SCA40910	16	48	Placebo	4
SCAA2010	15	43	Placebo	4
SCAB2001	5	35	Placebo	4

4.2.1 Analysis with RR

4.2.1.1 Definition

The ES for the RR of one treatment (such as "Experimental") to another (such as "Control") is defined as:

$$ES = \frac{p_E}{p_C} = \frac{x_E/n_E}{x_C/n_C} \tag{4.1}$$

where p_E is the so-called risk (or risk probability) for the experimental treatment (E) which is computed as the total number of events (x_E) divided by the total number of patients (n_E), i.e., $p_E = \frac{x_E}{n_E}$ with similar notations for control (C).

Corresponding to the statin data in Section 4.1.1, a RR of 1 means that the risk of death or MI was the same in both groups, while a RR less than 1.0 would mean that the risk was lower in the high-dose group, and a RR greater than 1.0 would mean that the risk was lower in the standard- dose group.

To construct an approximate CI based on the normal distribution, ES is transformed using the natural logarithm and then employing the delta-method where $lnES = ln(ES)$. The variance for $lnES$ can be shown to be

$$Var_{lnES} = \frac{1}{x_E} - \frac{1}{n_E} + \frac{1}{x_C} - \frac{1}{n_C} \tag{4.2}$$

This is accomplished by representing $lnES$ as the linear terms in a Taylor series expansion about its expected value as:

$$\begin{aligned}
lnES = lnES(x_E, x_C) &= ln(p_E) - ln(p_C) \\
&= ln(x_E) - ln(n_E) - ln(x_C) + ln(n_C) \\
&= lnES(\mu_{x_E}, \mu_{x_C}) + \left(\frac{\partial lnES}{\partial x_E}\right)_{\mu_E} (x_E - \mu_{x_E}) \\
&+ \left(\frac{\partial lnES}{\partial x_C}\right)_{\mu_C} (x_C - \mu_{x_C})
\end{aligned}$$

Then

$$\begin{aligned}
Var(lnES) &= \left(\frac{\partial lnES}{\partial x_E}\right)_{\mu_E}^2 Var(x_E) + \left(\frac{\partial lnES}{\partial x_C}\right)_{\mu_C}^2 Var(x_C) \\
&= \left(\frac{1}{n_E p_E}\right)^2 n_E p_E (1 - p_E) + \left(\frac{1}{n_C p_C}\right)^2 n_C p_C (1 - p_C) \\
&= \frac{1}{n_E p_E}(1 - p_E) + \frac{1}{n_C p_C}(1 - p_C) \\
&= \frac{1}{n_E p_E}(1 - p_E) - \frac{1}{n_E} + \frac{1}{n_C p_C}(1 - p_C) - \frac{1}{n_C}
\end{aligned}$$

which is simplified to be equation (4.2). Therefore, the approximated standard error (SE) is

$$SE_{lnES} = \sqrt{Var(lnES)} \tag{4.3}$$

With this, the 95% CI for $lnES$ can be expressed as

$$(lnES - 1.96 \times SE_{lnES}, lnES + 1.96 \times SE_{lnES}). \tag{4.4}$$

We then transform back to the original scale for RR as:

$$RR = exp(lnES)$$
$$L_{RR} = exp(lnES - 1.96 \times SE_{lnES})$$
$$U_{RR} = exp(lnES + 1.96 \times SE_{lnES})$$

For illustration with this data, the risks for experimental high-dose group are:

```
> # the events
> xE = dat$evhigh
> # the total number
> nE = dat$nhigh
> # the risk
> pE = xE/nE
> # print the risk
> pE
```

```
[1] 0.0700 0.0905 0.0669 0.0926
```

And the risks from the standard low-dose group are:

```
> xC = dat$evstd
> nC = dat$nstd
> pC = xC/nC
> pC
```

```
[1] 0.0834 0.1053 0.0835 0.1041
```

And we can see generally that the risk for the experimental high-dose group is lower than the standard low-dose group. Then the RRs are calculated as:

```
> # The risk-ratios
> ES = pE/pC
> # print the RR
> ES
```

```
[1] 0.840 0.860 0.801 0.890
```

Again the ratios are smaller than 1 for all four studies indicating the experimental treatment is descriptively better than the standard treatment.

4.2.1.2   Statistical Significance

With the definition and calculations above, we can assess whether the ESs are statistically significant. We have several ways to do this.

1. **CI Approach**

   The first way is to use a CI. The CI is usually started with the log RR to use the normal approximation. The log-ES and its variance can be calculated using R as follows:

   ```
   > # calculate the log risk-ratio
   > lnES = log(ES)
   > # print the log risk-ratio
   > lnES

   [1] -0.174 -0.151 -0.222 -0.117

   > # calculate the variance
   > VlnES = 1/dat$evhigh - 1/dat$nhigh + 1/dat$evstd
              - 1/dat$nstd
   > # print the variance
   > VlnES

   [1] 0.01166 0.00824 0.00499 0.00414
   ```

   With these calculations, we can construct the 95% CI for *lnES* as follows:

   ```
   > # upper CI
   > ciup  = lnES+1.96*sqrt(VlnES)
   > print(ciup)

   [1]    0.03724   0.02671 -0.08374   0.00927

   > # lower CI
   > cilow  = lnES-1.96*sqrt(VlnES)
   > print(cilow)

   [1] -0.386 -0.329 -0.361 -0.243

   > # then transform back to the original scale
   > cat("The low CI is:", exp(cilow),"\n\n")

   The low CI is: 0.68 0.719 0.697 0.784

   > cat("The upper CI is:", exp(ciup),"\n\n")

   The upper CI is: 1.04 1.03 0.92 1.01
   ```

We can see from the 95% CI that only the study TNT (i.e., the third study) is statistically significant and the other three are not. Corresponding to Figure 4.1, the ES for each study is represented by a square, with the location of the square representing both the direction and magnitude of the effect. Here, the ES for each study falls to the left of the center line (indicating a benefit for the high-dose group). The effect is strongest (most distant from the center) in the TNT study and weakest in the Ideal study.

2. **The p-value Approach**

The second way is to calculate the classical p-values. To calculate the p-values, we first calculate the z-values as follows:

```
> # The z-value
> z = lnES/sqrt(VlnES)
> z
```

```
[1] -1.62 -1.67 -3.15 -1.82
```

Then the p-values can be calculated as:

```
> pval = 2*(1-pnorm(abs(z)))
> cat("p-values = ", pval, sep=" ", "\n\n")
```

```
p-values =  0.106 0.0957 0.00166 0.0694
```

Again, only the study TNT is statistically significant at the 5% level.

3. **The Post-Power Approach**

Looking into the data, we can easily see that the sample sizes for TNT, $IDEAL$, *Prove It*, and *A-to-Z* are 10,001, 8,888, 4,162 and 4,497, respectively. The TNT has the largest sample size which would have greater power to detecting statistically significant effect. We can calculate a statistical postpower for these four studies using the R package `pwr` as follows:

```
> # load the pwr library
> library(pwr)
> # calculate the power
> pow.study = pwr.2p2n.test(ES.h(pE,pC),n1=dat$nhigh,
        n2=dat$nstd,sig.level=0.05)
> # print it
> pow.study
```

```
    difference of proportion power calculation for
            binomial distribution (arcsine transformation)
```

```
              h = 0.0502, 0.0498, 0.0632, 0.0386
             n1 = 2099, 2265, 4995, 4439
             n2 = 2063, 2232, 5006, 4449
      sig.level = 0.05
          power = 0.367, 0.386, 0.885, 0.444
    alternative = two.sided
```

NOTE: different sample sizes

We can see that the associated statistical power for Study TNT is 0.885 and the rest of the three studies are all about 40% indicating these studies are low-powered statistically.

4.2.1.3   The RR Meta-Analysis: Step-by-Step

To increase precision and statistical power to detect a clinically significant ES, we conduct a meta-analysis of the ESs across the individual studies. We first review some relevant concepts used in both fixed-effects and random-effects meta-analysis models and show step-by-step calculations in R.

The precision in meta-analysis can be addressed in two ways with one as the CI and another as the SE of the ES. Both are in fact related. As depicted in Figure 4.1, the ES for each study is bounded by a CI, reflecting the precision with which the ES has been estimated in that study. The CI for the last study (Ideal) is noticeably narrower than that for the first study (Prove-it), reflecting the fact that the Ideal study has greater precision. Another way is to observe the size of the variances or SEs. For these studies, the variances for the log RR of $lnES$ are:

```
> VlnES
```

```
[1] 0.01166 0.00824 0.00499 0.00414
```

Again, we can see the last two studies have the smallest variances indicating greater precision. Studies with greater precision should have larger weights when combining studies. This may be done by using a fixed-effects meta-analysis model and weighting each study by its inverse variance as:

$$w_i = \frac{1}{Var_i} \tag{4.5}$$

where $i = 1, \cdots, K = 4$. For these studies, the inverse weights are calculated as:

```
> w = 1/VlnES
> w
```

```
[1]   85.8 121.3 200.5 241.4
```

In Figure 4.1, the solid squares that are used to depict each of the studies vary in size, reflecting the weight that is assigned to the corresponding study in computing the summary effect. The *TNT* and *Ideal* studies are assigned relatively large weights, while a somewhat lower weight is assigned to the *A to Z* study and less still to the *Prove-It* study.

As one would expect, there is a relationship between a study's precision and that study's weight in the combined analysis. Studies with relatively good precision (TNT and Ideal) are assigned greater weights while studies with relatively poor precision (Prove-It) are assigned lesser weights. Since precision is driven primarily by sample size, we can think of the studies as being weighted by sample size, where the last two studies have the larger weights.

The fixed-effects weighted-average meta-analysis model to combine the studies is then derived as:

$$lnES = \frac{\sum_{i=1}^{4} lnES_i \times w_i}{\sum_{i=1}^{4} w_i} \tag{4.6}$$

with variance calculated by:

$$Var(lnES) = \frac{1}{\sum_{i=1}^{4} w_i} \tag{4.7}$$

The calculations can be performed step-by-step as follows:

```
> # the inverse of variance for each study
> fwi = 1/VlnES
> fwi

[1]   85.8 121.3 200.5 241.4

> # the total weight
> fw = sum(fwi)
> fw

[1] 649

> # the relative weight for each study
> rw = fwi/fw
> rw

[1] 0.132 0.187 0.309 0.372

> # the weighted mean
> flnES = sum(lnES*rw); flnES

[1] -0.163

> # the variance for the weighted mean
> var= 1/fw; var

[1] 0.00154
```

We then transform back to the original scale to estimate the RR as well as the CI as:

```
> # the RR
> exp(flnES)

[1] 0.849

> # the lower CI bound
> exp(flnES-1.96*sqrt(var))

[1] 0.786

> # the upper CI bound
> exp(flnES+1.96*sqrt(var))

[1] 0.917
```

This CI is below the RR of 1 which indicates that the high-dose regimen is statistically significantly more effective than the standard dose regimen.

To illustrate the random-effects meta-model, we first need to estimate the heterogeneity statistic Q in equation (3.18) as:

```
> # estimate heterogeneity statistic Q
> Q = sum(fwi*lnES^2)-(sum(fwi*lnES))^2/fw
> Q

[1] 1.24

> # Get the degrees of freedom
> K  = dim(dat)[1]
> df = K -1
> df

[1] 3

> # calculate the statistical significance: p-value
> pval4Q =  pchisq(Q, df, lower.tail=F)
> pval4Q

[1] 0.743
```

From this p-value, we can conclude that there is no statistically significant heterogeneity among these 4 studies. Furthermore since this estimated Q is less than the df of 3, the estimated τ^2 in equation (3.18) is then set to zero which would lead to the conclusion that the random-effects meta-analysis is exactly the same as the fixed-effects model.

4.2.1.4   RR Meta-Analysis with R package meta

All the above calculations can be summarized in the R package meta in this one-line code where Inverse weighting method is used for "summary method" sm="RR":

```
> # call "metabin" for RR meta-analysis
> RR.Statin = metabin(evhigh,nhigh,evstd,nstd,studlab=Study,
                 data=dat, method="Inverse", sm="RR")
> # print the analysis summary
> summary(RR.Statin)


Number of studies combined: k = 4

                        RR          95%-CI       z   p-value
Fixed effect model   0.8492 [0.7863; 0.9171] -4.16  < 0.0001
Random effects model 0.8492 [0.7863; 0.9171] -4.16  < 0.0001

Quantifying heterogeneity:
 tau^2 = 0 [0.0000; 0.0253]; tau = 0 [0.0000; 0.1589];
 I^2 = 0.0% [0.0%; 63.0%]; H = 1.00 [1.00; 1.64]

Test of heterogeneity:
    Q d.f. p-value
 1.24    3  0.7428

Details on meta-analytical method:
- Inverse variance method
- DerSimonian-Laird estimator for tau^2
- Jackson method for CI of tau^2 and tau
```

Readers can check the results from this output with the step-by-step calculations in Section 4.2.1.3 and should find the results to match exactly.

The forest plot in Figure 4.1 is then produced as follows:

```
> forest(RR.Statin)
```

4.2.1.5   RR Meta-Analysis with R package metafor

To meta-analyze this data with R package metafor, the first step is to load the package into R session as follows:

```
> # Load metafor package
> library(metafor)
```

With this package loaded, we need to calculate the ESs from each study using the function `escalc`:

```
> # Call escalc to calculate the ESs
> ES.RR.Statin = escalc(measure="RR",
                        ai=evhigh, bi=nhigh-evhigh,
                        ci=evstd,  di=nstd-evstd, data=dat)
> # Print the calculated ESs
> ES.RR.Statin

    Study nhigh evhigh nstd evstd  ntot evtot       yi      vi
1 Prove It  2099    147 2063   172  4162   319 -0.1744 0.0117
2   A-to-Z  2265    205 2232   235  4497   440 -0.1513 0.0082
3      TNT  4995    334 5006   418 10001   752 -0.2221 0.0050
4    IDEAL  4439    411 4449   463  8888   874 -0.1169 0.0041
```

In the above R code, we call the function `escalc` to calculate effect-size (i.e., `escalc`) for each study with option `measure="RR"` for log risk-ratio (denoted by `RR`, but in fact `RR` indicates log risk-ratio).

After this `escalc` calculation, two extra columns' data are added to the original data, where `yi` is the ESs as the log RR and `vi` is the associated sample variance for that study.

With these calculated ESs from each study, we can then call `rma` to meta-analyze the data from all studies together with fixed-effects and random-effects models.

The fixed-effects model can be implemented as follows:

```
> # Call rma for FE
> RR.Statin.FE = rma(yi, vi, data=ES.RR.Statin, method="FE")
> # Print the summary of FE analysis
> RR.Statin.FE

Fixed-Effects Model (k = 4)

I^2 (total heterogeneity / total variability):   0.00%
H^2 (total variability / sampling variability):   0.41

Test for Heterogeneity:
Q(df = 3) = 1.2425, p-val = 0.7428

Model Results:

estimate       se     zval     pval    ci.lb     ci.ub
 -0.1634   0.0393  -4.1635   <.0001  -0.2404   -0.0865   ***
---
Signif. codes:  0 *** 0.001 ** 0.01 * 0.05 . 0.1
```

To obtain the results in RR, we transform back to the original scale from the log RR as follows:

```
> # The overall risk-ratio
> exp(RR.Statin.FE$beta)

intrcpt 0.849

> # The lower bound of 95% confidence interval
> exp(RR.Statin.FE$ci.lb)

[1] 0.786

> # The upper bound of 95% confidence interval
> exp(RR.Statin.FE$ci.ub)

[1] 0.917
```

As seen from these calculations, we reproduced the results in the step-by-step meta-analysis as well as the results in the meta-analysis with meta package.

For random-effects meta-analysis with DerSimonian-Laird estimator, we can call rma as follows:

```
> # Call rma with DL for DL random-effects analysis
> RR.Statin.RE = rma(yi, vi, data=ES.RR.Statin, method="DL")
> # Print the summary of DL
> RR.Statin.RE

Random-Effects Model (k = 4; tau^2 estimator: DL)

tau^2 (estimated amount of total heterogeneity): 0 (SE = 0.0053)
tau (square root of estimated tau^2 value):       0
I^2 (total heterogeneity / total variability):   0.00%
H^2 (total variability / sampling variability):  1.00


Test for Heterogeneity:
Q(df = 3) = 1.2425, p-val = 0.7428


Model Results:

estimate      se     zval     pval     ci.lb     ci.ub
 -0.1634  0.0393  -4.1635   <.0001   -0.2404   -0.0865  ***


---
Signif. codes: 0 *** 0.001 ** 0.01 * 0.05 . 0.1

> # Tranform back to original RR
> exp(RR.Statin.RE$beta)
```

```
         [,1]
intrcpt 0.849

> # Transform back the lower bound
> exp(RR.Statin.RE$ci.lb)

[1] 0.786

> # Transform back the upper bound
> exp(RR.Statin.RE$ci.ub)

[1] 0.917
```

This reproduced the random-effects analysis from both the step-by-step illustration and the meta-analysis with `meta` package.

4.2.2   Analysis with Risk Difference

4.2.2.1   Definition

Even though the RR is the most commonly used in binomial data, the risk difference (RD) is a ES which is easily understandable. The definition of RD is simply the difference of the risks between two treatments as:

$$ES_{RD} = \hat{p}_E - \hat{p}_C = \frac{x_E}{n_E} - \frac{x_C}{n_C} \tag{4.8}$$

from the notations from previous section.

The variance of ES_{RD} can be estimated as:

$$Var\left(ES_{RD}\right) = \frac{\hat{p}_E(1 - \hat{p}_E)}{n_E} + \frac{\hat{p}_C(1 - \hat{p}_C)}{n_C} \tag{4.9}$$

and the SE is then calculated as $SE_{ES_{RD}} = \sqrt{Var\left(ES_{RD}\right)}$. With the point estimate from equation (4.8) and its variance in equation (4.9), we can frame the same procedure for statistical inference similar to those in Section 4.2.1.2.

4.2.2.2   Meta-Analysis with Step-by-Step Implementation

For the statin data in Section 4.1.1, an RD of 0 means that the risk of death or MI was the same in both groups, while a RR less than 0 means that the risk was lower in the high-dose group, and a RR greater than 0 means that the risk was lower in the standard-dose group. The RD can be calculated as:

```
> # the risk difference
> ESRD = pE-pC
> ESRD

[1] -0.0133 -0.0148 -0.0166 -0.0115
```

The differences are less than 0 for all four studies indicating that the experimental treatment is descriptively better than the standard treatment. The variance can be calculated as:

```
> # calculate the variance
> VarRD = pE*(1-pE)/nE + pC*(1-pC)/nC
> VarRD

[1] 6.81e-05 7.85e-05 2.78e-05 3.99e-05

> # calculate the standard error
> SERD = sqrt(VarRD)
> SERD

[1] 0.00825 0.00886 0.00527 0.00632
```

With this calculation, we leave the other steps for RD to interested readers for practice purposes. We now illustrate use of the R package meta.

4.2.2.3 Meta-Analysis in **R** Package meta

The same R function metabin is called with sm (i.e., "summary method") now set to RD:

```
> # call metabin for RD meta-analysis
> RD.Statin = metabin(evhigh,nhigh,evstd,nstd,studlab=Study,
  data=dat, method="Inverse", sm="RD")
> # print the summary
> summary(RD.Statin)

Number of studies combined: k = 4

                          RD          95%-CI      z  p-value
Fixed effect model   -0.0144 [-0.0209; -0.0078] -4.27 < 0.0001
Random effects model -0.0144 [-0.0209; -0.0078] -4.27 < 0.0001

Quantifying heterogeneity:
 tau^2 = 0 [0.0000; 0.0001]; tau = 0 [0.0000; 0.0082];
 I^2 = 0.0% [0.0%; 0.0%]; H = 1.00 [1.00; 1.00]

Test of heterogeneity:
    Q d.f. p-value
 0.41    3  0.9379

Details on meta-analytical method:
- Inverse variance method
- DerSimonian-Laird estimator for tau^2
- Jackson method for CI of tau^2 and tau
```

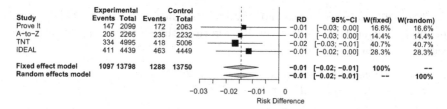

FIGURE 4.2
Meta-analysis with risk RD.

The conclusions from the meta-analysis of the RR are reached from the meta-analysis of the RD; i.e., the high-dose regimen is statistically more effective than the standard dose regimen. With this RD meta-analysis, the forest plot can be shown in Figure 4.2 as follows:

```
> forest(RD.Statin)
```

4.2.2.4 Meta-Analysis in R Package metafor

Similar to the meta-analysis with RR, we calculate the ESs (i.e., RD now) from each study using the function escalc:

```
> # Call escalc to calculate the ESs
> ES.RD.Statin = escalc(measure="RD",
             ai=evhigh, bi=nhigh-evhigh,
             ci=evstd,  di=nstd-evstd, data=dat)
> # Print the calculated ESs
> ES.RD.Statin
```

```
      Study nhigh evhigh nstd evstd  ntot evtot      yi      vi
1 Prove It  2099    147 2063   172  4162   319 -0.0133 0.0001
2   A-to-Z  2265    205 2232   235  4497   440 -0.0148 0.0001
3      TNT  4995    334 5006   418 10001   752 -0.0166 0.0000
4    IDEAL  4439    411 4449   463  8888   874 -0.0115 0.0000
```

Note that the only change from RR to RD is to change measure="RR" to measure="RD". Notice that there is a big different from the measure="RR" to calculate the log RR, measure="RD" is to calculate the actual RD, not the logged RD.

With these calculated RD ESs from each study, we can then call rma to meta-analyze the data from all studies together with fixed-effects and random-effects models.

The fixed-effects model can be implemented as follows:

```
> # Call rma for FE
> RD.Statin.FE = rma(yi, vi, data=ES.RD.Statin, method="FE")
```

```
> # Print the summary of FE analysis
> RD.Statin.FE

Fixed-Effects Model (k = 4)

I^2 (total heterogeneity / total variability):   0.00%
H^2 (total variability / sampling variability):  0.14

Test for Heterogeneity:
Q(df = 3) = 0.4115, p-val = 0.9379

Model Results:

estimate      se      zval     pval     ci.lb      ci.ub
 -0.0144  0.0034  -4.2717  <.0001  -0.0209   -0.0078  ***

---
Signif. codes:  0 *** 0.001 ** 0.01 * 0.05 . 0.1
```

For random-effects meta-analysis with DerSimonian-Laird estimator, we can call rma as follows:

```
> # Call rma with DL for DL random-effects analysis
> RD.Statin.RE = rma(yi, vi, data=ES.RD.Statin, method="DL")
> # Print the summary of DL
> RD.Statin.RE

Random-Effects Model (k = 4; tau^2 estimator: DL)

tau^2 (estimated amount of total heterogeneity): 0 (SE = 0.0000)
tau (square root of estimated tau^2 value):      0
I^2 (total heterogeneity / total variability):   0.00%
H^2 (total variability / sampling variability):  1.00

Test for Heterogeneity:
Q(df = 3) = 0.4115, p-val = 0.9379

Model Results:

estimate      se      zval     pval     ci.lb      ci.ub
 -0.0144  0.0034  -4.2717  <.0001  -0.0209   -0.0078  ***

---
Signif. codes:  0 *** 0.001 ** 0.01 * 0.05 . 0.1
```

Again, this reproduced the fixed-effects and random-effects analyses from both the step-by-step illustrations and the meta-analysis with meta package.

4.2.3 Meta-Analysis with OR

4.2.3.1 Data Structure

The definition of OR starts with a 2 by 2 table which is usually used to report the number of events and nonevents in two groups.

From a total of K studies, the data from the ith study ($i = 1, \cdots, K$) can be represented as cells A_i, B_i, C_i, and D_i, as shown in Table 4.3.

For example, the data from the TNT study can be seen in Table 4.4.

4.2.3.2 OR: Woolf's Method

The OR associated with an event is defined as the ratio of the odds of the event in one study group to the odds of the event in another study group. The odds of the event for the treatment group in the ith study as:

$$OddsE_i = \frac{p_{E_i}}{1 - p_{E_i}} = \frac{\frac{A_i}{A_i+B_i}}{1 - \frac{A_i}{A_i+B_i}} = \frac{\frac{A_i}{A_i+B_i}}{\frac{B_i}{A_i+B_i}} = \frac{A_i}{B_i} \tag{4.10}$$

Similarly the odds of the event for the control group in the ith study is

$$OddsC_i = \frac{p_{C_i}}{1 - p_{C_i}} = \frac{\frac{C_i}{C_i+D_i}}{1 - \frac{C_i}{C_i+D_i}} = \frac{\frac{C_i}{C_i+D_i}}{\frac{D_i}{C_i+D_i}} = \frac{C_i}{D_i} \tag{4.11}$$

Then the OR of the treatment group to the control group for ith study is as follows:

$$OR_i = \frac{OddsE_i}{OddsC_i} = \frac{\frac{A_i}{B_i}}{\frac{C_i}{D_i}} = \frac{A_i D_i}{B_i C_i} \tag{4.12}$$

For the statin studies, the odds of MI in the experimental high-dose group is

```
> oddsE = pE/(1-pE)
> oddsE
```

TABLE 4.3
Nomenclature for 2×2 Table of Outcome by Treatment

	Events	Non-Events	Total Event
Experimental (High dose)	A_i	B_i	n_1
Standard (Low dose)	C_i	D_i	n_2

TABLE 4.4
Data from TNT

	MI	No-MI	Total
High dose	334	4995-334	4995
Low dose	418	5006-418	5006

```
[1] 0.0753 0.0995 0.0717 0.1020
```

and the odds of MI in the standard low-dose group is

```
> oddsC = pC/(1-pC)
> oddsC
```

```
[1] 0.0910 0.1177 0.0911 0.1162
```

The OR would then be

```
> OR = oddsE/oddsC
> OR
```

```
[1] 0.828 0.846 0.787 0.878
```

Readers may find the OR intuitively less appealing than the RR or RD. However, the OR is used in many statistically sound analysis methods, especially in logistic regression. It is commonly used as a measure of ES in analyzing categorical data in the form of 2 by 2 tables including the meta-analyses of binomial data in this chapter. For the case when the risk of the event is low, the OR is close to the RR.

To better approximate the normal distribution in using ORs, we usually convert the OR to the log scale and estimate the log OR and its SE and use these numbers to perform the meta-analysis. Then we transform the results back into the original metric.

With this direction, the log OR is

$$LogOR = ln(OR) \tag{4.13}$$

The approximate variance can be derived from delta method from the definition as follows:

$$OR = \frac{AD}{BC} = \frac{\frac{\hat{P}_E}{1-\hat{P}_E}}{\frac{\hat{P}_C}{1-\hat{P}_C}} \tag{4.14}$$

and the log OR is

$$logOR = ln(OR)$$
$$= ln\left(\frac{\hat{P}_E}{1-\hat{P}_E}\right) - ln\left(\frac{\hat{P}_C}{1-\hat{P}_C}\right)$$
$$= f(\hat{P}_E) - f(\hat{P}_C) \tag{4.15}$$

where $f(x) = ln\left(\frac{x}{1-x}\right)$ with derivative as $f'(x) = -\frac{1}{x(1-x)}$

The approximate variance can be derived using the delta method to expand (via Taylor series) the log-odds for both treatment and control about their expected values as

$$logOR = ln\left(\frac{\hat{P}_E}{1 - \hat{P}_E}\right) - ln\left(\frac{\hat{P}_C}{1 - \hat{P}_C}\right)$$

$$\approx \left[f(P_E) + f'(P_E)(\hat{P}_E - P_E)\right] - \left[f(P_C) + f'(P_C)(\hat{P}_C - P_C)\right]$$

$$= \left[f(P_E) - \frac{1}{P_E(1 - P_E)}(\hat{P}_E - P_E)\right]$$

$$- \left[f(P_C) - \frac{1}{P_C(1 - P_C)}(\hat{P}_C - P_C)\right] \tag{4.16}$$

The variance can then be obtained as follows:

$$var(logOR) = \left[\frac{1}{P_E(1 - P_E)}\right]^2 var(\hat{P}_E - P_E)$$

$$+ \left[\frac{1}{P_C(1 - P_C)}\right]^2 var(\hat{P}_C - P_C)$$

$$= \left[\frac{1}{P_E(1 - P_E)}\right]^2 \frac{P_E(1 - P_E)}{n_E} + \left[\frac{1}{P_C(1 - P_C)}\right]^2 \frac{P_C(1 - P_C)}{n_C}$$

$$= \frac{1}{n_E P_E(1 - P_E)} + \frac{1}{n_C P_C(1 - P_C)}$$

$$= \frac{1}{n_E \frac{A}{n_E} \frac{B}{n_E}} + \frac{1}{n_C \frac{C}{n_C} \frac{D}{n_C}}$$

$$= \frac{n_T}{AB} + \frac{n_C}{CD} = \frac{1}{A} + \frac{1}{B} + \frac{1}{C} + \frac{1}{D} \tag{4.17}$$

Therefore, the approximate SE is:

$$SE_{logOR} = \sqrt{V_{logOR}} \tag{4.18}$$

With these calculations in the log-scale, we then transform them back to original scale for OR using

$$OR = exp(logOR) \tag{4.19}$$

$$LL_{OR} = exp(LL_{logOR}) \tag{4.20}$$

and

$$UL_{OR} = exp(LL_{logOR}) \tag{4.21}$$

where LL and UL represent the lower and upper limits, respectively.

Now we illustrate the calculations using the TNT study. For this study, the OR for the 4 studies are

```
> OR

[1] 0.828 0.846 0.787 0.878
```

and then the log odds ratios are

```
> LogOR= log(OR)
> LogOR
```

[1] -0.189 -0.168 -0.240 -0.130

The approximate variance can be calculated as $V_{LogOR} = \dfrac{1}{334} + \dfrac{1}{4995 - 334} + \dfrac{1}{418} + \dfrac{1}{5006 - 418}$ as:

```
> VLogOR = 1/334+ 1/(4995-334)+1/418+1/(5006-418)
> VLogOR
```

[1] 0.00582

and standard error

```
> SE.LogOR=sqrt(VLogOR)
> SE.LogOR
```

[1] 0.0763

The weightings from both fixed-effects and random-effects models can be easily implemented. We leave these as exercises for interested readers. We will now use the R package meta for meta-analysis of OR.

4.2.3.3 Meta-Analysis with R Package meta

The OR meta-analysis can be easily implemented in this package with the following code where sm="OR" is used to call "OR":

```
> OR.Statin = metabin(evhigh,nhigh,evstd,nstd,studlab=Study,
    data=dat, method="Inverse", sm="OR")
> summary(OR.Statin)
```

Number of studies combined: k = 4

```
                         OR          95%-CI      z  p-value
Fixed effect model    0.8355 [0.7679; 0.9090] -4.18 < 0.0001
Random effects model  0.8355 [0.7679; 0.9090] -4.18 < 0.0001
```

Quantifying heterogeneity:
  tau^2 = 0 [0.0000; 0.0269]; tau = 0 [0.0000; 0.1641];
  I^2 = 0.0% [0.0%; 59.7%]; H = 1.00 [1.00; 1.58]

Test of heterogeneity:
     Q d.f. p-value
  1.14   3 0.7673

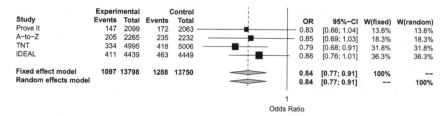

FIGURE 4.3
Meta-analysis with OR with inverse-weighting.

```
Details on meta-analytical method:
- Inverse variance method
- DerSimonian-Laird estimator for tau^2
- Jackson method for CI of tau^2 and tau
```

The forest plot can be shown as in Figure 4.3 as follows:

```
> forest(OR.Statin)
```

4.2.3.4   Meta-Analysis with R Package metafor

Similar to the meta-analysis with RR, we calculate the ESs (denoted by OR which is in fact the log odds-ratio) from each study using the function escalc:

```
> # Calculate OR
> ES.OR.Statin =escalc(measure="OR",
                    ai=evhigh, bi=nhigh-evhigh,
                    ci=evstd,  di=nstd-evstd, data=dat)
> # Print the OR calculation
> ES.OR.Statin
```

	Study	nhigh	evhigh	nstd	evstd	ntot	evtot	yi	vi
1	Prove It	2099	147	2063	172	4162	319	-0.1888	0.0137
2	A-to-Z	2265	205	2232	235	4497	440	-0.1676	0.0101
3	TNT	4995	334	5006	418	10001	752	-0.2401	0.0058
4	IDEAL	4439	411	4449	463	8888	874	-0.1296	0.0051

With these calculated log OR ESs from each study, we can then call rma to meta-analyze the data from all studies together with fixed-effects and random-effects models.

The fixed-effects model can be implemented as follows:

```
> # call rma
> OR.Statin.FE = rma(yi, vi, data=ES.OR.Statin, method="FE")
> # Print the meta-analysis result
> OR.Statin.FE
```

Fixed-Effects Model (k = 4)

I^2 (total heterogeneity / total variability):   0.00%
H^2 (total variability / sampling variability): 0.38

Test for Heterogeneity:
Q(df = 3) = 1.1406, p-val = 0.7673

Model Results:
```
estimate      se     zval    pval    ci.lb    ci.ub
 -0.1797  0.0430  -4.1779  <.0001  -0.2641  -0.0954  ***
```

Signif. codes: 0 *** 0.001 ** 0.01 * 0.05 . 0.1

```
> # Transform from the log OR to OR
> exp(OR.Statin.FE$beta)
```

intrcpt 0.835

```
> # Transform from log-OR to OR for the lower bound
> exp(OR.Statin.FE$ci.lb)
```

[1] 0.768

```
> # Transform from log-OR to OR for the upper bound
> exp(OR.Statin.FE$ci.ub)
```

[1] 0.909

The random-effects model can be implemented as follows:

```
> # Call rma with DL for random-effects
> OR.Statin.RE = rma(yi, vi, data=ES.OR.Statin, method="DL")
> # Print the summary
> OR.Statin.RE
```

Random-Effects Model (k = 4; tau^2 estimator: DL)

tau^2 (estimated amount of total heterogeneity): 0 (SE = 0.0063)
tau (square root of estimated tau^2 value):   0
I^2 (total heterogeneity / total variability):   0.00%
H^2 (total variability / sampling variability): 1.00

Test for Heterogeneity:
Q(df = 3) = 1.1406, p-val = 0.7673

Model Results:

```
estimate      se     zval    pval    ci.lb    ci.ub
 -0.1797  0.0430  -4.1779  <.0001  -0.2641  -0.0954  ***
```

```
---
```

Signif. codes: 0 *** 0.001 ** 0.01 * 0.05 . 0.1

```
> # Transform from the log OR to OR
> exp(OR.Statin.RE$beta)
```

intrcpt 0.835

```
> # Transform from log-OR to OR for the lower bound
> exp(OR.Statin.RE$ci.lb)
```

[1] 0.768

```
> # Transform from log-OR to OR for the upper bound
> exp(OR.Statin.RE$ci.ub)
```

[1] 0.909

Again, this reproduced the fixed-effects and random-effects analyses from both the step-by-step illustrations and the meta-analysis with `meta` package for the OR.

4.2.4　Meta-Analysis Using Mantel-Haenszel Method

4.2.4.1　Details of the Mantel-Haenszel Method

As an alternative, the Mantel-Haenszel(MH) method may be used to provide an estimate of the pooled OR across the studies (summarized as 2 by 2 tables) under a fixed-effects model. The MH pooled OR corresponding to data in Table 4.3 is defined as follows:

$$\widehat{OR}_{MH} = \frac{\sum_{i=1}^{K}\left(\frac{A_i D_i}{N_i}\right)}{\sum_{i=1}^{K}\left(\frac{B_i C_i}{N_i}\right)} \qquad (4.22)$$

where $N_i = A_i + B_i + C_i + D_i$

There are alternative fixed-effects methods, such as Woolf and inverse variance. However, the MH method is generally regarded as more robust, particularly when cell counts are small and the number of studies is large.

The pooled MH OR defined above is in fact a weighted average of the ORs from the individual studies. This can be seen from re-arranging the MH equation (4.22) and using the equation (4.12) as follows:

$$\widehat{OR}_{MH} = \frac{\sum_{i=1}^{K}\left(\frac{B_iC_i}{N_i}\frac{A_iD_i}{B_iC_i}\right)}{\sum_{i=1}^{K}\left(\frac{B_iC_i}{N_i}\right)} = \frac{\sum_{i=1}^{K}\left(\frac{B_iC_i}{N_i}\times OR_i\right)}{\sum_{i=1}^{K}\left(\frac{B_iC_i}{N_i}\right)}$$

$$= \sum_{i=1}^{K}\left(\frac{\frac{B_iC_i}{N_i}}{\sum_{i=1}^{K}\left(\frac{B_iC_i}{N_i}\right)}\right)\times OR_i$$

$$= \sum_{i=1}^{K} relWeight_i \times OR_i \qquad (4.23)$$

where the weight is defined as $wt_i = \frac{B_iC_i}{N_i}$ and the relative weight is defined as $relWeight_i = \frac{\frac{B_iC_i}{N_i}}{\sum_{i=1}^{K}\left(\frac{B_iC_i}{N_i}\right)}$ with total weight as $totalWeight = \frac{1}{\sum_{i=1}^{K}\left(\frac{B_iC_i}{N_i}\right)}$.

Note that the weight of $wt_i = \frac{B_iC_i}{N_i}$ is the inverse of the variance of OR_i for each study when the $OR = 1$ which is to say that the weight is related to the variance in a special form when there is no association. Because MH works well in many applications and is much simpler, it is often favored in the statistical analysis of binomial data.

Recall from the derivation of inverse-weighting, this total weight is in fact the variance of MH estimator as

$$Var\left(\widehat{OR}_{MH}\right) = totalWeight = \frac{1}{\sum_{i=1}^{K}\left(\frac{B_iC_i}{N_i}\right)} \qquad (4.24)$$

Therefore, the 95% CI for the Mantel-Haenszel OR may be calculated as:

$$\widehat{OR}_{MH} \pm 1.96\sqrt{Var\left(\widehat{OR}_{MH}\right)} \qquad (4.25)$$

Although the MH OR estimate has many advantages and statistical properties, it is used to estimate the OR instead of log OR. Its distribution is not symmetric and the normal distribution is not appropriate for constructing CIs. Emerson (1994) proposed to use the variance estimate from Robins et al. (1986) for the log-OR to provide a CI for this meta OR. Denote the $\hat{\theta}$ as the estimated log-OR where $\hat{\theta} = log(OR)$, then the variance estimate can be obtained as:

$$Var(\hat{\theta}) = \frac{1}{2}\sum_{i=1}^{K}\left(\frac{T_{1i}T_{3i}}{ST_3^2} + \frac{T_{1i}T_{4i}+T_{2i}T_{3i}}{ST_3ST_4} + \frac{T_{2i}T_{4i}}{ST_4^2}\right) \qquad (4.26)$$

where

$$T_{1i} = \frac{A_i + D_i}{N_i}$$

$$T_{2i} = \frac{B_i + C_i}{N_i}$$

$$T_{3i} = \frac{A_i D_i}{N_i}$$

$$T_{4i} = \frac{B_i C_i}{N_i}$$

$$ST_3 = \sum_{i=1}^{K} T_{3i}$$

$$ST_4 = \sum_{i=1}^{K} T_{4i}$$

4.2.4.2   Step-by-Step R Implementation

We have obtained the ORs from previous section as:

```
> OR
```

```
[1] 0.828 0.846 0.787 0.878
```

To calculate the relative weighting from each study, we first calculate $\frac{B_i C_i}{N_i}$ as:

```
> w0 = (dat$nhigh-dat$evhigh)*dat$evstd/(dat$nhigh+dat$nstd); w0
```

```
[1]   80.7 107.6 194.8 209.8
```

The total weights can then be calculated as:

```
> TotWeight = sum(w0); TotWeight
```

```
[1] 593
```

With this total weight, we can compute the relative weighting as:

```
> relWt = w0/TotWeight; relWt
```

```
[1] 0.136 0.182 0.329 0.354
```

The MH OR estimate across the studies is then calculated as:

```
> OR.MH = sum(relWt*OR); OR.MH
```

```
[1] 0.835
```

We will demonstrate both the naive and the Emerson approaches to calculate the variance.

As the naive approach to use the inverse of the total weight as the variance, the variance is:

```
> Var.ORMH1 = 1/TotWeight; Var.ORMH1
```

```
[1] 0.00169
```

Therefore, the 95% CI can be computed as:

```
> lowCI = OR.MH-1.96*sqrt(Var.ORMH1); lowCI
```

```
[1] 0.755
```

```
> upCI = OR.MH+1.96*sqrt(Var.ORMH1); upCI
```

```
[1] 0.916
```

```
> cat("MH estimate=", round(OR.MH,4),sep="", "\n\n")
```

```
MH estimate=0.835
```

```
> cat("The 95% CI for MH =(", round(lowCI, 4), ",",
round(upCI, 4), ")", sep="", "\n\n")
```

```
The 95% CI for MH =(0.755,0.916)
```

Since this approximation is not good as discussed, we will use Emerson's approximation. Let us first get the data:

```
> A = dat$evhigh
> B  = dat$nhigh-dat$evhigh
> C = dat$evstd
> D = dat$nstd - dat$evstd
> N = A+B+C+D
```

And then calculate the quantities from the Emerson approximation as follows:

```
> T1 = (A+D)/N
> T2 = (B+C)/N
> T3 = A*D/N
> T4 = B*C/N
> ST3 = sum(T3)
> ST4 = sum(T4)
```

Then the variance for each study can be obtained as:

```
> Var.lnOddsRatio = 0.5*(
 (T1*T3)/ST3^2+(T1*T4+T2*T3)/(ST3*ST4)+T2*T4/ST4^2)
> Var.lnOddsRatio
```

```
[1] 0.000250 0.000338 0.000590 0.000672
```

And the variance for the log OR is:

```
> Var.lnMH = sum(Var.lnOddsRatio)
> Var.lnMH
```

[1] 0.00185

With this variance, the 95% CI for the log OR is:

```
> lowCI.lnMH = log(OR.MH)-1.96*sqrt(Var.lnMH)
> upCI.lnMH = log(OR.MH)+1.96*sqrt(Var.lnMH)
> cat("The 95% CI for log-MH =(", round(lowCI.lnMH, 4), ",",
round(upCI.lnMH, 4), ")", sep="", "\n\n")
```

The 95% CI for log-MH =(-0.264,-0.0955)

Transforming back to the original scale, the 95% CI for the OR is:

```
> lowCI.MH = exp(lowCI.lnMH)
> upCI.MH  = exp(upCI.lnMH)
> cat("The 95% CI for MH =(", round(lowCI.MH, 4), ",",
round(upCI.MH, 4), ")", sep="", "\n\n")
```

The 95% CI for MH =(0.768,0.909)

4.2.4.3 Meta-Analysis Using R Library Meta

The implementation for MH OR method in R library can be done easily by calling function `metabin` as follows:

```
> # MH OR meta-analysis
> ORMH.Statin = metabin(evhigh,nhigh,evstd,nstd,studlab=Study,
                          data=dat, method="MH", sm="OR")
> # print the summary
> summary(ORMH.Statin)
```

Number of studies combined: k = 4

	OR	95%-CI	z	p-value
Fixed effect model	0.8354	[0.7679; 0.9089]	-4.18	< 0.0001
Random effects model	0.8355	[0.7679; 0.9090]	-4.18	< 0.0001

```
Quantifying heterogeneity:
 tau^2 = 0; tau = 0; I^2 = 0.0% [0.0%; 59.7%];
 H = 1.00 [1.00; 1.58]

Test of heterogeneity:
    Q d.f. p-value
 1.14    3  0.7673
```

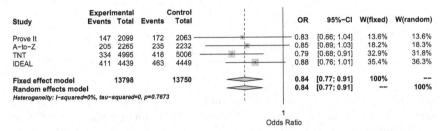

FIGURE 4.4
Meta-analysis with MH OR.

```
Details on meta-analytical method:
- MH method
- DerSimonian-Laird estimator for tau^2
- MH estimator used in calculation of Q
                        and tau^2 (like RevMan 5)
```

Interested readers can check the results from `metabin` with the results from previous section and find that they are identical.

The forest plot can be shown as in Figure 4.4 as follows:

```
> forest(ORMH.Statin)
```

4.2.5   Peto's Meta-Analysis Method

4.2.5.1   Peto's Odds Ratio

Another alternative to the MH method in analyzing ORs is Peto's method Yusuf et al. (1985). The Peto OR can be biased, especially when there is a substantial difference between treatment and control group sizes, but it performs well in many situations.

For each study i, the Peto's OR is defined as:

$$\hat{\Psi}_i = exp\left(\frac{O_i - E_i}{V_i}\right) \tag{4.27}$$

where

$$O_i = A_i$$

$$E_i = \frac{(A_i + B_i)(A_i + C_i)}{N_i}$$

$$V_i = \frac{(A_i + B_i)(C_i + D_i)(A_i + C_i)(B_i + D_i)}{N_i^2(N_i - 1)}$$

$$z_i = \frac{O_i - E_i}{\sqrt{V_i}}$$

$$CI_i = exp\left(\frac{(O_i - E_i) \pm z_{\alpha/2}\sqrt{V_i}}{V_i}\right)$$

Note that O_i and E_i are the observed and expected counts in the ith 2 by 2 table, z_i is the asymptotically normal test statistic for the ith study, CI_i is the CI where $z_{\alpha/2}$ as the quantile from the standard normal distribution. V_i is both the weighting factor and the variance for the difference between observed and expected $O_i - E_i$.

Then the pooled Peto OR is

$$\Psi_{pooled} = exp\left(\frac{\sum_{i=1}^{K}(O_i - E_i)}{\sum_{i=1}^{K} V_i}\right) \tag{4.28}$$

$$CI_{pooled} = exp\left(\frac{\sum_{i=1}^{K}(O_i - E_i) \pm z_{\alpha/2}\sqrt{\sum_{i=1}^{K} V_i}}{\sum_{i=1}^{K} V_i}\right) \tag{4.29}$$

4.2.5.2   Step-by-Step Implementation in R

First, Peto OR for each study can be calculated as follows:

```
> # the needed quantities of observed and expected
> Oi  = A
> Ei  = (A+B)*(A+C)/N
> Vi  = (A+B)*(C+D)/N*(A+C)/N*(B+D)/(N-1)
```

Then Peto's OR for each study can be calculated as:

```
> psii= exp( (Oi-Ei)/Vi ); psii

[1] 0.828 0.846 0.787 0.879
```

and the CI for each study can then be computed as follows:

```
> # lower bounds of CI
> lowCIi = exp( (Oi-Ei-1.96*sqrt(Vi))/Vi ); lowCIi

[1] 0.659 0.695 0.679 0.764
```

```
> # upper bounds of CI
> upCIi = exp( (Oi-Ei + 1.96*sqrt(Vi))/Vi );  upCIi

[1] 1.041 1.030 0.913 1.010
```

Again we can see that only the third study is significant based on this CI approach. To perform Peto's OR meta-analysis, we can calculate the pooled Peto's OR for the entire study as follows:

```
> # pooled Peto OR
> psi = exp( sum(Oi-Ei)/sum(Vi)) ; psi

[1] 0.836

> # lower bounds for CI
> lowCI = exp((sum(Oi-Ei)-1.96*sqrt(sum(Vi)))/sum(Vi)); lowCI

[1] 0.768

> # upper bounds for CI
> upCI = exp((sum(Oi-Ei)+1.96*sqrt(sum(Vi)))/sum(Vi)); upCI

[1] 0.909
```

Again, this 95% CI does not cover zero concluding again that the experimental high-dose scheme is statistically more effective than the standard dose scheme.

As an exercise, we encourage interested readers to compute the p-value and the (post) power for Peto's OR.

4.2.5.3   R Implementation in meta

The implementation of this Peto's OR meta-analysis in R library can be done easily as follows:

```
> # call "metabin" for Peto OR
> ORPeto.Statin =
  metabin(evhigh,nhigh,evstd,nstd,studlab=Study,
               data=dat, method="Peto", sm="OR")
> # print the summary
> summary(ORPeto.Statin)

                        OR        95%-CI     z  p-value
Fixed effect model    0.8357 [0.7684; 0.9090] -4.18 < 0.0001
Random effects model 0.8357 [0.7684; 0.9090] -4.18 < 0.0001


Quantifying heterogeneity:
 tau^2 = 0 [0.0000; 0.0265]; tau = 0 [0.0000; 0.1628];
 I^2 = 0.0% [0.0%; 59.5%]; H = 1.00 [1.00; 1.57]


Test of heterogeneity:
    Q d.f. p-value
 1.13    3  0.7692


Details on meta-analytical method:
- Peto method
- DerSimonian-Laird estimator for tau^2
- Jackson method for confidence CI of tau^2 and tau
```

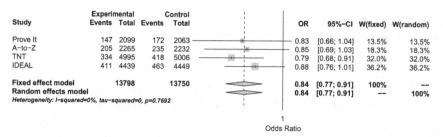

FIGURE 4.5
Meta-analysis with Peto's OR.

The forest plot can be shown as in Figure 4.5 as follows:

```
> forest(ORPeto.Statin)
```

4.3 Meta-Analysis of Lamotrigine Studies

As shown in Section 4.1.2, the data were read into R using `read.xls` and displayed in Table 4.2. The first category data can be printed using the following R code:

```
> head(Lamo, n=10)
```

```
# A tibble: 10 x 5
     Trial      Events Total Group        Category
     <chr>       <dbl> <dbl> <chr>           <dbl>
 1 SCA100223        59   111 lamotrigine         1
 2 SCA30924         47   131 lamotrigine         1
 3 SCA40910         51   133 lamotrigine         1
 4 SCAA2010         51   103 lamotrigine         1
 5 SCAB2001         32    63 lamotrigine         1
 6 SCA100223        44   109 placebo             1
 7 SCA30924         37   128 placebo             1
 8 SCA40910         39   124 placebo             1
 9 SCAA2010         45   103 placebo             1
10 SCAB2001         21    66 placebo             1
```

4.3.1 Risk Ratio

To reproduce the RR results in the Geddes et al.'s paper, we can call the `metabin` function for the category 1 data using following R code chunk as follows:

```
> # Get the Category 1 data
> d1      = Lamo[Lamo$Category==1,]
> evlamo = d1[d1$Group=="lamotrigine",]$Events
> nlamo  = d1[d1$Group=="lamotrigine",]$Total
> evcont = d1[d1$Group=="placebo",]$Events
> ncont  = d1[d1$Group=="placebo",]$Total
> trial  = d1[d1$Group=="placebo",]$Trial
> # Call metabin function for meta-analysis
> RR1.Lamo = metabin(evlamo,nlamo,evcont,ncont,studlab=trial,
 label.e="Lamotrigine", label.c="Placebo", method="MH",
 sm="RR")
> # print the RR fitting
> RR1.Lamo
```

	RR	95%-CI	%W(fixed)	%W(random)
SCA100223	1.3167	[0.9879; 1.7551]	23.7	26.4
SCA30924	1.2412	[0.8700; 1.7706]	19.9	17.3
SCA40910	1.2192	[0.8699; 1.7088]	21.5	19.1
SCAA2010	1.1333	[0.8451; 1.5198]	24.0	25.3
SCAB2001	1.5964	[1.0398; 2.4509]	10.9	11.9

	RR	95%-CI	z	p-value
Fixed effect model	1.2673	[1.0927; 1.4698]	3.13	0.0017
Random effects model	1.2650	[1.0914; 1.4663]	3.12	0.0018

```
Quantifying heterogeneity:
 tau^2 = 0; tau = 0; I^2 = 0.0% [0.0%; 53.9%];
 H = 1.00 [1.00; 1.47]

Test of heterogeneity:
    Q d.f. p-value
 1.80    4  0.7720

Details on meta-analytical method:
- MH method
- DerSimonian-Laird estimator for tau^2
- MH estimator used in calculation of Q and tau^2
```

This reproduces all the results. The figure 1a in the paper can be produced simply using forest from the meta package as seen in Figure 4.6 as follows:

```
> forest(RR1.Lamo)
```

Similarly, the meta-analysis for (i.e., Category 2) can be done using the following R code chunk:

```
> # Get the Category 2 data
> d2      = Lamo[Lamo$Category==2,]
```

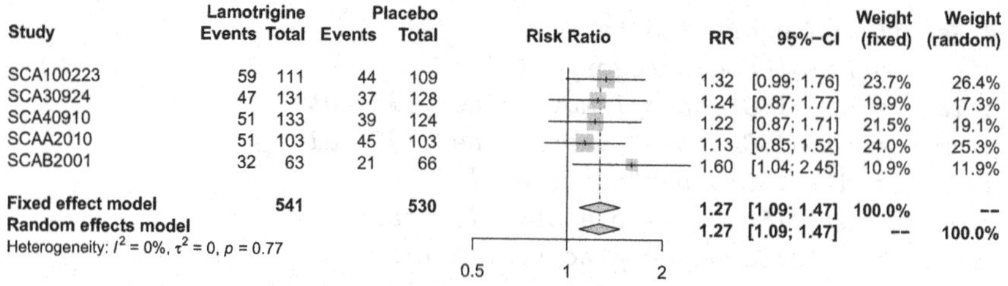

Study	Lamotrigine Events	Total	Placebo Events	Total	Risk Ratio	RR	95%-CI	Weight (fixed)	Weight (random)
SCA100223	59	111	44	109		1.32	[0.99; 1.76]	23.7%	26.4%
SCA30924	47	131	37	128		1.24	[0.87; 1.77]	19.9%	17.3%
SCA40910	51	133	39	124		1.22	[0.87; 1.71]	21.5%	19.1%
SCAA2010	51	103	45	103		1.13	[0.85; 1.52]	24.0%	25.3%
SCAB2001	32	63	21	66		1.60	[1.04; 2.45]	10.9%	11.9%
Fixed effect model		541		530		1.27	[1.09; 1.47]	100.0%	--
Random effects model						1.27	[1.09; 1.47]	--	100.0%

Heterogeneity: $I^2 = 0\%$, $\tau^2 = 0$, $p = 0.77$

0.5   1   2

FIGURE 4.6
Forest plot for category 1.

```
> evlamo = d2[d2$Group=="lamotrigine",]$Events
> nlamo  = d2[d2$Group=="lamotrigine",]$Total
> evcont = d2[d2$Group=="placebo",]$Events
> ncont  = d2[d2$Group=="placebo",]$Total
> trial  = d2[d2$Group=="placebo",]$Trial
> # Call metabin function for meta-analysis
> RR2.Lamo = metabin(evlamo,nlamo,evcont,ncont,studlab=trial,
  label.e="Lamotrigine", label.c="Placebo", method="MH",
  sm="RR")
> # print the RR fitting
> RR2.Lamo
```

```
                RR        95%-CI %W(fixed) %W(random)
SCA100223   1.3167 [0.9879; 1.7551]     22.0       24.2
SCA30924    1.2436 [0.9114; 1.6968]     22.0       20.7
SCA40910    1.0910 [0.8060; 1.4769]     24.1       21.8
SCAA2010    1.1087 [0.8294; 1.4821]     22.8       23.7
SCAB2001    1.7093 [1.0846; 2.6938]      9.2        9.7

Number of studies combined: k = 5
                        RR        95%-CI    z p-value
Fixed effect model    1.2350 [1.0722; 1.4226] 2.93  0.0034
Random effects model  1.2297 [1.0677; 1.4164] 2.87  0.0041

Quantifying heterogeneity:
 tau^2 = 0; tau = 0; I^2 = 0.0% [0.0%; 75.0%];
 H = 1.00 [1.00; 2.00]


Test of heterogeneity:
    Q d.f. p-value
 3.33    4  0.5045
```

Details on meta-analytical method:
- MH method
- DerSimonian-Laird estimator for tau^2
- MH estimator used in calculation of Q
                and tau^2 (like RevMan 5)

In comparing these results with those in the paper, we see there is a slight discrepancy for study SCA100223. In the paper, the RR was reported as 1.26 with CI of (0.95, 1.67) whereas the result from R is 1.32 with CI of (0.99, 1.76). This may be a good exercise for the reader to investigate and explain the nature of the discrepancy. In addition, we do not produce Figure 2a in the paper since readers can reproduce it using `forest` as we did for Figure 4.6.

Categories 3 and 4 reflect subsets of category 2 based on the mean baseline HRSD score being <24 or $\geq$ 24. The meta-analyses can be produced using the following R code chunks:

```
> # Get the Category 3 data
> d3    = Lamo[Lamo$Category==3,]
> evlamo = d3[d3$Group=="lamotrigine",]$Events
> nlamo = d3[d3$Group=="lamotrigine",]$Total
> evcont = d3[d3$Group=="placebo",]$Events
> ncont = d3[d3$Group=="placebo",]$Total
> trial = d3[d3$Group=="placebo",]$Trial
> # Call metabin function for meta-analysis
> RR3.Lamo = metabin(evlamo,nlamo,evcont,ncont,studlab=trial,
  label.e="Lamotrigine", label.c="Placebo", method="MH",
  sm="RR")
> # print the RR fitting for Category 3
> RR3.Lamo
```

	RR	95%-CI	%W(fixed)	%W(random)
SCA100223	0.9831	[0.6593; 1.4659]	20.6	18.9
SCA30924	1.1740	[0.8004; 1.7219]	20.3	20.6
SCA40910	0.9692	[0.6652; 1.4122]	25.0	21.3
SCAA2010	1.0714	[0.7630; 1.5044]	22.8	26.2
SCAB2001	1.2653	[0.7810; 2.0499]	11.3	13.0

Number of studies combined: k = 5

	RR	95%-CI	z	p-value
Fixed effect model	1.0703	[0.8991; 1.2741]	0.76	0.4450
Random effects model	1.0744	[0.9030; 1.2783]	0.81	0.4185

Quantifying heterogeneity:
  tau^2 = 0; tau = 0; I^2 = 0.0% [0.0%; 26.2%];
  H = 1.00 [1.00; 1.16]

Test of heterogeneity:
     Q d.f. p-value
  1.13   4 0.8900

Details on meta-analytical method:
- MH method
- DerSimonian-Laird estimator for tau^2
- MH estimator used in calculation of Q
                          and tau^2 (like RevMan 5)

```
> # Now analyze category 4
> # first get the Category 4 data
> d4      = Lamo[Lamo$Category==4,]
> evlamo = d4[d4$Group=="lamotrigine",]$Events
> nlamo  = d4[d4$Group=="lamotrigine",]$Total
> evcont = d4[d4$Group=="placebo",]$Events
> ncont  = d4[d4$Group=="placebo",]$Total
> trial  = d4[d4$Group=="placebo",]$Trial
> # Call metabin function for meta-analysis
> RR4.Lamo = metabin(evlamo,nlamo,evcont,ncont,studlab=trial,
 label.e="Lamotrigine", label.c="Placebo", method="MH",
 sm="RR")
> # print the RR fitting for Category 4
> RR4.Lamo
```

                    RR   95%-CI %W(fixed) %W(random)
SCA100223 1.6296 [1.0655; 2.4923]   25.8   30.8
SCA30924 1.3333 [0.8031; 2.2138]   24.8   21.6
SCA40910 1.3404 [0.8040; 2.2347]   21.8   21.2
SCAA2010 1.2199 [0.7206; 2.0650]   21.6   20.0
SCAB2001 2.7500 [1.0817; 6.9911]   6.1   6.4

Number of studies combined: k = 5
                          RR   95%-CI   z p-value
Fixed effect model   1.4734 [1.1640; 1.8650] 3.22 0.0013
Random effects model 1.4606 [1.1540; 1.8487] 3.15 0.0016

Quantifying heterogeneity:
 tau^2 = 0; tau = 0; I^2 = 0.0% [0.0%; 69.3%];
 H = 1.00 [1.00; 1.80]

Test of heterogeneity:
     Q d.f. p-value
  2.71   4 0.6076

```
Details on meta-analytical method:
- MH method
- DerSimonian-Laird estimator for tau^2
- MH estimator used in calculation of Q
                        and tau^2 (like RevMan 5)
```

The same conclusions are produced where lamotrigine was more beneficial than placebo in patients with severe depression at baseline but not in patients with moderate depression. We again encourage readers to reproduce Figure 2 in the paper by using `forest`.

We re-did the meta-analysis in this chapter using the MH weighting method (i.e., `method="MH"`) corresponding to the original paper. As an exercise, we encourage readers to use the inverse weighting (i.e., `method="Inverse"`) as an alternative meta-analysis.

4.3.2   Risk Difference

Further analysis for this data set can be performed using the RD as the treatment effect. We can use `metabin` function and change summary method (i.e., `sm`) from RR to RD. In addition, we replace the MH weighting scheme (i.e., `method="MH"`) with the inverse weighting scheme (i.e., `method="Inverse"`) in this analysis and leave the MH weighting scheme to interested readers (just replace `method="Inverse"` with `method="MH"`) as an exercise. We put all four categories into one R code chunk without producing the `forest`, but with detailed explanations in the code chunk as follows:

```
> #
> # meta-analysis for Category 1 HRSD data
> #
> evlamo = d1[d1$Group=="lamotrigine",]$Events
> nlamo  = d1[d1$Group=="lamotrigine",]$Total
> evcont = d1[d1$Group=="placebo",]$Events
> ncont  = d1[d1$Group=="placebo",]$Total
> trial  = d1[d1$Group=="placebo",]$Trial
> # Call metabin function for meta-analysis
> RD1.Lamo = metabin(evlamo,nlamo,evcont,ncont,studlab=trial,
          label.e="Lamotrigine", label.c="Placebo",
          method="Inverse", sm="RD")
> # print the result for category 1
> RD1.Lamo

              RD           95%-CI %W(fixed) %W(random)
SCA100223 0.1279 [-0.0029; 0.2586]      19.5       19.5
SCA30924  0.0697 [-0.0439; 0.1834]      25.8       25.8
```

```
SCA40910   0.0689  [-0.0473;  0.1852]      24.7        24.7
SCAA2010   0.0583  [-0.0778;  0.1943]      18.0        18.0
SCAB2001   0.1898  [ 0.0228;  0.3567]      12.0        12.0


                            RD          95%-CI     z p-value
Fixed effect model     0.0932 [0.0354;  0.1509] 3.16  0.0016
Random effects model   0.0932 [0.0354;  0.1509] 3.16  0.0016


Quantifying heterogeneity:
  tau^2 = 0 [0.0000; 0.0180]; tau = 0 [0.0000; 0.1340];
  I^2 = 0.0% [0.0%; 61.1%]; H = 1.00 [1.00; 1.60]


Test of heterogeneity:
    Q d.f. p-value
  2.14    4  0.7100


Details on meta-analytical method:
- Inverse variance method
- DerSimonian-Laird estimator for tau^2
- Jackson method for CI of tau^2 and tau

> #
> # meta-analysis for Category 2 MADRS data
> #
> evlamo = d2[d2$Group=="lamotrigine",]$Events
> nlamo  = d2[d2$Group=="lamotrigine",]$Total
> evcont = d2[d2$Group=="placebo",]$Events
> ncont  = d2[d2$Group=="placebo",]$Total
> trial  = d2[d2$Group=="placebo",]$Trial
> # Call metabin function for meta-analysis
> RD2.Lamo = metabin(evlamo,nlamo,evcont,ncont,studlab=trial,
  label.e="Lamotrigine", label.c="Placebo", method="Inverse",
  sm="RD")
> # print the result for category 2
> RD2.Lamo

             RD          95%-CI %W(fixed) %W(random)
SCA100223 0.1279 [-0.0029;  0.2586]      20.1        20.1
SCA30924  0.0837 [-0.0344;  0.2018]      24.7        24.7
SCA40910  0.0345 [-0.0851;  0.1541]      24.0        24.0
SCAA2010  0.0485 [-0.0876;  0.1847]      18.5        18.5
SCAB2001  0.2042 [ 0.0393;  0.3690]      12.7        12.7

Number of studies combined: k = 5
```

```
                        RD           95%-CI      z p-value
Fixed effect model    0.0895 [0.0308; 0.1481] 2.99  0.0028
Random effects model  0.0895 [0.0308; 0.1481] 2.99  0.0028
```

```
Quantifying heterogeneity:
 tau^2 = 0 [0.0000; 0.0305]; tau = 0 [0.0000; 0.1746];
 I^2 = 0.0% [0.0%; 75.2%]; H = 1.00 [1.00; 2.01]
```

```
Test of heterogeneity:
    Q d.f. p-value
 3.36    4  0.4996
```

```
Details on meta-analytical method:
- Inverse variance method
- DerSimonian-Laird estimator for tau^2
- Jackson method for CI of tau^2 and tau
```

```
> #
> # meta-analysis for category 3
> # i.e. moderate depressed individuals at baseline
> #
> evlamo = d3[d3$Group=="lamotrigine",]$Events
> nlamo  = d3[d3$Group=="lamotrigine",]$Total
> evcont = d3[d3$Group=="placebo",]$Events
> ncont  = d3[d3$Group=="placebo",]$Total
> trial  = d3[d3$Group=="placebo",]$Trial
> # Call metabin function for meta-analysis
> RD3.Lamo = metabin(evlamo,nlamo,evcont,ncont,studlab=trial,
 label.e="Lamotrigine", label.c="Placebo", method="Inverse",
 sm="RD")
> # print the result for category 3
> RD3.Lamo
```

```
               RD         95%-CI %W(fixed) %W(random)
SCA100223 -0.0076 [-0.1842; 0.1691]    20.4       20.4
SCA30924   0.0730 [-0.0998; 0.2457]    21.3       21.3
SCA40910  -0.0125 [-0.1638; 0.1387]    27.8       27.8
SCAA2010   0.0369 [-0.1446; 0.2184]    19.3       19.3
SCAB2001   0.1198 [-0.1201; 0.3597]    11.1       11.1
```

```
Number of studies combined: k = 5
```

```
                        RD           95%-CI      z p-value
Fixed effect model    0.0309 [-0.0489; 0.1107] 0.76  0.4476
Random effects model  0.0309 [-0.0489; 0.1107] 0.76  0.4476
```

Quantifying heterogeneity:
 tau^2 = 0 [0.0000; 0.0150]; tau = 0 [0.0000; 0.1226];
 I^2 = 0.0% [0.0%; 33.9%]; H = 1.00 [1.00; 1.23]

Test of heterogeneity:
    Q d.f. p-value
 1.26   4 0.8684

Details on meta-analytical method:
- Inverse variance method
- DerSimonian-Laird estimator for tau^2
- Jackson method for CI of tau^2 and tau

```
> #
> # meta-analysis for category 4:
> #        i.e. severe depressed individuals at baseline
> #
> evlamo = d4[d4$Group=="lamotrigine",]$Events
> nlamo  = d4[d4$Group=="lamotrigine",]$Total
> evcont = d4[d4$Group=="placebo",]$Events
> ncont  = d4[d4$Group=="placebo",]$Total
> trial  = d4[d4$Group=="placebo",]$Trial
> # Call metabin function for meta-analysis
> RD4.Lamo = metabin(evlamo,nlamo,evcont,ncont,studlab=trial,
  label.e="Lamotrigine", label.c="Placebo", method="Inverse",
  sm="RD")
> # print the result for category 4
> RD4.Lamo
```

	RD	95%-CI	%W(fixed)	%W(random)
SCA100223	0.2433	[0.0502; 0.4364]	19.2	19.2
SCA30924	0.0909	[-0.0672; 0.2491]	28.6	28.6
SCA40910	0.1135	[-0.0814; 0.3084]	18.9	18.9
SCAA2010	0.0767	[-0.1240; 0.2774]	17.8	17.8
SCAB2001	0.2500	[0.0351; 0.4649]	15.5	15.5

Number of studies combined: k = 5

	RD	95%-CI	z	p-value
Fixed effect model	0.1466	[0.0620; 0.2312]	3.39	0.0007
Random effects model	0.1466	[0.0620; 0.2312]	3.39	0.0007

Quantifying heterogeneity:
 tau^2 = 0 [0.0000; 0.0485]; tau = 0 [0.0000; 0.2203];
 I^2 = 0.0% [0.0%; 71.4%]; H = 1.00 [1.00; 1.87]

```
Test of heterogeneity:
    Q d.f. p-value
 2.91    4  0.5737
```

```
Details on meta-analytical method:
- Inverse variance method
- DerSimonian-Laird estimator for tau^2
- Jackson method for CI of tau^2 and tau
```

From the outputs, we see that with the exception of study SCAB2001, the first four studies (i.e., SCA100223, SCA30924, SCA40910, SCAA2010) have a 95% CI covering zero for all four categories indicating that lamotrigine was not more beneficial than the placebo if analyzed individually. However, when combined, a statistically significant result is found for categories of 1,2, and 4. This result is similar to the finding from RR indicated in the previous section as well as in the Geddes et al's paper.

In this analysis of RD, both the fixed-effects and random-effects meta-analysis gave the same inferential results because of statistically insignificant heterogeneity as seen from the Q-statistic with estimated between-study variance $\hat{\tau}^2 = 0$.

4.3.3 Odds Ratio

OR is a commonly used metric in the analysis of binomial data. We illustrate the meta-analysis using OR for the lamotrigine data. There are several methods implemented for OR in the R package meta as described in Section 4.2. To control the number of pages in this chapter, we only illustrate the MH weighting scheme (i.e., method="MH") here and leave the inverse weighting scheme (i.e., method="Inverse") and the Peto method (i.e., method="Peto") to interested readers as exercises. In addition, we encourage readers to produce the forest plots for each analysis.

The implementation of the OR with MH weighting scheme can be done with the following code chunk:

```
> #
> # meta-analysis for Category 1 HRSD data
> #
> evlamo = d1[d1$Group=="lamotrigine",]$Events
> nlamo  = d1[d1$Group=="lamotrigine",]$Total
> evcont = d1[d1$Group=="placebo",]$Events
> ncont  = d1[d1$Group=="placebo",]$Total
> trial  = d1[d1$Group=="placebo",]$Trial
> # Call metabin function for meta-analysis
> OR1.Lamo = metabin(evlamo,nlamo,evcont,ncont,studlab=trial,
  label.e="Lamotrigine", label.c="Placebo", method="MH",
  sm="OR")
```

```
> # print the result for category 1
> OR1.Lamo
```

```
               OR          95%-CI %W(fixed) %W(random)
SCA100223 1.6761 [0.9824; 2.8597]      20.3       21.6
SCA30924  1.3761 [0.8157; 2.3216]      23.4       22.6
SCA40910  1.3555 [0.8094; 2.2701]      24.3       23.2
SCAA2010  1.2641 [0.7305; 2.1876]      22.2       20.5
SCAB2001  2.2120 [1.0813; 4.5250]       9.8       12.1
```

```
Number of studies combined: k = 5
```

```
                          OR          95%-CI   z p-value
Fixed effect model    1.4895 [1.1623; 1.9088] 3.15  0.0016
Random effects model  1.4892 [1.1615; 1.9092] 3.14  0.0017
```

```
Quantifying heterogeneity:
 tau^2 = 0; tau = 0; I^2 = 0.0% [0.0%; 56.7%];
 H = 1.00 [1.00; 1.52]
```

```
Test of heterogeneity:
    Q d.f. p-value
 1.92    4  0.7504
```

```
Details on meta-analytical method:
- MH method
- DerSimonian-Laird estimator for tau^2
- MH estimator used in calculation of Q
                        and tau^2 (like RevMan 5)
```

```
> #
> # meta-analysis for Category 2 MADRS data
> #
> evlamo = d2[d2$Group=="lamotrigine",]$Events
> nlamo  = d2[d2$Group=="lamotrigine",]$Total
> evcont = d2[d2$Group=="placebo",]$Events
> ncont  = d2[d2$Group=="placebo",]$Total
> trial  = d2[d2$Group=="placebo",]$Trial
> # Call metabin function for meta-analysis
> OR2.Lamo = metabin(evlamo,nlamo,evcont,ncont,studlab=trial,
  label.e="Lamotrigine", label.c="Placebo", method="MH",
  sm="OR")
> # print the result for category 2
> OR2.Lamo
```

```
                  OR              95%-CI %W(fixed) %W(random)
SCA100223 1.6761 [0.9824; 2.8597]     19.4        21.0
SCA30924  1.4255 [0.8621; 2.3569]     23.7        23.7
SCA40910  1.1552 [0.7002; 1.9060]     26.5        23.9
SCAA2010  1.2153 [0.7027; 2.1018]     21.6        20.0
SCAB2001  2.3964 [1.1588; 4.9556]      8.8        11.4


Number of studies combined: k = 5


                       OR        95%-CI    z p-value
Fixed effect model   1.4420 [1.1296; 1.8407] 2.94  0.0033
Random effects model 1.4411 [1.1281; 1.8410] 2.92  0.0035


Quantifying heterogeneity:
 tau^2 = 0; tau = 0; I^2 = 0.0% [0.0%; 74.9%];
 H = 1.00 [1.00; 2.00]


Test of heterogeneity:
    Q d.f. p-value
 3.31    4  0.5070


Details on meta-analytical method:
- MH method
- DerSimonian-Laird estimator for tau^2
- MH estimator used in calculation of Q
              and tau^2 (like RevMan 5)

> #
> # meta-analysis for category 3:
> #         (moderate depressed individuals at baseline)
> #
> evlamo = d3[d3$Group=="lamotrigine",]$Events
> nlamo  = d3[d3$Group=="lamotrigine",]$Total
> evcont = d3[d3$Group=="placebo",]$Events
> ncont  = d3[d3$Group=="placebo",]$Total
> trial  = d3[d3$Group=="placebo",]$Trial
> # Call metabin function for meta-analysis
> OR3.Lamo = metabin(evlamo,nlamo,evcont,ncont,studlab=trial,
  label.e="Lamotrigine", label.c="Placebo", method="MH",
  sm="OR")
> # print the result for category 3
> OR3.Lamo

                  OR              95%-CI %W(fixed) %W(random)
SCA100223 0.9698 [0.4739; 1.9848]     22.3        20.7
SCA30924  1.3427 [0.6663; 2.7055]     19.8        21.6
```

```
SCA40910   0.9491  [0.5058;  1.7810]        29.1        26.7
SCAA2010   1.1600  [0.5586;  2.4088]        19.5        19.8
SCAB2001   1.6190  [0.6113;  4.2878]         9.3        11.2
```

```
Number of studies combined: k = 5
```

```
                              OR           95%-CI     z p-value
Fixed effect model     1.1351 [0.8203;  1.5708] 0.76  0.4444
Random effects model   1.1349 [0.8196;  1.5716] 0.76  0.4460
```

```
Quantifying heterogeneity:
 tau^2 = 0; tau = 0; I^2 = 0.0% [0.0%; 32.4%];
 H = 1.00 [1.00; 1.22]
```

```
Test of heterogeneity:
   Q d.f. p-value
 1.23   4  0.8730
```

```
Details on meta-analytical method:
- MH method
- DerSimonian-Laird estimator for tau^2
- MH estimator used in calculation of Q
               and tau^2 (like RevMan 5)
```

```
> #
> # meta-analysis for category 4
> #        (severe depressed individuals at baseline)
> #
> evlamo = d4[d4$Group=="lamotrigine",]$Events
> nlamo  = d4[d4$Group=="lamotrigine",]$Total
> evcont = d4[d4$Group=="placebo",]$Events
> ncont  = d4[d4$Group=="placebo",]$Total
> trial  = d4[d4$Group=="placebo",]$Trial
> # Call metabin function for meta-analysis
> OR4.Lamo = metabin(evlamo,nlamo,evcont,ncont,studlab=trial,
 label.e="Lamotrigine", label.c="Placebo", method="MH",
 sm="OR")
> # print the result for category 4
> OR4.Lamo
```

```
              OR           95%-CI %W(fixed) %W(random)
SCA100223 2.7000 [1.1885;  6.1337]      17.9       21.8
SCA30924  1.5238 [0.7283;  3.1881]      29.5       26.9
SCA40910  1.6154 [0.7036;  3.7089]      22.5       21.2
SCAA2010  1.3827 [0.5892;  3.2448]      23.2       20.1
SCAB2001  3.8824 [1.1542; 13.0594]       6.9       10.0
```

```
Number of studies combined: k = 5

                        OR           95%-CI      z p-value
Fixed effect model    1.8857 [1.2894; 2.7577] 3.27  0.0011
Random effects model 1.8809 [1.2826; 2.7583] 3.23  0.0012

Quantifying heterogeneity:
 tau^2 = 0; tau = 0; I^2 = 0.0% [0.0%; 72.8%];
 H = 1.00 [1.00; 1.92]

Test of heterogeneity:
    Q d.f. p-value
 3.06    4  0.5482

Details on meta-analytical method:
- MH method
- DerSimonian-Laird estimator for tau^2
- MH estimator used in calculation of Q
             and tau^2 (like RevMan 5)
```

Again, the results from the analyses of OR are similar to those of RR and of RD further confirming that lamotrigine was statistically better than the placebo in treating bipolar depression.

4.4 Discussions

In this chapter, we illustrated meta-analysis methods for binomial data using published results from two clinical trials programs. The first data set was from clinical trials designed to compare intensive statin therapy to moderate statin therapy in the reduction of cardiovascular outcomes. The other data set was from clinical trials of lamotrigine designed for treating depression in patients with bipolar disorder. Both data sets were used to illustrate meta-analyses using the R packages meta and metafor. The cardiovascular data set was used primarily to illustrate meta-analysis methods with step-by-step implementation in R along with the mathematical formula as discussed in Section 4.2. The lamotrigine data set further illustrated the R implementation in package meta. We leave the meta-analysis of lamotrigine data set with R package metafor to interested readers as an exercise. The results with the metafor package should be the same as the results in step-by-step illustration and results with the meta package.

For studies with binary or binomial outcome measures, we focused on the most commonly used measures of treatment effect; i.e., RD, RR, and OR.

The arcsine (AS) difference can also be used as a measure of treatment effect, although it rarely appears in the medical literature. It is implemented in R package `meta` as `sm="AS"` as one of the summary methods. As discussed in Rucker et al. (2009), the AS has considerable promise in handling zeros and its asymptotic variance does not depend on the event probability. We encourage interested readers to experiment with `sm="AS"` for their own data.

Appendix: Stata Programs for Meta-Analysis with Binary Data by Manyun Liu

The `Stata` program below corresponds to the R program.

```
/*### Reproduce R Results in Subsection 4.1.1 ###*/
/* You can use the following command to load the excel file */
cd "your file path"
import excel using dat4Meta.xls, sheet("Data_Statin2006")
        firstrow clear

/*  present the data */
browse

/*  Or we can use list command to present the data */
list

/*### Reproduce R Results in Subsection 4.1.1 ###*/
list

/*### Reproduce R Results in Subsection 4.1.2 ###*/
/* You can use the following command to load the excel file */
import excel using dat4Meta.xls, sheet("Data_Lamo")
        firstrow clear

/*  present the data */
browse

/*### Reproduce R Results in Subsection 4.2.1.1 ###*/
/* You can use the following command to reload the excel file
        from Subsection 4.1.1 */
import excel using dat4Meta.xls, sheet("Data_Statin2006")
        firstrow clear
```

```
/* For the risk high dose group, the events evhigh,
   the total number nhigh, the risk pE= evhigh/nhigh */
generate pE = evhigh/nhigh

/* present the risk pE */
 list pE

/* For the risk low dose group, the events evstd,
   the total number nstd, the risk pC= evstd/nstd */
generate pC= evstd/nstd

/* present the risk pC */
 list pC

/* The risk-ratios */
generate ES = pE/pC

/* present the risk RR */
 list ES

/*### Reproduce R Results in Subsection 4.2.1.2 ###*/
/* calculate the log risk-ratio */
generate lnES = log(ES)

/*  print the log risk-ratio */
list lnES

/*  calculate the variance */
generate VlnES = 1/evhigh - 1/nhigh + 1/evstd - 1/nstd

/*  print the variance */
list VlnES

/* upper CI */
generate ciup  = lnES+1.96*sqrt(VlnES)
list ciup

/*  lower CI */
generate cilow  = lnES-1.96*sqrt(VlnES)
list cilow

/* then transform back to the original scale */
forvalues i = 1/4 {
   display "The low CI is:" exp(cilow[`i'])
 }
```

```
/* The z-value */
generate z = lnES/sqrt(VlnES)
list z

generate pval = 2*(1- normal(abs(z)))
forvalues i = 1/4 {
   display "p-values =" pval[`i']
 }

generate rhigh=evhigh/nhigh
generate rstd=evstd/nstd
list rhigh rstd nhigh nstd

/* Input the data to calcuate the power */
power twoproportions 0.0700333    0.0833737, n1(2099) n2(2063)
power twoproportions 0.0905077    0.1052867, n1(2265) n2(2232)
power twoproportions 0.0668669    0.0834998, n1(4995) n2(5006)
power twoproportions 0.0925884    0.1040683, n1(4439) n2(4449)

/*### Reproduce R Results in Subsection 4.2.1.3 ###*/
list VlnES

generate w = 1/VlnES
list w

/*  the inverse of variance for each study */
generate fwi = 1/VlnES
list fwi

/*  the total weight */
egen fw = total(fwi)
display fw

/*  the relative weight for each study */
generate rw = fwi/fw
list rw

/*  the weighted mean */
egen flnES = total(lnES*rw)
display flnES

/*  the variance for the weighted mean */
generate var= 1/fw
display var
```

```
/* the RR */
display exp(flnES)

/* the lower CI bound */
display exp(flnES-1.96*sqrt(var))

/* the upper CI bound */
display exp(flnES+1.96*sqrt(var))

/* estimate heterogeneity statistic Q */
egen Q1 = total(fwi*lnES^2)
egen Q2= total(fwi*lnES)
generate Q=Q1-Q2^2/fw
display Q

/* Get the degrees of freedom */
generate K= r(N)
generate df = K -1
display df

/* calculate the statistical significance: p-value */
generate pval4Q =  chi2tail(df, Q)
display pval4Q

/*### Reproduce R Results in Subsection 4.2.1.4 ###*/
/* Generate two new variables, which are the non-event
      number of patients of each group */
 generate nonhigh = nhigh-evhigh
 generate nonstd = nstd-evstd

/* For the fixed-effects model, print the results and also
            automatically produces the forest plot */
metan evhigh nonhigh evstd nonstd, label(namevar=Study)
      fixedi rr

/* For the random-effects model, print the results and
        automatically produces the forest plot */
metan evhigh nonhigh evstd nonstd, label(namevar=Study)
      randomi rr

/*### Reproduce R Results in Subsection 4.2.1.5 ###*/
/* These parts are specific to R, which utilize alternative
    R metafor and rmeta packages to reproduce previous rr
    meta-analysis results. Here, we utilize similar function
```

```
      Stata code to produce similar results. */
/* For the fixed model. */
meta esize evhigh nonhigh evstd nonstd, esize(lnrratio)
            fixed(mhaenszel)
list Study _meta_es _meta_se
meta summarize, fixed(mhaenszel)

/* For the random model. */
meta esize evhigh nonhigh evstd nonstd, esize(lnrratio)
    random(dlaird)
meta summarize, random(dlaird)

/*### Reproduce R Results in Subsection 4.2.2.2 ###*/
/* the risk difference */
generate ESRD = pE-pC
list ESRD

/* calculate the variance: nE=nhigh, nC=nstd */
generate VarRD = pE*(1-pE)/nhigh + pC*(1-pC)/nstd
list VarRD

/* calculate the standard error */
generate SERD = sqrt(VarRD)
list SERD

/*### Reproduce R Results in Subsection 4.2.2.3 ###*/

/* For the fixed-effects model, print the results
   and automatically produces the forest plot */
metan evhigh nonhigh evstd nonstd, label(namevar=Study)
      fixedi rd

/* For the random-effects model, print the results and
    also automatically produces the forest plot */
metan evhigh nonhigh evstd nonstd, label(namevar=Study)
      randomi rd

/*### Reproduce R Results in Subsection 4.2.2.4 ###*/
/* These parts are specific to R, which utilize
   alternative R metafor and rmeta packages to reproduce
   previous rd meta-analysis results. Here, we utilize
   similar function Stata code to produce similar results. */

/* For the fixed model. */
meta esize evhigh nonhigh evstd nonstd, esize(rdiff)
```

```
      fixed(mhaenszel)
list Study _meta_es _meta_se
meta summarize, fixed(mhaenszel)


/* For the random model. */
meta esize evhigh nonhigh evstd nonstd, esize(rdiff)
      random(dlaird)
meta summarize, random(dlaird)


/*#### Reproduce R Results in Subsection 4.2.3.2 ###*/
generate oddsE = pE/(1-pE)
list oddsE

generate oddsC = pC/(1-pC)
list oddsC

generate OR = oddsE/oddsC
list OR

generate LogOR= log(OR)
list LogOR

generate VLogOR = 1/334+ 1/(4995-334)+1/418+1/(5006-418)
display VLogOR

generate SE_LogOR=sqrt(VLogOR)
display SE_LogOR


/*#### Reproduce R Results in Subsection 4.2.3.3 ###*/
/* For the fixed-effects model, print the results
  and also automatically produces the forest plot */
metan evhigh nonhigh evstd nonstd, label(namevar=Study)
      fixedi or


/* For the random-effects model, print the results
      and also automatically produces the forest plot */
metan evhigh nonhigh evstd nonstd, label(namevar=Study)
      randomi or


/*#### Reproduce R Results in Subsection 4.2.3.4 ###*/
/* For the fixed model. */
meta esize evhigh nonhigh evstd nonstd, esize(lnorpeto)
      fixed
list Study _meta_es _meta_se
meta summarize, fixed(invvariance)
```

```
/* For the random model. */
meta esize evhigh nonhigh evstd nonstd, esize(lnorpeto)
     random(dlaird)
meta summarize, random(dlaird)

/*### Reproduce R Results in Subsection 4.2.4.2 ###*/
list OR

generate w0 = (nhigh-evhigh)*evstd/(nhigh+nstd)
list w0

egen TotWeight = total(w0)
display TotWeight

generate relWt = w0/TotWeight
list relWt

egen OR_MH = total(relWt*OR)
display OR_MH

generate Var_ORMH1 = 1/TotWeight
display Var_ORMH1

generate lowCI = OR_MH-1.96*sqrt(Var_ORMH1)
display lowCI
generate upCI = OR_MH+1.96*sqrt(Var_ORMH1)
display upCI
display "MH estimate=" round(OR_MH,0.0001)
display "The 95% CI for MH =(" round(lowCI, 0.0001) ","
     round(upCI, 0.0001) ")"

generate A = evhigh
generate B  = nhigh-evhigh
generate C  = evstd
generate D = nstd-evstd
generate N = A+B+C+D
generate T1 = (A+D)/N
generate T2 = (B+C)/N
generate T3 = A*D/N
generate T4 = B*C/N
egen ST3 = total(T3)
egen ST4 = total(T4)
```

```
generate Var_lnOddsRatio = 0.5*((T1*T3)/ST3^2+
       (T1*T4+T2*T3)/(ST3*ST4)+T2*T4/ST4^2)
list Var_lnOddsRatio

egen Var_lnMH = total(Var_lnOddsRatio)
display Var_lnMH

generate lowCI_lnMH = log(OR_MH)-1.96*sqrt(Var_lnMH)
generate upCI_lnMH = log(OR_MH)+1.96*sqrt(Var_lnMH)
display "The 95% CI for log-MH =(" round(lowCI_lnMH, 0.0001) ","
       round(upCI_lnMH, 0.0001) ")"

generate lowCI_MH = exp(lowCI_lnMH)
generate upCI_MH  = exp(upCI_lnMH)
display "The 95% CI for MH =(" round(lowCI_MH, 0.0001) ","
       round(upCI_MH, 0.0001) ")"

/*### Reproduce R Results in Subsection 4.2.4.3 ###*/
/* These parts are specific to R, which utilize
   alternative R metabin package MH method to reproduce
   or meta-analysis results. Here, we still utilize
   Stata metan to produce similar results. */

/* For the fixed model. */
metan evhigh nonhigh evstd nonstd, label(namevar=Study)
       fixed or

/* For the random model. */
metan evhigh nonhigh evstd nonstd, label(namevar=Study)
       random or

/*### Reproduce R Results in Subsection 4.2.5.2 ###*/
/*  the needed quantities of observed and expected */
generate Oi  = A
generate Ei  = (A+B)*(A+C)/N
generate Vi  = (A+B)*(C+D)/N*(A+C)/N*(B+D)/(N-1)

generate psii= exp( (Oi-Ei)/Vi)
list psii

/*  lower bounds of CI */
generate lowCIi = exp( (Oi-Ei-1.96*sqrt(Vi))/Vi )
list lowCIi
```

```
/* upper bounds of CI */
generate upCIi = exp( (Oi-Ei + 1.96*sqrt(Vi))/Vi )
list upCIi

/* pooled Peto OR */
egen sumOiEi= total(Oi-Ei)
egen sumVi= total(Vi)
generate psi = exp(sumOiEi/sumVi)
display psi

/* lower bounds for CI */
generate lowCI = exp( (sumOiEi - 1.96*sqrt(sumVi))/sumVi )
display lowCI

/* upper bounds for CI */
generate upCI = exp( ( sumOiEi + 1.96*sqrt(sumVi))/sumVi )
display upCI

/* For the peto model, Stata specifies Peto's assumption
   free method to pool odds ratios. It prints the results
   and also automatically produces the forest plot */
metan evhigh nonhigh evstd nonstd, or peto label(namevar=Study)

/*### Reproduce R Results in Subsection 4.3 ###*/
/* You can use the following command to load the excel file */
import excel using dat4Meta.xls, sheet("Data_Lamo") firstrow clear

/* present the top 10 rows of data */
list in 1/10

/*### Reproduce R Results in Subsection 4.3.1 ###*/
/* Get the Category 1 data */
/* Generate a new table to only contain only Category 1 data*/
import excel using dat4Meta.xls, sheet("Data_Lamo")
     firstrow clear

keep if Category==1 & Group=="lamotrigine"
rename Events evlamo
rename Total nlamo
generate nonevlamo=nlamo-evlamo
drop Group
save Category1_lamotrigine.dta, replace

import excel using dat4Meta.xls, sheet("Data_Lamo")
         firstrow clear
```

```
keep if Category==1 & Group=="placebo"
rename Events evcont
rename Total ncont
generate nonevcont=ncont-evcont
drop Group
save Category1_placebo.dta, replace

merge 1:1 Trial using Category1_lamotrigine.dta
list
save Category1.dta, replace

/* For the fixed-effects model, print the results
      and also automatically produces the forest plot */
 metan evlamo nonevlamo evcont nonevcont, label(namevar=Trial)
       fixed rr

/* For the random-effects model, print the results
    and also automatically produces the forest plot */
metan evlamo nonevlamo evcont nonevcont, label(namevar=Trial)
       random rr

/* Get the Category 2 data */
/* Generate a new table to only contain only Category 2 data */
import excel using dat4Meta.xls, sheet("Data_Lamo")
    firstrow clear
keep if Category==2 & Group=="lamotrigine"
rename Events evlamo
rename Total nlamo
generate nonevlamo=nlamo-evlamo
drop Group
save Category2_lamotrigine.dta, replace

import excel using dat4Meta.xls, sheet("Data_Lamo")
        firstrow clear
keep if Category==2 & Group=="placebo"
rename Events evcont
rename Total ncont
generate nonevcont=ncont-evcont
drop Group
save Category2_placebo.dta, replace

merge 1:1 Trial using Category2_lamotrigine.dta
list
save Category2.dta, replace
```

```
/* For the fixed-effects model, print the results
    and also automatically produces the forest plot */
 metan evlamo nonevlamo evcont nonevcont, label(namevar=Trial)
    fixed rr

/* For the random-effects model, print the results and
    also automatically produces the forest plot */
metan evlamo nonevlamo evcont nonevcont, label(namevar=Trial)
    random rr

/* Get the Category 3 data */
/* Generate a new table to only contain only Category 3 data */
import excel using dat4Meta.xls, sheet("Data_Lamo")
        firstrow clear
keep if Category==3 & Group=="lamotrigine"
rename Events evlamo
rename Total nlamo
generate nonevlamo=nlamo-evlamo
drop Group
save Category3_lamotrigine.dta, replace

import excel using dat4Meta.xls, sheet("Data_Lamo")
        firstrow clear
keep if Category==3 & Group=="placebo"
rename Events evcont
rename Total ncont
generate nonevcont=ncont-evcont
drop Group
save Category3_placebo.dta, replace

merge 1:1 Trial using Category3_lamotrigine.dta
list
save Category3.dta, replace

/* For the fixed-effects model, print the results and
    also automatically produces the forest plot */
metan evlamo nonevlamo evcont nonevcont, label(namevar=Trial)
    fixed rr

/* For the random-effects model, print the results and
    also automatically produces the forest plot */
metan evlamo nonevlamo evcont nonevcont, label(namevar=Trial)
    random rr
```

```
/* Get the Category 4 data */
/* Generate a new table to only contain only Category 4 data */
import excel using dat4Meta.xls, sheet("Data_Lamo")
      firstrow clear
keep if Category==4 & Group=="lamotrigine"
rename Events evlamo
rename Total nlamo
generate nonevlamo=nlamo-evlamo
drop Group
save Category4_lamotrigine.dta, replace

import excel using dat4Meta.xls, sheet("Data_Lamo")
      firstrow clear
keep if Category==4 & Group=="placebo"
rename Events evcont
rename Total ncont
generate nonevcont=ncont-evcont
drop Group
save Category4_placebo.dta, replace

merge 1:1 Trial using Category4_lamotrigine.dta
list
save Category4.dta, replace

/* For the fixed-effects model, print the results
      and also automatically produces the forest plot */
metan evlamo nonevlamo evcont nonevcont, label(namevar=Trial)
      fixed rr

/* For the random-effects model, print the results and
        also automatically produces the forest plot */
metan evlamo nonevlamo evcont nonevcont, label(namevar=Trial)
      random rr

/*### Reproduce R Results in Subsection 4.3.2 ###*/
/* meta-analysis for Category 1 HRSD data */

use Category1.dta, clear
/* For the fixed-effects model, print the results and
      also automatically produces the forest plot */
metan evlamo nonevlamo evcont nonevcont, label(namevar=Trial)
      fixedi rd
```

```
/* For the random-effects model, print the results
      and also automatically produces the forest plot */
metan evlamo nonevlamo evcont nonevcont, label(namevar=Trial)
      randomi rd

/* meta-analysis for Category 2 MADRS data */
use Category2.dta, clear
metan evlamo nonevlamo evcont nonevcont, label(namevar=Trial)
      fixedi rd
metan evlamo nonevlamo evcont nonevcont, label(namevar=Trial)
      randomi rd

/* meta-analysis for Category 3 */
use Category3.dta, clear
metan evlamo nonevlamo evcont nonevcont, label(namevar=Trial)
      fixedi rd
metan evlamo nonevlamo evcont nonevcont, label(namevar=Trial)
      randomi rd

/* meta-analysis for Category 4 */
use Category4.dta, clear
metan evlamo nonevlamo evcont nonevcont, label(namevar=Trial)
      fixedi rd
metan evlamo nonevlamo evcont nonevcont, label(namevar=Trial)
      randomi rd

/*### Reproduce R Results in Subsection 4.3.3 ###*/
/* meta-analysis for Category 1 HRSD data */

use Category1.dta, clear
/* For the fixed-effects model, print the results and also
      automatically produces the forest plot */
metan evlamo nonevlamo evcont nonevcont, label(namevar=Trial)
      fixed or

/* For the random-effects model, print the results and
      also automatically produces the forest plot */
metan evlamo nonevlamo evcont nonevcont, label(namevar=Trial)
      random or

/* meta-analysis for Category 2 MADRS data */
use Category2.dta, clear
metan evlamo nonevlamo evcont nonevcont, label(namevar=Trial)
      fixed or
```

```
metan evlamo nonevlamo evcont nonevcont, label(namevar=Trial)
      random or

/* meta-analysis for Category 3 */
use Category3.dta, clear
metan evlamo nonevlamo evcont nonevcont, label(namevar=Trial)
        fixed or
metan evlamo nonevlamo evcont nonevcont, label(namevar=Trial)
        random or

/* meta-analysis for Category 4 */
use Category4.dta, clear
metan evlamo nonevlamo evcont nonevcont, label(namevar=Trial)
        fixed or
metan evlamo nonevlamo evcont nonevcont, label(namevar=Trial)
        random or
```

5

Meta-Analysis for Continuous Data

Continuous data are commonly reported as endpoints in clinical trials and other studies. In this chapter, we discuss the meta-analysis methods for this type of data. For continuous data, the typical reported summary statistics are the means and standard deviations (or standard errors) along with the sample sizes for each study.

Meta-analyses of means for continuous data are usually performed on the mean differences (MDs) across studies in reference to the pooled variance. Similarly to Chapter 4, we introduce two published data sets in Section 5.1 with the first meta-data on impact of intervention in Section 5.1.1 and then the second meta-data on clinical trials to compare tubeless vs standard percutaneous nephrolithotomy (PCNL) for patients with stones of the kidney or upper ureter in Section 5.1.2. We then describe the meta-analysis models for continuous data to facilitate analyses in Section 5.2.

In Section 5.3, we use the first data set to illustrate the step-by-step R implementation of the methods in Section 5.2 to facilitate the understanding of these methods and compare the results to the meta-analyses from R packages `meta` and `metafor`. The second data set is used in Section 5.4 to illustrate the application of R package `meta` corresponding to the meta-analysis methods detailed in Section 5.2. Discussion appears in Section 5.5.

Note to readers: You need to install R packages `readxl` to read in the excel data file, and `meta` and `metafor` to perform the meta-analysis.

5.1 Two Published Data Sets

5.1.1 Impact of Intervention

Table 5.1 is reproduced from Table 14.1 in Borenstein et al. (2009). Interested readers can refer to the book for details. In this chapter, we use this data set to illustrate the step-by-step calculations using R for continuous data methods.

TABLE 5.1

Impact of Intervention: Continuous Data

Study	Treated			Control		
	Mean	SD	N	Mean	SD	N
Carroll	94	22	60	92	20	60
Grant	98	21	65	92	22	65
Peck	98	28	40	88	26	40
Donat	94	19	200	82	17	200
Stewart	98	21	50	88	22	45
Young	96	21	85	92	22	85

5.1.2   Tubeless vs Standard PCNL

To systematically review and compare tubeless PCNL with standard PCNL for stones of the kidney or the upper ureter, Wang et al. (2011) conducted a meta-analysis from all English language literature on studies from randomized controlled trials to obtain definitive conclusions for clinical practice. The paper can be accessed from http://www.ncbi.nlm.nih.gov/pubmed/21883839.

The authors found 127 studies from the first search. After initial screening of the title and abstract, 20 studies met the inclusion criteria. Upon further screening the full text of these 20 studies, 7 studies were included in their meta-analysis.

To reproduce the results from this paper, we entered all the data as seen in Table 5.2 from these seven studies into the excel databook dat4Meta which can be loaded into R using following R code chunk:

```
> # Load the library
> require(readxl)
> # Get the data path
> datfile = "Path to your data file 'dat4Meta.xls'"
> # Call "read_excel" to read the Excel data in data sheet
> dat  = read_excel(datfile, sheet="Data_tubeless")
```

Note that in this table, column Outcome lists the four outcome measures considered in the paper which are operation duration (abbreviated by "duration"), length of hospital stay (abbreviated by "LOS"), analgesic requirement after tubeless (abbreviated by "analgesic"), and the pre- and postoperative hematocrit changes (abbreviated by "hematocrit"). Column Study denotes the selected clinical studies for this meta-analysis. The remaining columns Mean.E, SD.E, n.E, Mean.C, SD.C, and n.C denote the means, standard deviations, and total observations from the experimental and control arms, respectively.

The authors performed their meta-analysis using the Cochrane Review Manager (REVMAN 5.0) software. In this chapter, we use the R package meta to reanalyze this data set.

TABLE 5.2
Data from PCNL Studies

Outcome	Study	Mean.E	SD.E	n.E	Mean.C	SD.C	n.C
Duration	Ahmet Tefekli 2007	60	9	17	76	10	18
Duration	B.Lojanapiwat 2010	49	24	45	57	20	59
Duration	Hemendra N. Shah 2008	51	10	33	47	16	32
Duration	Hemendra Shah 2009	52	23	454	68	34	386
Duration	J. Jun-Ou 2010	47	17	43	59	18	52
Duration	Michael Choi 2006	82	18	12	73	15	12
LOS	Ahmet Tefekli 2007	38	10	17	67	22	18
LOS	B.Lojanapiwat 2010	85	23	45	129	54	59
LOS	Hemendra N. Shah 2008	35	11	33	44	22	32
LOS	Hemendra Shah 2009	34	17	454	56	62	386
LOS	J. Jun-Ou 2010	82	24	43	106	35	52
LOS	Madhu S. Agrawal 2008	22	4	101	54	5	101
LOS	Michael Choi 2006	37	24	12	38	24	12
Analgesic	B.Lojanapiwat 2010	39	35	45	75	32	59
Analgesic	Hemendra N. Shah 2008	150	97	33	246	167	32
Analgesic	Hemendra Shah 2009	103	116	454	250	132	386
Analgesic	J. Jun-Ou 2010	37	31	43	70	36	52
Analgesic	Madhu S. Agrawal 2008	82	24	101	126	33	101
Haematocrit	Ahmet Tefekli 2007	2	1	17	1	0	18
Haematocrit	Hemendra N. Shah 2008	0	0	33	0	1	32
Haematocrit	Hemendra Shah 2009	1	1	454	1	2	386
Haematocrit	Madhu S. Agrawal 2008	0	0	101	0	0	202

5.2   Methods for Continuous Data

First suppose that the objective of a study is to compare two groups, such as Treated (referenced as 1) and Control (referenced as 2), in terms of their means. Let μ_1 and μ_2 be the true (population) means of the two groups. The population MD is defined as

$$\Delta = \mu_1 - \mu_2 \qquad (5.1)$$

and the standardized mean difference (SMD)

$$\delta = \frac{\mu_1 - \mu_2}{\sigma} \qquad (5.2)$$

which is usually used as the effect size.

5.2.1   Estimate the MD Δ

For multiple studies that report outcome measures in the same scales or units, a meta-analysis can be carried out directly on the differences in means and preserve the original scales. In this situation, all calculations are relatively straightforward. For each study, we estimate Δ directly from the reported means as follows. Let $\bar{X}_1$ and $\bar{X}_2$ be the reported sample means of the two groups. Then the estimate of the population MD Δ is the difference in sample means:

$$D = \hat{\Delta} = \bar{X}_1 - \bar{X}_2 \qquad (5.3)$$

For further statistical inference, we need to calculate the standard deviation of D which is easily done from the reported sample standard errors from the study. Let S_1 and S_2, n_1 and n_2 denote the corresponding sample standard errors and sample sizes in the two groups. Then the variance of D can be obtained as:

$$V_D = \frac{S_1^2}{n_1} + \frac{S_2^2}{n_2}, \qquad (5.4)$$

if we do not assume homogeneity of variances for the two groups, i.e., $\sigma_1 \neq \sigma_2$. With the assumption of homogeneity of variance (i.e., $\sigma_1 = \sigma_2 = \sigma$) in the two groups, the variance of D is calculated using the pooled sample variance as:

$$V_D = \frac{n_1 + n_2}{n_1 n_2} S_{pooled}^2, \qquad (5.5)$$

where

$$S_{pooled} = \sqrt{\frac{(n_1 - 1)S_1^2 + (n_2 - 1)S_2^2}{n_1 + n_2 - 2}}. \qquad (5.6)$$

In either case, the standard deviation of D can be obtained by the square root of V_D as:

$$SE_D = \sqrt{V_D}. \qquad (5.7)$$

Meta-analysis would then proceed by combining the differences (Ds) in sample means of the two groups across the individual studies and using the appropriate function of the variances (V_D) for statistical inference.

5.2.2   Estimate the SMD δ

When different measurement scales (e.g., different instruments in different laboratories or different clinical sites) are used in individual studies, it is meaningless to try to combine MDs in the original scales using meta-analysis techniques. In such cases, a meaningful measure to be used for meta-analysis is the SMD δ as suggested by Cohen (1988) as the effect size in statistical power analysis.

Again, denote the population means of two groups by μ_1 and μ_2 and their corresponding variances by σ_1^2 and σ_2^2, respectively. Then the SMD or effect size (ES) δ is defined as the difference between μ_1 and μ_2 divided by their standard deviation which is denoted by

$$\delta = \frac{\mu_1 - \mu_2}{\sigma} \tag{5.8}$$

where σ is the associated standard deviation from either the population control group or a pooled population standard deviation.

To estimate the ES of δ, two commonly proposed measures are as follows. One of the measures is known as Cohen's d (Cohen, 1988) and is given by:

$$d = \frac{\bar{X}_1 - \bar{X}_2}{S} \tag{5.9}$$

where the standardized quantity S is the pooled sample standard error as $S = \sqrt{S^2}$ where

$$S^2 = \frac{(n_1 - 1)S_1^2 + (n_2 - 1)S_2^2}{n_1 + n_2}.$$

The second measure of δ is known as Hedges' g (Hedges, 1982) defined as

$$g = \frac{\bar{X}_1 - \bar{X}_2}{S_*} \tag{5.10}$$

where

$$S_*^2 = \frac{(n_1 - 1)S_1^2 + (n_2 - 1)S_2^2}{n_1 + n_2 - 2}.$$

It is shown in Hedges and Olkin (1985) that

$$E(g) \approx \delta + \frac{3\delta}{4N - 9} \tag{5.11}$$

$$Var(g) \approx \frac{1}{\tilde{n}} + \frac{\delta^2}{2(N - 3.94)} \tag{5.12}$$

where

$$N = n_1 + n_2, \tilde{n} = \frac{n_1 n_2}{n_1 + n_2}$$

With the assumptions of equal variances in both groups and normality of the data, Hedges (1981) showed that $\sqrt{\tilde{n}}g$ follows a noncentral t-distribution with noncentrality parameter $\sqrt{\tilde{n}}\theta$ and $n_1 + n_2 - 2$ degrees of freedom. Based on this conclusion, the exact mean and variance of Hedges' g are given by

$$E(g) = \sqrt{\frac{N-2}{2}} \frac{\Gamma[(N-3)/2]}{\Gamma[(N-2)/2]} \delta \tag{5.13}$$

$$Var(g) = \frac{N-2}{N-4}(1+\delta^2) - \delta^2 \frac{N-2}{2} \frac{\{\Gamma[(N-3)/2]\}^2}{\{\Gamma[(N-2)/2]\}^2} \tag{5.14}$$

where $\Gamma()$ is the gamma function.

It should be noted that g is *biased* as an estimator for the population ES δ. However, this bias can be easily corrected by multiplication with a factor since the exact mean in equation (5.13) is well approximated by equation (5.11) so that an approximately unbiased SMD g^* is given by

$$g^* \approx \left(1 - \frac{3}{4N-9}\right)g = J \times g \tag{5.15}$$

It can be seen that the correction factor J above is always less than 1 which would lead to g^* always being less than g in absolute value. However, J will be very close to 1 when N is large.

We denoted this unbiased estimator as g^* in this book to avoid confusion. Confusion about the notations has resulted since Hedges and Olkin (1985) in their seminal book referred to this unbiased estimator as d – which is not the same as Cohen's d.

With this unbiased form of g^*, the estimated variance is approximated using equation (5.12) as follows:

$$\widehat{Var}(g^*) \approx \frac{1}{\tilde{n}} + \frac{g^{*2}}{2(N-3.94)} \tag{5.16}$$

For statistical inference of ES δ for $H_0 : \delta = 0$ versus $H_1 : \delta \neq 0$ based on Hedges g, the typical standardized normal statistic can be constructed as follows:

$$Z = \frac{\hat{\delta}}{\widehat{Var}(\hat{\delta})} = \frac{g^*}{\widehat{Var}(g^*)} \tag{5.17}$$

where g^* is from equation (5.11) and $\widehat{Var}(g^*)$ is from equation (5.16). H_0 is rejected if $|Z|$ exceeds $z_{\alpha/2}$, the upper $\alpha/2$ cut-off point of the standard normal distribution. A confidence interval for δ can be constructed as

$$1 - \alpha \approx Pr\left[g^* - z_{\alpha/2}\sqrt{\widehat{Var}(g^*)} \leq \delta \leq g^* + z_{\alpha/2}\sqrt{\widehat{Var}(g^*)}\right] \tag{5.18}$$

Note that the Cohen's d in equation (5.9) is proportional to Hedges' g in equation (5.10) as

$$d = \frac{n_1 + n_2}{n_1 + n_2 - 2} g = \frac{n_1 + n_2}{n_1 + n_2 - 2} \frac{g^*}{J}. \tag{5.19}$$

the results from Hedges g can be easily transformed to provide the mean and variance of Cohen's d.

Readers may be aware that there are several slightly different calculations for the variance of g in the literature. We used (5.16) to comply with the R **meta** package. In Borenstein et al. (2009), $2N$, instead of $2(N - 3.94)$, is used at the denominator of the second term of the variance formula (5.16). Another commonly used alternative is $2(N - 2)$. All these calculations are almost identical in practice unless n_1 and n_2 are very small which is usually not the case in meta-analysis.

5.3 Meta-Analysis of the Impact of Intervention

To illustrate the methods in Section 5.2 for continuous data, we make use of the impact of intervention data from Borenstein et al. (2009) as seen in Table 5.1.

The estimation using Δ for the MD as discussed in Section 5.2.1 is straight-forward and is left to interested readers. We illustrate Hedges' method in this section for the SMD as seen in Section 5.2.2 with three approaches with (1) meta-analysis implemented with **meta** to get the readers familiar with continuous data, (2) step-by-step implementation to get the readers familiar with the theoretical methods described in Section 5.2, and (3) meta-analysis implemented with **metafor** for readers to compare results from this the **metafor** package to the **meta** package and the step-by-step implementation. They should be the same!

5.3.1 Load the Data Into R

Let us illustrate the data management from scratch by typing the data into R as follows:

```
> # Type the data
> Carroll = c(94, 22,60,92, 20,60)
> Grant   = c(98, 21,65, 92,22, 65)
> Peck    = c(98, 28, 40,88 ,26, 40)
> Donat   = c( 94,19, 200, 82,17, 200)
> Stewart = c( 98, 21,50, 88,22 , 45)
> Young   = c(96,21,85, 92 ,22, 85)
```

```
> # Make a data frame
> dat.Int = as.data.frame(rbind(Carroll, Grant, Peck,
                          Donat, Stewart,Young))
> colnames(dat.Int) = c("m.t","sd.t","n.t","m.c","sd.c","n.c")
> # Print the data
> dat.Int
```

```
         m.t sd.t n.t m.c sd.c n.c
Carroll   94   22  60  92   20  60
Grant     98   21  65  92   22  65
Peck      98   28  40  88   26  40
Donat     94   19 200  82   17 200
Stewart   98   21  50  88   22  45
Young     96   21  85  92   22  85
```

This reproduces Table 5.1.

5.3.2   Meta-Analysis Using **R** Library meta

We first illustrate the application using R library **meta** with a simple code **metacont**. To do this, we first load the library as:

```
> library(meta)
```

Since the data are continuous, we call the R function **metacont** for this meta-analysis using the build-in summary function (**sm**) of SMD (i.e., SMD) with Hedges' adjusted g. The R code chunk is as follows:

```
> # call the metacont
> mod = metacont(n.t,m.t,sd.t,n.c,m.c,sd.c,
        data=dat.Int,studlab=rownames(dat.Int),sm="SMD")
> # print the meta-analysis
> mod
```

```
             SMD            95%-CI %W(fixed) %W(random)
Carroll   0.0945 [-0.2635; 0.4526]      12.4       15.8
Grant     0.2774 [-0.0681; 0.6229]      13.3       16.3
Peck      0.3665 [-0.0756; 0.8087]       8.1       12.6
Donat     0.6644 [ 0.4630; 0.8658]      39.2       23.3
Stewart   0.4618 [ 0.0535; 0.8701]       9.5       13.8
Young     0.1852 [-0.1161; 0.4865]      17.5       18.3
```

```
Number of studies combined: k = 6
                          SMD            95%-CI     z  p-value
Fixed effect model     0.4150 [0.2889; 0.5410]  6.45 < 0.0001
Random effects model   0.3585 [0.1518; 0.5652]  3.40   0.0007
```

Quantifying heterogeneity:
```
tau^2 = 0.0372 [0.0000; 0.2903]; tau = 0.1930 [0.0000; 0.5388];
I^2 = 58.0% [0.0%; 83.0%]; H = 1.54 [1.00; 2.43]
```

Test of heterogeneity:
```
         Q d.f. p-value
    11.91   5  0.0360
```

Details on meta-analytical method:
- Inverse variance method
- DerSimonian-Laird estimator for tau^2
- Jackson method for confidence interval of tau^2 and tau
- Hedges' g (bias corrected standardised mean difference)

Notice that by changing sm="MD" in the above code chunk, the simple MD Δ in Section 5.2.1 is obtained. We leave this as practice for interested readers (Figure 5.1).

The forest plot can be generated by calling forest as follows:

```
> forest(mod)
```

5.3.3 Step-by-Step Implementation in R

To add to the understanding of the methods in this section, we make use of R to illustrate the step-by-step calculations to check against the output from Section 5.3.2.

The first step in pooling the studies is to calculate the pooled variance or the pooled standard deviation:

```
> # First get the pooled sd to calculate the SMD
> pooled.sd = sqrt(((dat.Int$n.t-1)*dat.Int$sd.t^2
```

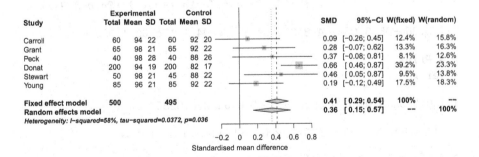

FIGURE 5.1
Forest plot for the continuous data.

```
 +(dat.Int$n.c-1)*dat.Int$sd.c^2)/(dat.Int$n.t+dat.Int$n.c-2))
> # Print the SD
> pooled.sd
```

[1] 21.0 21.5 27.0 18.0 21.5 21.5

With the pooled SD, we then calculate the SMD as:

```
> # The SMD
> g = (dat.Int$m.t-dat.Int$m.c)/pooled.sd; g
```

[1] 0.0951 0.2790 0.3701 0.6656 0.4656 0.1860

Since this SMD is biased, Hedges' correction should be used to adjust for the bias. The correction factor is calculated as follows:

```
> # Hedges correction factor
> N = dat.Int$n.t+dat.Int$n.c; J = 1- 3/(4*N-9)
> # Print the correction factor J
> J
```

[1] 0.994 0.994 0.990 0.998 0.992 0.996

We see that these values are very close to 1. With these correction factors, we adjust the SMD for Hedges' g as follows:

```
> # now the Hedges g*
> gstar = J*g; gstar
```

[1] 0.0945 0.2774 0.3665 0.6644 0.4618 0.1852

The variance for g^* is calculated as follows:

```
> # Variance of SMD
> var.gstar = (dat.Int$n.t+dat.Int$n.c)/(dat.Int$n.t*dat.Int$n.c)
>                    + gstar^2/(2*(dat.Int$n.t+dat.Int$n.c-3.94))
```

[1] 3.85e-05 3.05e-04 8.83e-04 5.57e-04 1.17e-03 1.03e-04

```
> # Print it
> var.gstar
```

[1] 0.0333 0.0308 0.0500 0.0100 0.0422 0.0235

Therefore, the 95% CI for the 6 studies is constructed as:

```
> lowCI.gstar = gstar-1.96*sqrt(var.gstar)
> upCI.gstar  = gstar+1.96*sqrt(var.gstar)
> # Print the CIs and the SMD
> cbind(lowCI.gstar, gstar, upCI.gstar)
```

```
        lowCI.gstar  gstar upCI.gstar
[1,]       -0.2633 0.0945     0.452
[2,]       -0.0665 0.2774     0.621
[3,]       -0.0717 0.3665     0.805
[4,]        0.4684 0.6644     0.860
[5,]        0.0591 0.4618     0.865
[6,]       -0.1155 0.1852     0.486
```

Readers can check these results with the output from R **meta** and should find that they are exactly the same.

To combine the studies with fixed-effects model, we first calculate the weights as:

```
> # The individual weight
> w = 1/var.gstar; w

[1]   30.0  32.5  20.0 100.0  23.7  42.5

> # The total weight
> tot.w = sum(w); tot.w

[1] 249

> # And the relative weight
> rel.w = w/tot.w; rel.w

[1] 0.1206 0.1307 0.0804 0.4021 0.0952 0.1709
```

With these weights, we calculate the meta-estimate as:

```
> # Meta-estimate
> M = sum(rel.w*gstar); M

[1] 0.42
```

The variance and CI for the meta-estimate are computed as follows:

```
> # The variance of M
> var.M = 1/tot.w; var.M

[1] 0.00402

> # The SE
> se.M = sqrt(var.M); se.M

[1] 0.0634

> # The lower 95% CI bound
> lowCI.M = M-1.96*se.M; lowCI.M
```

[1] 0.296

```
> # The upper 95% CI bound
> upCI.M = M+1.96*se.M; upCI.M
```

[1] 0.544

The 95% CI does not cover zero, and we conclude that the pooled effect is statistically significant. We calculate the z-value and the associated p-value as follows:

```
> # Compute z
> z = M/se.M; z
```

[1] 6.62

```
> # Compute p-value
> pval = 2*(1-pnorm(abs(z))); pval
```

[1] 3.54e-11

The result is statistically significant as noted from the p-value and confirms the conclusion from the 95% CI.

For meta-analysis using the random-effects model, we calculate the estimate for τ^2 from the Q-statistic as follows:

```
> # The Q statistic
> Q = sum(w*gstar^2)-(sum(w*gstar))^2/tot.w; Q
```

[1] 12.3

```
> # The degrees of freedom from 6 studies
> df= 6-1
> # C quantity
> C = tot.w - sum(w^2)/tot.w; C
```

[1] 189

```
> # The tau-square estimate
> tau2 = (Q-df)/C; tau2
```

[1] 0.0383

With this estimate, we then calculate the weightings in the random-effects model as follows:

```
> # Now compute the weights incorporating heterogeneity
> wR = 1/(var.gstar+tau2); wR
```

```
[1] 14.0 14.5 11.3 20.7 12.4 16.2

> # The total weight
> tot.wR = sum(wR); tot.wR

[1] 89.1

> # The relative weight
> rel.wR = wR/tot.wR; rel.wR

[1] 0.157 0.163 0.127 0.232 0.139 0.182
```

Then we calculate the random-effects meta-estimate, its variance, and 95% CI as follows:

```
> # The meta-estimate
> MR = sum(rel.wR*gstar); MR

[1] 0.359

> # The variance of MR
> var.MR = 1/tot.wR; var.MR

[1] 0.0112

> # The SE of MR
> se.MR = sqrt(var.MR); se.MR

[1] 0.106

> # The lower bound of 95% CI
> lowCI.MR = MR - 1.96*se.MR; lowCI.MR

[1] 0.151

> # The upper 95% CI
> upCI.MR = MR + 1.96*se.MR; upCI.MR

[1] 0.567

> # The z value
> zR = MR/se.MR; zR

[1] 3.39

> # The p-value
> pval.R = 2*(1-pnorm(abs(zR))); pval.R

[1] 0.000703
```

The summary table for the Hedges' estimate and weightings can be printed as:

```
> # The summary table
> sumTab = data.frame(SMD=round(gstar,4),
        lowCI= round(lowCI.gstar,4),
        upperCI=round(upCI.gstar,4),
        pctW.fixed = round(rel.w*100,2),
        pctW.random= round(rel.wR*100,2))
> rownames(sumTab) = rownames(dat.Int)
> # Print it
> sumTab
```

	SMD	lowCI	upperCI	pctW.fixed	pctW.random
Carroll	0.0945	-0.2633	0.452	12.06	15.7
Grant	0.2774	-0.0665	0.621	13.07	16.3
Peck	0.3665	-0.0717	0.805	8.04	12.7
Donat	0.6644	0.4684	0.860	40.21	23.2
Stewart	0.4618	0.0591	0.865	9.52	13.9
Young	0.1852	-0.1155	0.486	17.09	18.2

Interested readers should see now that all results from Section 5.3.2 using R library meta are reproduced.

5.3.4   Meta-Analysis Using R Library metafor

To further assure that same results can be produced by different R packages, we further illustrate the meta-analysis of this data with the metafor package.

To use this package, we first load the package into R as follows:

```
> library(metafor)
```

We then calculate the standardized mean-difference, i.e., ES, for all studies by calling the R function of escalc as follows:

```
> # Call escalc to calculate ES
> ES.Int = escalc(measure="SMD",
                n1i=n.t,m1i=m.t,sd1i=sd.t,
                n2i=n.c,m2i=m.c,sd2i=sd.c,
                data=dat.Int,slab=rownames(dat.Int) )
> # Print the ES
> ES.Int
```

	m.t	sd.t	n.t	m.c	sd.c	n.c	yi	vi
Carroll	94	22	60	92	20	60	0.0945	0.0334
Grant	98	21	65	92	22	65	0.2774	0.0311
Peck	98	28	40	88	26	40	0.3665	0.0508

```
Donat     94   19 200   82    17 200 0.6644 0.0106
Stewart   98   21  50   88    22  45 0.4618 0.0433
Young     96   21  85   92    22  85 0.1852 0.0236
```

Notice that in the dataframe ES.Int above, the column yi is the calculated standardized mean-difference and the column vi is the corresponding within-study sampling variance. With the ESs, we can then perform meta-analysis. The fixed-effects meta-analysis is implemented as follows:

```
> # Call rma to perform FE-MA
> metafor.FE.Int = rma(yi, vi, data=ES.Int, method="FE")
> # Print the summary of FE-MA
> metafor.FE.Int

Fixed-Effects Model (k = 6)
I^2 (total heterogeneity / total variability):   58.03%
H^2 (total variability / sampling variability):  2.38

Test for Heterogeneity: Q(df = 5) = 11.9138, p-val = 0.0360

Model Results:
estimate      se     zval     pval    ci.lb    ci.ub
  0.4150  0.0643   6.4557   <.0001   0.2890   0.5410  ***
```

Similar implementation can be done for DL random-effects meta-analysis as follows:

```
> # Call rma for DL RE-MA
> metafor.RE.Int = rma(yi, vi, data=ES.Int, method="DL")
> # Print the summary of RE-MA
> metafor.RE.Int

Random-Effects Model (k = 6; tau^2 estimator: DL)

tau^2 (estimated amount of total heterogeneity):0.0372(SE=0.0421)
tau (square root of estimated tau^2 value):       0.1930
I^2 (total heterogeneity / total variability):   58.03%
H^2 (total variability / sampling variability): 2.38

Test for Heterogeneity: Q(df = 5) = 11.9138, p-val = 0.0360

Model Results:
estimate      se     zval     pval    ci.lb    ci.ub
  0.3585  0.1055   3.3996   0.0007   0.1518   0.5652  ***
```

Interested readers can check these results with the meta-analysis results from the meta and the step-by-step implementation. The results are the same!

5.4 Meta-Analysis of Tubeless vs Standard PCNL

As seen from Section 5.1.2, the PCNL data are loaded into R from the external excel file `dat4Meta` and named as `dat` as seen from Table 5.2.

5.4.1 Comparison of Operation Duration

To compare the operation duration for tubeless PCNL and standard PCNL, six of the seven studies were selected for this outcome measure. The authors used MD Δ for their meta-analysis. This analysis can be reproduced using the following R code chunk:

```
> # Call metacont for meta analysis
> duration = metacont(n.E,Mean.E, SD.E, n.C, Mean.C, SD.C,
          studlab=Study, data=dat[dat$Outcome=="duration",],
          sm="MD", label.e="Tubeless", label.c="Standard")
> # Print the analysis
> duration
```

```
                            MD            95%-CI %W(fixed)%W(random)
Ahmet Tefekli2007   -16.7000[-23.0626;-10.3374]   16.5       17.7
B.Lojanapiwat2010    -8.2300[-16.8816;  0.4216]    8.9       16.0
Hemendra N.Shah 2008  3.6400[ -2.9698; 10.2498]   15.3       17.5
Hemendra Shah2009   -16.0000[-19.9736;-12.0264]   42.3       19.1
J. Jun-Ou 2010      -11.4700[-18.5960; -4.3440]   13.2       17.1
Michael Choi 2006     9.1400[ -4.1380; 22.4180]    3.8       12.5


                            MD          95%-CI      z  p-value
Fixed effect model  -10.8689[-13.4539; -8.2839] -8.24  <0.0001
Random effects model -7.5130[-15.1555;  0.1295] -1.93   0.0540

Quantifying heterogeneity:
 tau^2=75.4491[24.2384;604.8121]; tau=8.6861[4.9233;24.5929];
 I^2 = 86.6% [73.0%; 93.3%]; H = 2.73 [1.92; 3.87]
Test of heterogeneity:    Q d.f.  p-value
                      37.25     5 < 0.0001
```

This reproduces all the results. These studies demonstrate statistically significant heterogeneity with $Q = 37.25$ and $d.f. = 5$, which gives a p-value < 0.0001. The authors thus used the random-effects model. From the random-effects model, the estimated MD $= -7.51$ and the 95% CI is ($-$15.2, 0.13) which covers zero indicating a nonstatistically significant difference between tubeless PCNL and standard PCNL in terms of operation duration. The z-statistic is -1.93 with p-value of 0.054 again indicating statistical nonsignificance at the 5% significance level (Figure 5.2).

Figure 1 in the paper can be produced simply using `forest` from the `meta` package as follows:

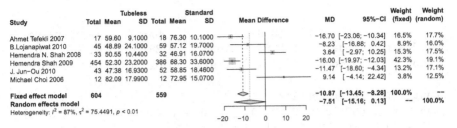

FIGURE 5.2
Forest plot for operation duration.

```
> forest(duration)
```

We are compelled to inject a word of caution concerning the conclusion from this meta-analysis. Among the six studies, three of them (i.e., Ahmet Tefekli 2007, Hemendra Shah 2009, J. Jun-Ou 2010) in fact yielded statistically significant results. In view of this and the fact that the random-effects meta-model yielded a p-value of 0.054 which is marginally statistically insignificant, the weight of evidence does not strongly support lack of a real difference between the two interventions in terms of operation duration. In fact, if the SMD using Hedges' g is used for meta-analysis, a statistically significant result is revealed as the estimated SMD $= -0.410$ with 95% CI of $(-0.798, -0.0229)$ and the z-statistic of -2.08 with p-value of 0.0379. The corresponding R code chunk is as follows:

```
> # Call metacont for meta analysis with SMD
> SMD.duration = metacont(n.E,Mean.E, SD.E, n.C, Mean.C, SD.C,
          studlab=Study, data=dat[dat$Outcome=="duration",],
          sm="SMD", label.e="Tubeless", label.c="Standard")
> # Print the analysis
> SMD.duration
```

```
                         SMD              95%-CI
Ahmet Tefekli 2007    -1.6948 [-2.4803; -0.9093]
B.Lojanapiwat 2010    -0.3763 [-0.7677;  0.0151]
Hemendra N. Shah 2008  0.2663 [-0.2223;  0.7548]
Hemendra Shah 2009    -0.5618 [-0.7001; -0.4235]
J. Jun-Ou 2010        -0.6397 [-1.0542; -0.2252]
Michael Choi 2006      0.5318 [-0.2851;  1.3487]
                      %W(fixed) %W(random)
Ahmet Tefekli 2007        2.3       11.9
B.Lojanapiwat 2010        9.1       18.8
Hemendra N. Shah 2008     5.8       17.0
Hemendra Shah 2009       72.7       22.6
J. Jun-Ou 2010            8.1       18.4
```

```
Michael Choi 2006              2.1        11.4
                           SMD            95%-CI      z  p-value
Fixed effect model    -0.5058 [-0.6237; -0.3878] -8.41 < 0.0001
Random effects model  -0.4104 [-0.7979; -0.0229] -2.08   0.0379

Quantifying heterogeneity:
 tau^2 = 0.1682 [0.0792; 2.2991]; tau = 0.4102 [0.2814; 1.5163];
 I^2 = 80.8% [58.7%; 91.1%]; H = 2.28 [1.56; 3.35]

Test of heterogeneity:
          Q d.f.  p-value
       26.04    5 < 0.0001
```

5.4.2   Comparison of Length of Hospital Stay

To compare the length of hospital stay between tubeless PCNL and tube PCNL, all seven studies are used. The meta-analysis can be performed using the following R code chunk:

```
> LOS = metacont(n.E,Mean.E, SD.E, n.C, Mean.C, SD.C,
               studlab=Study, data=dat[dat$Outcome=="LOS",],
               sm="MD", label.e="Tubeless", label.c="Standard")
> # Print the analysis
> LOS
```

```
                            MD                95%-CI
Ahmet Tefekli 2007      -28.8000 [-39.7725; -17.8275]
B.Lojanapiwat 2010      -44.6400 [-60.1162; -29.1638]
Hemendra N. Shah 2008    -9.0800 [-17.4691;  -0.6909]
Hemendra Shah 2009      -22.7000 [-29.0671; -16.3329]
J. Jun-Ou 2010          -23.9200 [-35.7828; -12.0572]
Madhu S. Agrawal 2008   -32.4000 [-33.6367; -31.1633]
Michael Choi 2006        -1.2000 [-20.3927;  17.9927]
                       %W(fixed) %W(random)
Ahmet Tefekli 2007          1.2        14.2
B.Lojanapiwat 2010          0.6        11.5
Hemendra N. Shah 2008       2.0        15.7
Hemendra Shah 2009          3.4        16.8
J. Jun-Ou 2010              1.0        13.6
Madhu S. Agrawal 2008      91.4        18.5
Michael Choi 2006           0.4         9.5

Number of studies combined: k = 7

                          MD              95%-CI       z p-value
Fixed effect model  -31.4289[-32.6115;-30.2463] -52.09       0
```

```
Random effects model-23.8569[-32.3533;-15.3605]   -5.50 <0.0001

Quantifying heterogeneity:
 tau^2 = 101.0369 [33.3714; 803.0417];
  tau = 10.0517 [5.7768; 28.3380];
  I^2 = 88.2% [78.1%; 93.7%];
   H = 2.91 [2.14; 3.97]

Test of heterogeneity:
    Q d.f.  p-value
 50.94    6 < 0.0001
```

Similar to the authors, we use the "MD" for this meta-analysis. It can be seen that the test of heterogeneity yields $Q = 50.94$ with $df = 6$ resulting in a p-value < 0.001 from χ^2-test. This indicates statistically significant heterogeneity which leads to the random-effects model. Using the random-effects model, the combined MD is $MD = -23.86$ hours with 95% of $(-32.35, -15.36)$ which is statistically significant with p-value < 0.0001. This indicates that the mean length of hospital stay for the tubeless PCNL group was statistically significantly shorter than that for standard the PCNL group by an estimate of 23.86 hours (Figure 5.3).

Figure 2 in the paper can be reproduced simply by using `forest` from the `meta` package as follows:

```
> forest(LOS)
```

We note that the results from this analysis match the results from the authors' Figure 2. We note that there is an obvious typo from the 95% CI reported in the paper as $(-39.77, -17.83)$ which is different from their Figure 2 as well as from the results of our analysis.

The same conclusion may be produced using Hedges' g, and we leave this analysis to interested readers.

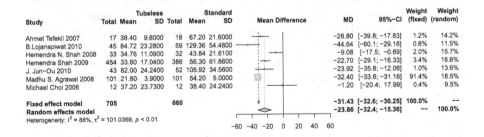

FIGURE 5.3
Forest plot for the length of hospital stay.

5.4.3   Comparison of Postoperative Analgesic Requirement

We now compare the tubeless and standard PCNL groups in terms of postoperative analgesic requirement (diclofenac sodium or morphine). As discussed in the chapter, the authors selected five of the seven studies for this meta-analysis based on the available data. The meta-analysis is implemented in R with code chunk as follows:

```
> analgesic = metacont(n.E,Mean.E, SD.E, n.C, Mean.C, SD.C,
        studlab=Study, data=dat[dat$Outcome=="analgesic",],
        sm="MD", label.e="Tubeless", label.c="Standard")
> # Print the summary
> analgesic
```

```
                          MD          95%-CI %W(fixed) %W(random)
B.Lojanapiwat 2010   -36.0000[ -49.0861; -22.9139]   19.2       21.7
Hemendra N.Shah 2008 -96.0900[-162.9421; -29.2379]    0.7       13.4
Hemendra Shah 2009  -147.2000[-164.1294;-130.2706]   11.5       21.3
J. Jun-Ou 2010       -33.0000[ -46.4756; -19.5244]   18.1       21.6
Madhu S.Agrawal 2008 -44.8000[ -52.8626; -36.7374]   50.5       22.0
```

```
                          MD           95%-CI      z p-value
Fixed effect model   -53.0909 [ -58.8222; -47.3595] -18.16 <0.0001
Random effects model -69.0160 [-107.6687; -30.3633]  -3.50  0.0005
```

```
Quantifying heterogeneity:
 tau^2 = 1749.7704 [681.0863; >21743.1624];
   tau = 41.8303 [26.0976; >147.4556];
   I^2 = 97.1% [95.3%; 98.3%];
     H = 5.90 [4.61; 7.56]
```

```
Test of heterogeneity:
     Q d.f.  p-value
 139.45    4 < 0.0001
```

We note from the analysis that the test of heterogeneity is statistically significant with p-value < 0.0001 ($Q = 139.45$, $df = 4$), and the random-effects model showed that the mean analgesic requirement for the tubeless PCNL was statistically significantly lower than that from the standard PCNL with a combined MD of 69.02 mg, postoperative analgesic requirement p-value < 0.05 and associated 95% CI of $(-107.67, -30.36)$.

Interested readers are encouraged to reproduce the **forest** plot for this analysis as well as the meta-analysis using Hedges g for SMD modifying the corresponding R code.

5.4.4   Comparison of Postoperative Hematocrit Change

To compare the two PCNL groups in terms of postoperative hematocrit changes, the authors selected four of the seven studies based on the available data for their meta-analysis using the "MD." The implementation in R is as follows:

```
> hematocrit = metacont(n.E,Mean.E, SD.E, n.C, Mean.C, SD.C,
        studlab=Study,data=dat[dat$Outcome=="haematocrit",],
        sm="MD", label.e="Tubeless", label.c="Standard")
> # Print the summary
> hematocrit
```

	MD	95%-CI	%W(fixed)	%W(random)
Ahmet Tefekli 2007	0.4000[0.1002;0.6998]		2.1	18.5
Hemendra N. Shah 2008	-0.0600[-0.4658;0.3458]		1.1	12.7
Hemendra Shah 2009	-0.1500[-0.3281;0.0281]		5.9	28.7
Madhu S. Agrawal 2008	-0.0300[-0.0755;0.0155]		90.8	40.1

	MD	95%-CI	z	p-value
Fixed effect model	-0.0285	[-0.0718; 0.0149]	-1.29	0.1984
Random effects model	0.0113	[-0.1625; 0.1851]	0.13	0.8988

```
Quantifying heterogeneity:
 tau^2 = 0.0191 [0.0000; 0.6190]; tau = 0.1382 [0.0000; 0.7868];
 I^2 = 68.9% [10.3%; 89.3%]; H = 1.79 [1.06; 3.05]

Test of heterogeneity:
    Q d.f. p-value
 9.66   3  0.0217
```

From the analysis, there is statistically significant heterogeneity among the 4 studies with p-value = 0.0217 ($Q = 9.66$, df = 3). With the random-effects model, the results showed that the difference in the hematocrit change between the tubeless group and the standard PCNL group was not statistically significant (p-value = 0.8988); the combined MD $MD = 0.0113$ with a 95% CI of $(-0.1625, 0.1851)$.

5.4.5   Conclusions and Discussion

We reanalyzed the data from Wang et al. (2011) to compare tubeless vs standard PCNL using the R package `meta` and reproduced the results from the paper.

This analysis demonstrated that tubeless PCNL is a good option to standard PCNL with the advantages of significantly reduced hospital stay and less need for postoperative analgesia. The analysis also showed that there was no significant difference between the groups in terms of hematocrit change after surgery. The authors concluded that there was no difference in operation duration based on the MD with a very marginally statistically insignificant p-value of 0.054. We reanalyzed the data using the Hedges' g using the SMD and revealed a statistically significant difference of -0.4104 with p-value of 0.0379.

For this reanalysis, we made use of the `meta` package, the meta-analysis using `metafor` can be similarly implemented, and we leave this as an exercise to interested readers.

5.5 Discussion

In this chapter, we illustrated meta-analysis methods for endpoints or summary statistics of continuous data arising in clinical trials and other studies. Two commonly used methods were described based on synthesizing the MD and Hedges' SMD g. Two data sets were used to illustrate the meta-analysis using R. More specifically, we used the first meta-data to show detailed step-by-step implementation of these methods in comparison with the meta-analysis with R packages `meta` and `metafor`. The second data were meta-analyzed by `meta`, and we left the analysis using `metafor` to interested readers due to its easy implementation.

The first data set reflecting the impact of some intervention on reading scores in children from Borenstein et al. (2009) was used to illustrate the methods with step-by-step implementation in R in comparison with the R packages `meta` and `metafor` so that readers may understand the methods in depth. The second data set from Wang et al. (2011) provided endpoints reflecting a set of seven studies that compared the effects of tubeless vs standard PCNL on several continuous measures. We illustrated meta-analyses of this data set using the R package `meta` to reproduce the results from this paper.

Appendix: Stata Programs for Meta-Analysis for Continuous Data by Manyun Liu

The `Stata` program below corresponds to the R program.

```
/*### Reproduce R Results in Section 5.1.2 ###*/
/* You can use the following command to load the excel file */
cd "your file path"
import excel using dat4Meta.xls,sheet("Data_tubeless")
 firstrow clear
list

/*### Reproduce R Results in Section 5.3.1 ###*/
/*  Type the data */
```

```
clear
input str10 name m_t sd_t n_t m_c sd_c n_c
Carroll 94 22 60 92 20 60
Grant 98 21 65 92 22 65
Peck 98 28 40 88 26 40
Donat  94 19 200 82 17 200
Stewart  98 21 50, 88 22 45
Young 96 21 85 92 22 85
end
/*  List the data */
list

/*### Reproduce R Results in Section 5.3.2 ###*/
ssc install metan

/* For the fixed-effects model. */
metan n_t m_t sd_t n_c m_c sd_c,label(namevar=name) fixed hedges
/* For the random-effects model. */
metan n_t m_t sd_t n_c m_c sd_c,label(namevar=name) random
    hedges

/*### Reproduce R Results in Section 5.3.3 ###*/
/* First get the pooled sd to calculate the SMD */
generate pooled_sd = sqrt(((n_t-1)*sd_t^2+
      (n_c-1)*sd_c^2)/(n_t+n_c-2))
/*  Print the SD */
list pooled_sd

/*  The standardized mean difference(SMD) */
generate g = (m_t-m_c)/pooled_sd
/*  Print the SMD */
list g
/*  Hedges correction factor */
generate N = n_t+n_c
generate J = 1- 3/(4*N-9)
/* Print the correction factor J */
list J
/*  now the Hedges g*  */
generate gstar = J*g
/*  Print it */
list gstar
/*  Variance of SMD */
generate var_gstar = (n_t+n_c)/(n_t*n_c)
      + gstar^2/(2*(n_t+n_c-3.94))
/*  Print it */
```

```
list var_gstar

generat lowCI_gstar = gstar-1.96*sqrt(var_gstar)
generate upCI_gstar = gstar+1.96*sqrt(var_gstar)

/*  Print the CIs and the SMD */
list lowCI_gstar gstar upCI_gstar

/*  The individual weight */
generate w = 1/var_gstar
list w

/*   The total weight */
egen tot_w = total(w)
display tot_w

/*  And the relative weight */
generate rel_w = w/tot_w
list rel_w

/*   Meta-estimate */
egen M = total(rel_w*gstar)
display M

/*  The variance of M */
generate var_M = 1/tot_w
display var_M

/*  The SE */
generate se_M = sqrt(var_M)
display se_M

/*  The lower 95% CI bound */
generate lowCI_M = M-1.96*se_M
display lowCI_M

/*  The upper 95% CI bound */
generate upCI_M = M+1.96*se_M
display upCI_M

/* Compute z */
generate z = M/se_M
display z

/* Compute p-value */
```

```
generate pval = 2*(1-normal(abs(z)))
display pval

/* The Q statistic */
egen Q1=total(w*gstar^2)
egen Q2=total(w*gstar)
generate Q = Q1-Q2^2/tot_w
display Q

/* The degrees of freedom from 6 studies */
generate df= 6-1

/* C quantity */
egen C1=total(w^2)
generate C = tot_w - C1/tot_w
display C

/* The tau-square estimate */
generate tau2 = (Q-df)/C
display tau2

/* Now compute the weights incorporating heterogeneity */
generate wR = 1/(var_gstar+tau2)
list wR

/* The total weight */
egen tot_wR = total(wR)
display tot_wR

/* The relative weight */
generate rel_wR = wR/tot_wR
list rel_wR

/* The meta-estimate */
egen MR = total(rel_wR*gstar)
display MR

/* The variance of MR */
generate var_MR = 1/tot_wR
display var_MR

/* The SE of MR */
generate se_MR = sqrt(var_MR)
display se_MR
```

```
/* The lower bound of 95% CI */
generate lowCI_MR = MR - 1.96*se_MR
display lowCI_MR

/* The upper 95% CI */
generate upCI_MR = MR + 1.96*se_MR
display upCI_MR

/* The z value */
generate zR = MR/se_MR
display zR

/* The p-value */
generate pval_R = 2*(1-normal(abs(zR)))
display pval_R

/* Print the summary table */
generate SMD=round(gstar,0.0001)
generate lowCI=round(lowCI_gstar,0.0001)
generate upperCI=round(upCI_gstar,0.0001)
generate pctW_fixed=round(rel_w*100,0.01)
generate pctW_random=round(rel_wR*100,0.01)
list name SMD lowCI upperCI pctW_fixed pctW_random

/*### Reproduce R Results in Section 5.3.4 ###*/
/* These parts are specific to R, which utilize
alternative metafor and rmeta to produce MA.
We utilize Stata code to produce similar results. */
/* For the fixed-effects model. */
meta esize n_t m_t sd_t n_c m_c sd_c, fixed
list name _meta_es _meta_se
meta summarize, fixed(invvariance)
/* For the random-effects model. */
 meta esize n_t m_t sd_t n_c m_c sd_c, random(dlaird)
meta summarize, random(dlaird)

/*### Reproduce R Results in Section 5.4 ###*/
import excel using dat4Meta.xls,sheet("Data_tubeless")
     firstrow clear
/*  present the data */
browse

/*### Reproduce R Results in Section 5.4.1 ###*/
keep if Outcome=="duration"
/* For the fixed model. */
```

```
metan nE MeanE SDE nC MeanC SDC, label(namevar=Study)
            fixed nostandard
/* For the random model. */
metan nE MeanE SDE nC MeanC SDC, label(namevar=Study)
            random nostandard
/* For the fixed-effects model. */
 metan nE MeanE SDE nC MeanC SDC, label(namevar=Study)
            fixed hedges
/* For the random-effects model. */
metan nE MeanE SDE nC MeanC SDC, label(namevar=Study)
            random hedges


/*### Reproduce R Results in Section 5.4.2 ###*/
import excel using dat4Meta.xls, sheet("Data_tubeless")
            firstrow clear
keep if Outcome=="LOS"
/* For the fixed-effects model. */
metan nE MeanE SDE nC MeanC SDC, label(namevar=Study)
            fixed nostandard
/* For the random-effects model. */
metan nE MeanE SDE nC MeanC SDC, label(namevar=Study)
            random nostandard


/*### Reproduce R Results in Section 5.4.3 ###*/
import excel using dat4Meta.xls, sheet("Data_tubeless")
            firstrow clear
keep if Outcome=="analgesic"
/* For the fixed model. */
metan nE MeanE SDE nC MeanC SDC, label(namevar=Study)
            fixed nostandard
/* For the random model. */
metan nE MeanE SDE nC MeanC SDC, label(namevar=Study)
            random nostandard


/*### Reproduce R Results in Section 5.4.4 ###*/
import excel using dat4Meta.xls, sheet("Data_tubeless")
            firstrow clear
keep if Outcome=="haematocrit"
/* For the fixed-effects model. */
metan nE MeanE SDE nC MeanC SDC, label(namevar=Study)
            fixed nostandard
/* For the random-effects model. */
metan nE MeanE SDE nC MeanC SDC, label(namevar=Study)
            random nostandard
```

6

Heterogeneity in Meta-Analysis

So far we have illustrated all the concepts in the output from meta-analysis using R except heterogeneity measures. Discerning readers may have noticed that whenever we called `metabin` or `metacont` from R package `meta`, and `rma` from the `metafor` package for meta-analysis as seen in Chapters 4 and 5, two other items appeared in the output as `Quantifying Heterogeneity` and `Test of heterogeneity`. We are using this chapter to discuss these heterogeneity measures in detail.

In Section 3.2.3 for the random-effects meta-analysis model, we briefly introduced a quantity Q to be used to estimate the between-study variance τ^2; i.e., Q is a measure of heterogeneity. In this chapter, we will go much further to discuss this measure, used for `Test of heterogeneity` in Section 6.1 along with other heterogeneity measures τ^2, H and I^2 from R output `Quantifying Heterogeneity` in Section 6.2. To enhance the understanding of these heterogeneity measures, we will use the Cochrane Collaboration Logo data to illustrate how to calculate these measures for Binomial data in Section 6.3 and percutaneous nephrolithotomy (PCNL) meta-data for continuous data in Section 6.4. These illustrations will be implemented in a step-by-step fashion to compare with the results in R packages `meta` and `metafor`. Discussion appears in Section 6.5.

Note to readers: You need to install R packages `readxl` to read in the excel data file, and `meta` and `metafor` to perform the meta-analysis.

6.1 Heterogeneity Quantity Q and the `Test of heterogeneity`

Introduced in Section 3.2.3, Q is used to quantify the heterogeneity across all studies and included both the true effect sizes and the random errors from the random-effects model of (3.11). As seen in Section 3.2.3, Q is defined as follows:

$$Q = \sum_{i=1}^{K} w_i(\hat{\delta}_i - \hat{\delta})^2 \tag{6.1}$$

where w_i is the weight from the ith study, $\hat{\delta}_i$ is the ith study effect size, and $\hat{\delta}$ is the summary effect. It can be seen that Q is calculated as follows: (1) compute the deviations of each effect size from the meta-estimate and square them (i.e., $(\hat{\delta}_i - \hat{\delta})^2$), (2) weight these values by the inverse-variance for each study, and (3) then sum these values across all K studies to produce a weighted sum of squares (WSS) to obtain the heterogeneity measure Q.

From equation (3.25), we have shown that the expected value of Q (i.e., (DerSimonian and Laird, 1986)) is:

$$E(Q) = (K - 1) + \tau^2 \left[\sum_{i=1}^{K} w_i - \frac{\sum_{i=1}^{K} w_i^2}{\sum_{i=1}^{K} w_i} \right] \qquad (6.2)$$

Under the assumption of no heterogeneity (all studies have the same effect size), then τ^2 would be zero and $E(Q) = df = K - 1$.

Based on this heterogeneity measure Q, the `Test of heterogeneity` is conducted and addresses the null hypothesis that the effect sizes δ_i from all studies share a common effect size δ (i.e., the assumption of homogeneity) and then test this hypothesis where the test statistic is constructed using Q as a central χ^2 distribution with degrees of freedom of $df = K - 1$ as defined by Cochran (1952, 1954). Under this testing procedure, the associated p-value for the calculated Q is reported in the R output to test for the existence of heterogeneity. The typical significance level for this test is α at 0.05. If the p-value is less than α, we reject the null hypothesis and conclude heterogeneity that all the studies do not share a common effect size.

The reader should be cautioned that there is a disadvantage of the χ^2-test using the Q-statistic; i.e., it has poor statistical power to detect true heterogeneity for a meta-analysis with a small number of studies, but excessive power to detect negligible variability with a large number of studies – as discussed in Harwell (1997) and Hardy and Thompson (1998). Thus, a nonsignificant Q-test from a small number of studies can lead to an erroneous selection of a fixed-effects model when there is possible true heterogeneity among the studies, and vice versa. The inability to conclude statistically significant heterogeneity in a meta-analysis of a small number of studies at the 0.05 level of significance is similar to failing to detect statistically significant treatment-by-center interaction in a multicenter clinical trial. In these settings, many analysts will conduct the test of homogeneity at the 0.10 level, as a means of increasing power of the test.

6.2   Quantifying Heterogeneity

We used the Q-statistic to test the existence of heterogeneity in the above section and report the p-value for the test. However, this test only informs us about the presence versus the absence of heterogeneity, but it does not report the extent of such heterogeneity. We will discuss other measures of the "extent" and magnitude of this heterogeneity using the Q-statistic and quantify heterogeneity of the true dispersion among the studies. As seen from the R output, several heterogeneity indices, τ^2, H and I^2, are commonly used to describe and report the magnitude of the dispersion of true effect sizes.

6.2.1 The τ^2 Index

The τ^2 index is defined as the variance of the true effect sizes as seen in the random-effects model (3.11). Since it is impossible to observe the true effect sizes, we cannot calculate this variance directly, but we can estimate it from the observed data using equation (6.1) as follows:

$$\hat{\tau}^2 = \frac{Q - (K-1)}{U} \tag{6.3}$$

which is the well-known DerSimonian-Laird method of moments for τ^2 in equation (3.18) and U is defined in equation (3.20). Since the true variance τ^2 can never be less than zero even though the estimated variance $\hat{\tau}^2$ can sometimes be due to the sampling error leading to $Q < df = K - 1$. When this happens, the estimated $\hat{\tau}^2$ is set to zero.

As used in the random-effects model, the τ^2 index is also an estimate for the between-studies variance in the meta-analysis of the true effects.

6.2.2 The H Index

Another index or measure of heterogeneity is the H, proposed in Higgins and Thompson (2002), and is defined as follows:

$$H = \sqrt{\frac{Q}{K-1}} \tag{6.4}$$

This index is based on the fact that $E[Q] = K - 1$ when there is no heterogeneity. In this case, H should be 1.

The confidence interval (CI) for the H index is derived in Higgins and Thompson (2002) based on the assumption that the natural logarithm of $\ln(H)$ follows a standard normal distribution. Accordingly,

$$LL_H = \exp\left\{\ln(H) - |z_{\alpha/2}| \times SE\left[\ln(H)\right]\right\} \tag{6.5}$$

$$UL_H = \exp\left\{\ln(H) + |z_{\alpha/2}| \times SE\left[\ln(H)\right]\right\} \tag{6.6}$$

where LL and UL denote the lower and upper limits of the CI, $z_{\alpha/2}$ is the $\alpha/2$-quantile of the standard normal distribution, and $SE[\ln(H)]$ is the standard error of $\ln(H)$ and is estimated by

$$SE\left[\ln(H)\right] = \begin{cases} \dfrac{1}{2}\dfrac{\ln(Q)-\ln(K-1)}{\sqrt{2Q}-\sqrt{2K-3}} & \text{if } Q > K \\[4mm] \sqrt{\dfrac{1}{2(K-2)}\left(1-\dfrac{1}{3(K-2)^2}\right)} & \text{if } Q \le K \end{cases} \qquad (6.7)$$

Since $E(Q) \approx K - 1$ as seen in equation (6.2), the H index should be greater than 1 to measure the relative magnitude of heterogeneity among all the studies. If the lower limit of this interval is greater than 1, the H is statistically significant and the `Test of heterogeneity` should also be significant.

6.2.3   The I^2 Index

To measure the proportion of observed heterogeneity from the real hetero-geneity, Higgins and Thompson (2002) and Higgins et al. (2003) proposed the I^2 index as follows:

$$I^2 = \left(\frac{Q-(K-1)}{Q}\right) \times 100\%, \qquad (6.8)$$

which again represents the ratio of excess dispersion to total dispersion and is similar to the well-known R^2 in classical regression which represents the proportion of the total variance that can be explained by the regression variables.

As suggested from Higgins et al. (2003), a value of the I^2 index around 25%, 50%, and 75% could be considered as *low-, moderate-,* and *high*-heterogeneity, respectively. As noted in their article, about half of the meta-analyses of clin-ical trials in the *Cochrane Database of Systematic Reviews* reported an I^2 index of zero and the rest reported evenly distributed I^2 indices between 0% and 100%.

Mathematically, the I^2 index can be represented using the H index as follows:

$$I^2 = \frac{H^2-1}{H^2} \times 100\% \qquad (6.9)$$

This expression allows us to use the results from the H index to give a CI for the I^2 index using the expressions in equations (6.5) and (6.6) as follows:

$$LL_{I^2} = \left[\frac{\left(LL_H\right)^2-1}{\left(LL_H\right)^2}\right] \times 100\%$$

$$UL_{I^2} = \left[\frac{\left(UL_H\right)^2-1}{\left(UL_H\right)^2}\right] \times 100\%$$

Since I^2 represents the percentage, any of these limits which is computed as negative is set to zero. In the case that the lower limit of I^2 is greater than zero, then the I^2 is regarded as statistically significant and the `Test of heterogeneity` should also be significant.

6.3 Illustration with Cochrane Collaboration Logo Data – Binomial Data

For further understanding of these heterogeneity measures, we reuse the Cochrane Collaboration Logo data from Chapter 3 as a binomial data to illustrate the step-by-step calculations to obtain these measures. We expect that readers should have deeper mastery of these concepts if they can go with these detailed calculations.

6.3.1 Cochrane Collaboration Logo Data

The data from Table 3.1 can be accessed from the R library **rmeta** as follows:

```
> # Load the rmeta
> library(rmeta)
> # load the data
> data(cochrane)
```

This is a binary data set and we only illustrate the step-by-step implementation in R for the risk-ratio (RR). The computations using the risk difference and odds-ratio can be easily done following the code in this chapter and is left for interested readers as practice.

6.3.2 Illustration Using R Package meta

For comparison, we first output the results using the R library **meta** in this subsection as reference for the next subsection in R step-by-step implementation.

The implementation in the R library **meta** can be easily done using the following R code chunk:

```
> # RE-MA with risk-ratio using "inverse weighting"
> RR.Cochrane = metabin(ev.trt,n.trt,ev.ctrl,n.ctrl,studlab=name,
                data=cochrane, method="Inverse", sm="RR")
> # Print the result
> RR.Cochrane
```

	RR	95%-CI	%W(fixed)	%W(random)
Auckland	0.6068	[0.4086; 0.9011]	53.0	42.2
Block	0.1768	[0.0212; 1.4719]	1.8	2.6
Doran	0.2828	[0.0945; 0.8463]	6.9	9.2
Gamsu	0.7321	[0.3862; 1.3878]	20.3	22.6
Morrison	0.3774	[0.1022; 1.3938]	4.9	6.7
Papageorgiou	0.1509	[0.0190; 1.1959]	1.9	2.8
Tauesch	1.0143	[0.4287; 2.3997]	11.2	14.0

Number of studies combined: k = 7

                                    RR   95%-CI   z   p-value
Fixed effect model   0.5889 [0.4415; 0.7853] -3.60   0.0003
Random effects model 0.5722 [0.4032; 0.8120] -3.13   0.0018

Quantifying heterogeneity:
 tau^2 = 0.0349 [0.0000; 1.6708]; tau = 0.1869 [0.0000; 1.2926];
 I^2 = 15.1% [0.0%; 58.8%]; H = 1.09 [1.00; 1.56]

Test of heterogeneity:
    Q d.f. p-value
 7.06   6 0.3150

Details on meta-analytical method:
- Inverse variance method
- DerSimonian-Laird estimator for tau^2
- Jackson method for CI of tau^2 and tau

From the output, we see that the RR from the fixed-effects model is RR = 0.589 with 95% CI of (0.442, 0.785) and the value of the z-statistic is -3.60 with a p-value of 0.0003, whereas the RR from the random-effects model is RR=0.572 with 95% CI of (0.403, 0.812) and the value of the z-statistic is -3.13 with a p-value of 0.0018. This again indicates that there was a significant overall effect for steroid treatment in reducing neonatal death.

For Test of heterogeneity, the Q-statistic = 7.06 with df = 6 which yields a p-value from the χ^2 distribution of 0.315, indicating there is no statistically significant heterogeneity among the seven studies. From Quantifying heterogeneity, the estimated between-study variance is $\tau^2 = 0.0349$, which is very small; the H index is 1.09 with 95% CI of (1, 1.56) with lower limit of 1, which indicates insignificant heterogeneity. Finally $I^2 = 15.1\%$ with 95% CI of (0%, 58.8%) where the lower limit of 0 again indicates insignificant heterogeneity.

6.3.3   Implementation in R: Step by Step

Now we come to the step-by-step illustration on how to calculate these heterogeneity measures. We hope interested readers can follow these step-by-step calculations to enhance the understanding of these measures.

For calculating the RR using R, we proceed as follows:

```
> # Calculate the risks from the treatment group
> pE = cochrane$ev.trt/cochrane$n.trt
> pE
```

[1] 0.0677 0.0145 0.0494 0.1069 0.0448 0.0141 0.1429

```
> # Calculate the risks from the control group
> pC = cochrane$ev.ctrl/cochrane$n.ctrl
> pC

[1] 0.1115 0.0820 0.1746 0.1460 0.1186 0.0933 0.1408

> # Then calculate the risk-ratio as effect size
> ES = pE/pC
> ES

[1] 0.607 0.177 0.283 0.732 0.377 0.151 1.014
```

For the RR, it is a common practice to use its natural logarithm to calculate the CI and then transform back to get the CI for the RR. This process can be implemented as follows:

```
> # Calculate the log risk ratio
> lnES = log(ES)
> lnES

[1] -0.4996 -1.7327 -1.2629 -0.3119 -0.9745 -1.8911
[7]  0.0142

> # Calculate the variance of the logged RR
> VlnES = 1/cochrane$ev.trt - 1/cochrane$n.trt
>          + 1/cochrane$ev.ctrl - 1/cochrane$n.ctrl

[1] 0.0148 0.1836 0.0750 0.0427 0.1259 0.1295 0.0859

> VlnES

[1] 0.0259 0.9855 0.2377 0.0638 0.3184 0.9859 0.1071

> # Then the upper CI limit
> ciup  = lnES+1.96*sqrt(VlnES)
> ciup

[1] -0.184  0.213 -0.307  0.183  0.132  0.055  0.656

> # The lower CI limit
> cilow  = lnES-1.96*sqrt(VlnES)
> cilow

[1] -0.815 -3.678 -2.218 -0.807 -2.080 -3.837 -0.627

> # Then transform back to the original scale
> cat("The low CI is:", exp(cilow),"\n\n")

The low CI is: 0.443 0.0253 0.109 0.446 0.125 0.0216 0.534
```

```
> cat("The upper CI is:", exp(ciup),"\n\n")
```

The upper CI is: 0.832 1.24 0.735 1.2 1.14 1.06 1.93

This reproduces the summary statistics from the R output in Section 6.3.2. We now calculate the statistics from the fixed-effects model as follows:

```
> # The inverse of variance for each study
> fwi = 1/VlnES
> fwi
```

[1] 38.61   1.01   4.21 15.68   3.14   1.01   9.33

```
> # The total weight
> fw  = sum(fwi)
> fw
```

[1] 73

```
> # The relative weight for each study
> rw  = fwi/fw
> rw
```

[1] 0.5290 0.0139 0.0576 0.2147 0.0430 0.0139 0.1279

```
> # The fixed-effects weighted mean estimate
> flnES = sum(lnES*rw)
> flnES
```

[1] -0.495

```
> # The variance for the weighted mean
> var = 1/fw
> var
```

[1] 0.0137

```
> # Then the fixed-effects meta-estimate of RR
> fRR = exp(flnES)
> fRR
```

[1] 0.61

```
> # The lower limit
> fLL = exp(flnES-1.96*sqrt(var))
> fLL
```

[1] 0.485

```
> # The upper limit
> fUL = exp(flnES+1.96*sqrt(var)); fUL
```

[1] 0.767

Again this reproduces the weightings and the meta-estimate from the fixed-effects model in the R output in Section 6.3.2. The statistics from the random-effects model can be calculated as follows:

```
> # Calculate the Q-statistic
> Q  = sum(fwi*lnES^2)-(sum(fwi*lnES))^2/fw
> Q
```

[1] 9.68

```
> # The number of studies and df
> K  = dim(cochrane)[1]
> df = K -1
> # The U-statistic
> U = fw - sum(fwi^2)/fw
> U
```

[1] 47.6

```
> # Then the estimate tau-square
> tau2  = ifelse(Q > K-1,(Q-df)/U,0)
> tau2
```

[1] 0.0773

This reproduces the between-study variance of $\hat{\tau}^2$=0.0773. With this estimate of τ^2, we can reproduce the statistics from random-effects model as follows:

```
> # Compute the weights from random-effects model
> wR = 1/(VlnES+tau2)
> wR
```

[1] 9.689 0.941 3.175 7.087 2.527 0.941 5.421

```
> # The total weight
> tot.wR = sum(wR)
> # The relative weight
> rel.wR = wR/tot.wR
> rel.wR
```

[1] 0.3253 0.0316 0.1066 0.2380 0.0849 0.0316 0.1820

```
> # Then the weighted mean from random-effects model
> rlnES = sum(lnES*rel.wR)
> rlnES

[1] -0.566

> # The variance for the weighted mean
> var    = 1/tot.wR
> var

[1] 0.0336

> # Transform back to the original scale
> rRR    =  exp(rlnES)
> rRR

[1] 0.568

> # The lower limits
> rLL  = exp(rlnES-1.96*sqrt(var))
> rLL

[1] 0.396

> # The upper limits
> rUL = exp(rlnES+1.96*sqrt(var))
> rUL

[1] 0.813

> # The z-statistic
> zR = rlnES/sqrt(var); zR

[1] -3.09

> # The p-value
> pval.R = 2*(1-pnorm(abs(zR))); pval.R

[1] 0.00201
```

This reproduces the weightings and the meta-estimate from the random-effects model in the R output in Section 6.3.2.

Now we consider the measures of heterogeneity. For Test of heterogeneity, we found that $Q = 9.6808$ with $df = 6$ above. The associated p-value can be then calculated as follows:

```
> pval4Q =  pchisq(Q, df, lower.tail=F)
> pval4Q

[1] 0.139
```

which indicates that there is no statistically significant heterogeneity. We found the estimate of $\hat{\tau}^2 = 0.0773$ above. The H index and its 95% CI can be calculated as follows:

```
> # The H index
> H = sqrt(Q/df)
> H

[1] 1.27

> # The SE for logH
> se.logH = ifelse(Q>K,
        0.5*(log(Q)-log(K-1))/(sqrt(2*Q)-sqrt(2*K-3)),
        sqrt(1/(2*(K-2))*(1-1/(3*(K-2)^2)))))
> se.logH

[1] 0.221

> # The lower limit
> LL.H  = max(1,exp(log(H) -1.96*se.logH))
> LL.H

[1] 1

> # The upper limit
> UL.H  = exp(log(H) +1.96*se.logH)
> UL.H

[1] 1.96
```

The I^2 index and its 95% CI are then calculated as follows:

```
> # The I-square
> I2 = (Q-df)/Q*100
> I2

[1] 38

> # The lower limit for I-square
> LL.I2 = max(0,(LL.H^2-1)/LL.H^2*100)
> LL.I2

[1] 0

> # The upper limit for I-square
> UL.I2 = max(0,(UL.H^2-1)/UL.H^2*100)
> UL.I2

[1] 73.9
```

This reproduces all the measures from Quantifying heterogeneity from R library meta in Section 6.3.2.

6.3.4   Meta-Analysis Using **R** Package metafor

To further enhance learning, we illustrate the meta-analysis of this data with the metafor package to meta-analyze this data.

To use this package, we load the package into R as follows:

```
> library(metafor)
```

We then calculate the effect-size (ES) using measure="RR", which is to calculate the (log)RR, for all studies by calling the R function of escalc as follows:

```
> # Call escalc to calculate the ESs
> ES.RR.Cochrane = escalc(measure="RR",
                    ai=ev.trt, bi=n.trt-ev.trt,
                    ci=ev.ctrl, di=n.ctrl-ev.ctrl,
                    data=cochrane)
> # Print the calculated ESs
> ES.RR.Cochrane
```

	name	ev.trt	n.trt	ev.ctrl	n.ctrl	yi	vi
1	Auckland	36	532	60	538	-0.4996	0.0407
2	Block	1	69	5	61	-1.7327	1.1691
3	Doran	4	81	11	63	-1.2629	0.3127
4	Gamsu	14	131	20	137	-0.3119	0.1065
5	Morrison	3	67	7	59	-0.9745	0.4443
6	Papageorgiou	1	71	7	75	-1.8911	1.1154
7	Tauesch	8	56	10	71	0.0142	0.1931

Notice that in the dataframe ES.RR.Cochrane above, the column yi is the calculated (log)RR as implemented in metafor and the column vi is the corresponding within-study sampling variance for (log)RR. With the ESs, we can then perform meta-analysis. The fixed-effects meta-analysis is implemented as follows:

```
> # Call rma for FE
> RR.Cochrane.FE = rma(yi, vi, data=ES.RR.Cochrane, method="FE")
> # Print the summary of FE analysis
> RR.Cochrane.FE

Fixed-Effects Model (k = 7)

I^2 (total heterogeneity / total variability):   15.06%
H^2 (total variability / sampling variability):  1.18

Test for Heterogeneity:
Q(df = 6) = 7.0638, p-val = 0.3150
```

Model Results:

```
estimate      se      zval     pval     ci.lb     ci.ub
 -0.5296   0.1469  -3.6048   0.0003   -0.8175   -0.2416   ***
```

```
---
Signif. codes:  0 *** 0.001 ** 0.01 * 0.05 . 0.1
```

To obtain the results in RR, we transform back to the original scale from the log RR as follows:

```
> # The overall risk-ratio
> exp(RR.Cochrane.FE$beta)
```

```
intrcpt 0.589
```

```
> # The lower bound of 95% confidence interval
> exp(RR.Cochrane.FE$ci.lb)
```

```
[1] 0.442
```

```
> # The upper bound of 95% confidence interval
> exp(RR.Cochrane.FE$ci.ub)
```

```
[1] 0.785
```

Similar implementation can be done for DL random-effects meta-analysis as follows:

```
> # Call rma with DL for DL random-effects analysis
> RR.Cochrane.RE = rma(yi, vi, data=ES.RR.Cochrane, method="DL")
> # Print the summary of DL
> RR.Cochrane.RE
```

```
Random-Effects Model (k = 7; tau^2 estimator: DL)
```

```
tau^2 (estimated amount of total heterogeneity): 0.0349
                                                 (SE = 0.1353)
tau (square root of estimated tau^2 value):      0.1869
I^2 (total heterogeneity / total variability):   15.06%
H^2 (total variability / sampling variability):  1.18
```

```
Test for Heterogeneity:
Q(df = 6) = 7.0638, p-val = 0.3150
```

```
Model Results:
estimate      se      zval     pval     ci.lb     ci.ub
```

```
 -0.5583   0.1786   -3.1257   0.0018   -0.9084   -0.2082  **

 ---

Signif. codes:   0 *** 0.001 ** 0.01 * 0.05 . 0.1

> # Transform back to original RR
> exp(RR.Cochrane.RE$beta)

intrcpt 0.572

> # Transform back the lower bound
> exp(RR.Cochrane.RE$ci.lb)

[1] 0.403

> # Transform back the upper bound
> exp(RR.Cochrane.RE$ci.ub)

[1] 0.812
```

As seen from these calculations with the `metafor` package, we reproduced the results in the step-by-step meta-analysis as well as the results in the meta-analysis with `meta` package.

6.4   Illustration with PCNL Meta-Data – Continuous Data

We now illustrate the concept and calculation of heterogeneity in meta-analysis for continuous data using the tubeless vs standard PCNL data from Chapter 5.

6.4.1   Tubeless vs Standard PCNL Data

In Chapter 5, we made use of the meta-analysis from Wang et al. (2011) on tubeless PCNL with standard PCNL for stones of the kidney or upper ureter. In this paper, several outcome measures were used including the operation duration, length of hospital stay, analgesic requirement pre- and postoperative tubeless PCNL hematocrit changes. We reproduced all the results in this paper using R in Section 5.4 except finding a slightly different conclusion in operation duration in Section 5.4.1 if the analysis is performed using the standardized mean difference (i.e., SMD).

In this section, we use this analysis to illustrate the presentation of heterogeneity for continuous data. As seen from Section 5.4, the PCNL data are loaded into R from the external excel file `dat4Meta` and named as `dat` for R implementation. To reuse the data and R code, we subset the `duration` data and again name this subset as `dat.duration` for analysis in this section and those that follow.

6.4.2 Implementation in R Library `meta`

For comparison, we first output the results using the R library in this section as reference for the next section in R step-by-step implementation. The implementation in the R library `meta` can be done easily using the following R code chunk:

```
> # Call "metacont" for meta-analysis
> SMD.duration = metacont(n.E,Mean.E, SD.E, n.C, Mean.C, SD.C,
                studlab=Study, data=dat.duration, sm="SMD",
                label.e="Tubeless", label.c="Standard")
> # Print the summary
> SMD.duration
```

```
                          SMD            95%-CI
Ahmet Tefekli 2007     -1.6948  [-2.4803;  -0.9093]
B.Lojanapiwat 2010     -0.3763  [-0.7677;   0.0151]
Hemendra N. Shah 2008   0.2663  [-0.2223;   0.7548]
Hemendra Shah 2009     -0.5618  [-0.7001;  -0.4235]
J. Jun-Ou 2010         -0.6397  [-1.0542;  -0.2252]
Michael Choi 2006       0.5318  [-0.2851;   1.3487]
                       %W(fixed)  %W(random)
Ahmet Tefekli 2007         2.3        11.9
B.Lojanapiwat 2010         9.1        18.8
Hemendra N. Shah 2008      5.8        17.0
Hemendra Shah 2009        72.7        22.6
J. Jun-Ou 2010             8.1        18.4
Michael Choi 2006          2.1        11.4


Number of studies combined: k = 6

                          SMD            95%-CI       z   p-value
Fixed effect model     -0.5058  [-0.6237;  -0.3878]  -8.41  < 0.0001
Random effects model   -0.4104  [-0.7979;  -0.0229]  -2.08    0.0379


Quantifying heterogeneity:
  tau^2 = 0.1682 [0.0792; 2.2991]; tau = 0.4102 [0.2814; 1.5163];
  I^2 = 80.8% [58.7%; 91.1%]; H = 2.28 [1.56; 3.35]

Test of heterogeneity:
     Q d.f.  p-value
  26.04    5 < 0.0001
```

```
Details on meta-analytical method:
```

```
- Inverse variance method
- DerSimonian-Laird estimator for tau^2
- Jackson method for CI of tau^2 and tau
- Hedges' g (bias-corrected standardised mean difference)
```

From this output, we can see that the Test of heterogeneity has a Q-statistic value of 26.04 with $df = 5$ and a p-value < 0.0001, indicating statistically significant heterogeneity among the six studies. The measures of heterogeneity in Quantifying heterogeneity are $\tau^2 = 0.1682$, $H = 2.28$ with 95% CI (1.56, 3.35) and $I^2 = 80.8\%$ with 95% CI (58.7%, 91.1%), respectively. From the CIs of H and I^2, we can also conclude the existence of statistically significant heterogeneity.

From the fixed-effects model, the SMD from all 6 studies is $SMD = -0.506$ with 95% CI of $(-0.624, -0.388)$, the estimated $\hat{\tau}^2 = 0.1682$, and the estimated $SMD = -0.410$ with 95% CI of $(-0.798, -0.0229)$ – which are statistically significant.

6.4.3   Implementation in R: Step by Step

To be consistent with the notation used in the R library meta, we rename the variables as follows:

```
> dat.duration$n.t = dat.duration$n.E
> dat.duration$n.c = dat.duration$n.C
> dat.duration$m.t = dat.duration$Mean.E
> dat.duration$m.c = dat.duration$Mean.C
> dat.duration$sd.t = dat.duration$SD.E
> dat.duration$sd.c = dat.duration$SD.C
```

Then we calculate the pooled standard deviation as follows:

```
> # Get the pooled sd to calculate the SMD
> pooled.sd = sqrt((((dat.duration$n.t-1)*dat.duration$sd.t^2+
        (dat.duration$n.c-1)*dat.duration$sd.c^2)
        /(dat.duration$n.t+dat.duration$n.c-2))
> pooled.sd
```

```
[1]   9.63 21.71 13.51 28.45 17.79 16.59
```

With the pooled SD, we then calculate Hedges' SMD with correction for unbiased estimate as follows:

```
> # Calculate the standardized mean difference(SMD)
> g = (dat.duration$m.t-dat.duration$m.c)/pooled.sd
> g
```

```
[1] -1.735 -0.379  0.269 -0.562 -0.645  0.551

> # Hedges' correction factor
> N = dat.duration$n.t+dat.duration$n.c
> J = 1- 3/(4*N-9)
> J

[1] 0.977 0.993 0.988 0.999 0.992 0.966

> # Now the Hedges's gstar
> gstar = J*g
> gstar

[1] -1.695 -0.376  0.266 -0.562 -0.640  0.532
```

We compute the variance of this SMD as follows:

```
> # Calculate the variance of Hedges's SMD
> var.gstar = (dat.duration$n.t+dat.duration$n.c)
>          /(dat.duration$n.t*dat.duration$n.c)
>    + gstar^2/(2*(dat.duration$n.t+dat.duration$n.c-3.94))

[1] 0.046238 0.000708 0.000581 0.000189 0.002247 0.007049

> # Print the variance
> var.gstar

[1] 0.11438 0.03917 0.06155 0.00479 0.04249 0.16667
```

Therefore, the 95% CI for all 6 studies can be constructed as:

```
> # The lower limit
> lowCI.gstar = gstar-1.96*sqrt(var.gstar)
> lowCI.gstar

[1] -2.358 -0.764 -0.220 -0.698 -1.044 -0.268

> # The upper limit
> upCI.gstar = gstar+1.96*sqrt(var.gstar)
> upCI.gstar

[1] -1.0319  0.0116  0.7525 -0.4261 -0.2357  1.3320
```

The above calculations reproduce the summary statistics from Section 6.4.2. For the fixed-effects model, we first calculate the weights using following R code chunk:

```
> # Calculate the individual weight
> w = 1/var.gstar
> w
```

```
[1]    8.74   25.53   16.25 208.62   23.54    6.00

> # The total weight
> tot.w = sum(w)
> tot.w

[1] 289

> # Then the relative weight
> rel.w = w/tot.w
> rel.w

[1] 0.0303 0.0884 0.0563 0.7227 0.0815 0.0208
```

With these weights, we calculate the meta-estimate as:

```
> # The meta-estimate
> M = sum(rel.w*g)
> M

[1] -0.518
```

Then the variance and CI computed as:

```
> # The variance of M
> var.M = 1/tot.w
> var.M

[1] 0.00346

> # The SE
> se.M = sqrt(var.M)
> se.M

[1] 0.0589

> # The 95% CI
> lowCI.M = M-1.96*se.M
> lowCI.M

[1] -0.634

> upCI.M = M+1.96*se.M
> upCI.M

[1] -0.403
```

The 95% CI does not cover zero and we conclude that the pooled effect is statistically significant. We can also calculate the z-value and the associated p-value as follows:

```
> # compute z
> z = M/se.M
> z

[1] -8.81

> # compute p-value
> pval = 2*(1-pnorm(abs(z)))
> pval

[1] 0
```

Again this reproduces the summary statistics from Section 6.4.2. For the random-effects model, we calculate the estimate of between-study variance τ^2 which is estimated from the Q-statistic as follows:

```
> # Calculate the heterogeneity Q statistic
> Q  = sum(w*gstar^2)-(sum(w*gstar))^2/tot.w
> Q

[1] 30

> # The number of studies
> K  = 6
> # The degrees of freedom
> df = K-1
> # The U quantity
> U  = tot.w - sum(w^2)/tot.w
> U

[1] 132

> # Now we can calculate the tau-square estimate
> tau2 = (Q-df)/U
> tau2

[1] 0.189
```

With this estimate, we can then calculate the weightings in the random-effects model as follows:

```
> # Compute the weights in the random-effects model
> wR = 1/(var.gstar+tau2)
> wR

[1] 3.30 4.39 4.00 5.17 4.33 2.81

> # The total weight
> tot.wR = sum(wR)
> tot.wR
```

```
[1] 24

> # The relative weight
> rel.wR = wR/tot.wR
> rel.wR

[1] 0.138 0.183 0.167 0.215 0.180 0.117
```

Then we calculate the meta-estimate, its variance, and 95% CI as follows:

```
> # The meta-estimate from the random-effects model
> MR = sum(rel.wR*gstar)
> MR

[1] -0.432

> # The var and SE of MR
> var.MR = 1/tot.wR
> var.MR

[1] 0.0417

> se.MR = sqrt(var.MR)
> se.MR

[1] 0.204

> # The 95% CI
> lowCI.MR = MR - 1.96*se.MR
> lowCI.MR

[1] -0.832

> upCI.MR = MR + 1.96*se.MR
> upCI.MR

[1] -0.0315

> # The z value
> zR = MR/se.MR
> zR

[1] -2.11

> # The p-value
> pval.R = 2*(1-pnorm(abs(zR)))
> pval.R

[1] 0.0345
```

These calculations reproduce the summary statistics for both fixed-effect and random-effect models from Section 6.4.2.

We now consider the `Test of heterogeneity`. We know that the Q-statistic is:

```
> Q
```

```
[1] 30
```

With $df = K - 1 = 6\text{-}1 = 5$, the p-value can be calculated as:

```
> pval.HG = 1-pchisq(Q,df)
> pval.HG
```

```
[1] 1.49e-05
```

which is less than 0.05 and we reject the null hypothesis that all studies share a common effect size and conclude that the true effect is not the same in all studies. With this conclusion, we compute other heterogeneity indices in `Quantifying heterogeneity` as follows:

```
> # Calculate the H index
> H = sqrt(Q/df)
> H
```

```
[1] 2.45
```

```
> # The standard error of log(H)
> se.logH = ifelse(Q > K, 0.5*((log(Q)-log(K-1)))
              /(sqrt(2*Q)-sqrt(2*K-3)),
              sqrt(1/(2*(K-2))*(1-1/(3*(k-2)^2)))))
> se.logH
```

```
[1] 0.189
```

```
> # The lower limit of 95% CI
> LL.H = max(1,exp(log(H) -1.96*se.logH))
> LL.H
```

```
[1] 1.69
```

```
> # The upper limit of 95% CI
> UL.H  = exp(log(H) +1.96*se.logH)
> UL.H
```

```
[1] 3.54
```

```
> # Calculate the heterogeneity I-square index
> I2 = (Q-df)/Q*100
> I2
```

```
[1] 83.3

> # The lower limit of I-square index
> LL.I2 = max(0,(LL.H^2-1)/LL.H^2*100)
> LL.I2

[1] 65

> # The upper limit of I-square index
> UL.I2 = max(0,(UL.H^2-1)/UL.H^2*100)
> UL.I2

[1] 92
```

Again these calculations reproduce the summary statistics for heterogeneity from Section 6.4.2.

6.4.4   Implementation in R Library `metafor`

Since the R package `metafor` was loaded in Section 6.3.4, we will then call the function `escalc` to calculate the standardized mean-difference for all studies as follows:

```
> # Call escalc to calculate ES
> ES.duration = escalc(measure="SMD",
                n1i=n.E,m1i=Mean.E,sd1i=SD.E,
                n2i=n.C,m2i=Mean.C,sd2i=SD.C,
                data=dat.duration,slab=rownames(dat.duration) )
> # Print the ES
> ES.duration
```

```
     Outcome                  Study Mean.E SD.E n.E Mean.C
1 duration      Ahmet Tefekli 2007   59.6  9.1  17   76.3
2 duration      B.Lojanapiwat 2010   48.9 24.1  45   57.1
3 duration Hemendra N. Shah 2008   50.5 10.4  33   46.9
4 duration      Hemendra Shah 2009   52.3 23.2 454   68.3
5 duration            J. Jun-Ou 2010   47.4 16.9  43   58.9
6 duration      Michael Choi 2006   82.1 18.0  12   73.0
  SD.C n.C n.t n.c  m.t  m.c sd.t sd.c      yi     vi
1 10.1  18  17  18 59.6 76.3  9.1 10.1 -1.6947 0.1554
2 19.7  59  45  59 48.9 57.1 24.1 19.7 -0.3763 0.0399
3 16.1  32  33  32 50.5 46.9 10.4 16.1  0.2663 0.0621
4 33.6 386 454 386 52.3 68.3 23.2 33.6 -0.5618 0.0050
5 18.5  52  43  52 47.4 58.9 16.9 18.5 -0.6397 0.0446
6 15.1  12  12  12 82.1 73.0 18.0 15.1  0.5318 0.1726
```

Similarly, the fixed-effects meta-analysis is implemented as follows:

```
> # Call rma to perform FE-MA
> metafor.FE.duration = rma(yi, vi, data=ES.duration,
                            method="FE")
> # Print the summary of FE-MA
> metafor.FE.duration

Fixed-Effects Model (k = 6)

I^2 (total heterogeneity / total variability):   81.05%
H^2 (total variability / sampling variability):  5.28


Test for Heterogeneity:
Q(df = 5) = 26.3853, p-val < .0001

Model Results:

estimate       se     zval     pval    ci.lb    ci.ub
 -0.5065   0.0601  -8.4238   <.0001  -0.6244  -0.3887  ***


---
Signif. codes:  0 *** 0.001 ** 0.01 * 0.05 . 0.1
```

Similar implementation can be done for DL random-effects meta-analysis as follows:

```
> # Call rma for DL RE-MA
> metafor.RE.duration = rma(yi, vi, data=ES.duration,
                            method="DL")
> # Print the summary of RE-MA
> metafor.RE.duration

Random-Effects Model (k = 6; tau^2 estimator: DL)

tau^2 (estimated amount of total heterogeneity): 0.1703
                                            (SE = 0.1660)
tau (square root of estimated tau^2 value):      0.4127
I^2 (total heterogeneity / total variability):   81.05%
H^2 (total variability / sampling variability):  5.28


Test for Heterogeneity:
Q(df = 5) = 26.3853, p-val < .0001
```

Model Results:

```
estimate       se     zval    pval    ci.lb    ci.ub
 -0.4124   0.1984  -2.0789  0.0376  -0.8013  -0.0236   *
```

```
---
Signif. codes:  0 *** 0.001 ** 0.01 * 0.05 . 0.1
```

Interested readers can check these results with the meta-analysis results from the **meta** and the step-by-step implementation. The results are the same!

6.5   Discussions

In this chapter, we discussed and illustrated measures of heterogeneity used in meta-analysis. The test of heterogeneity is based on the quantity Q which is distributed as a χ^2 with degrees of freedom $K - 1$. Three other heterogeneity indices were discussed. These are τ^2 to estimate the between-study variance which will be incorporated into random-effects model, H to estimate a standardized heterogeneity index on Q, and I^2 to estimate the proportion of true dispersion from the total dispersion.

The step-by-step implementation in R was illustrated using two data sets. This illustration should help readers understand the methods when they perform their own meta-analyses.

We did not specifically provide detailed calculations for the 95% CI of τ^2 and τ in this chapter. The CI can be easily obtained from the relationship between τ^2 and the H index. From the equation (6.3), we obtain

$$\hat{\tau}^2 = \frac{df\left(H^2 - 1\right)}{U} \tag{6.10}$$

Then the CI limits for H from equations (6.5) and (6.6) can be used to construct the CI for τ^2 as follows:

$$LL_{\tau^2} = \frac{df\left(LL_H^2 - 1\right)}{U}$$

$$UL_{\tau^2} = \frac{df\left(UL_H^2 - 1\right)}{U}$$

and consequently the 95% CI for τ can be constructed as follows:

$$LL_\tau = \sqrt{LL_{\tau^2}}$$

$$UL_\tau = \sqrt{UL_{\tau^2}}.$$

We have concentrated our attention to reproducing the output from R. Interested readers can refer to Bohning et al. (2002) for a more general discussion in estimating heterogeneity with the DerSimonian-Laird estimator. This estimator is commonly used in meta-analysis. More detailed derivation of these heterogeneity indices can be found from Higgins and Thompson (2002).

We indicated in Section 3.5 of Chapter 3 that the choice between a fixed-effects model or random-effects model should not be based on a test of heterogeneity. Rather the choice should be based on a detailed inspection of all aspects of the individual studies for which we desire synthesizing the treatment effects. Following this review, if it is reasonable to believe "a priori" that each study would provide an estimate of the same (or common) treatment effect, then a fixed-effects model should be used. Else, use a random-effects model. Further, we noted that in practice both models are usually used and the results reported.

So the practical utility of the methods presented in this chapter to assess heterogeneity is to additionally inform the consumer of the meta-analytic results. Following the presentation of synthesized results from a random-effects model, the assessment of heterogeneity using methods described in this chapter would be presented. The consumer would then know the extent to which differences in the observed treatment effects among individual studies were due not only to within study sampling error but also due to between study variability – as pointed out in Hedges and Vevea (1998) and Field (2003).

Another way to deal with between-study heterogeneity is to link the heterogeneity with other moderators such as meta-regression which is the focus of the next chapter.

Appendix: Stata Programs for Heterogeneity Assessment by Manyun Liu.

The Stata program below corresponds to the R program.

```
/*### Reproduce R Results in Section 6.3.1 ###*/
/* Load the rmeta */
ssc install metan

/* load the data */
/* Changes the wd */
cd "your file path"
import excel using dat4Meta.xls, sheet("Data_cochrane")
   firstrow clear

/*### Reproduce R Results in Section 6.3.2 ###*/
/* Generate two new variables, which are the survival
   number of patients of each group */
```

```
generate strt = ntrt-evtrt
generate sctrl = nctrl-evctrl

/* RE-MA with risk-ratio using "inverse weighting" */
/* For the fixed model. */
metan evtrt strt evctrl sctrl, label(namevar=name) fixedi rr

/* For the random model. */
metan evtrt strt evctrl sctrl, label(namevar=name) randomi rr

/*### Reproduce R Results in Section 6.3.3 ###*/
/*Calculate the risks from the treatment group*/
generate pE = evtrt/ntrt
list pE

/*Calculate the risks from the control group */
generate pC = evctrl/nctrl
list pC

/*Then calculate the risk-ratio as effect size*/
generate ES = pE/pC
list ES

/*Calculate the log risk ratio*/
generate lnES = log(ES)
list lnES

/*Calculate the variance of the logged RR*/
generate VlnES = 1/evtrt - 1/ntrt + 1/evctrl - 1/nctrl
list VlnES

/*Then the upper CI limit*/
generate ciup  = lnES+1.96*sqrt(VlnES)
list ciup

/*The lower CI limit*/
generate cilow  = lnES-1.96*sqrt(VlnES)
list cilow

/* then transform back to the original scale */
forvalues i = 1/7 {
   display "The low CI is:" exp(cilow[`i'])
 }
```

```
forvalues i = 1/7 {
   display "The upper CI is:" exp(ciup[`i'])
 }

/*The inverse of variance for each study*/
generate fwi      = 1/VlnES
list fwi

/*The total weight*/
egen fw       = total(fwi)
display fw

/*The relative weight for each study*/
generate rw       = fwi/fw
list rw

/*The fixed-effects weighted mean estimate*/
egen flnES   = total(lnES*rw)
display flnES

/*The variance for the weighted mean*/
generate var      = 1/fw
display var

/*Then the fixed-effects meta-estimate of RR*/
generate fRR      = exp(flnES)
display fRR

/*The lower limit*/
generate fLL      = exp(flnES-1.96*sqrt(var))
display fLL

/*The upper limit*/
generate fUL      = exp(flnES+1.96*sqrt(var))
display fUL

/*Calculate the Q-statistic*/
egen Q1 = total(fwi*lnES^2)
egen Q2= total(fwi*lnES)
generate Q=Q1-Q2^2/fw
display Q

/*The number of studies and df*/
generate K= r(N)
generate df = K -1
```

```
display df
/*The U-statistic*/
egen U1= total(fwi^2)
generat U      = fw - U1/fw
display U


/*Then the estimate tau-square*/

if Q > K-1 {
      generate tau2 = (Q-df)/U
      }
else if Q <= K-1 {
      generate tau2 = 0
      }
display tau2

/*Compute the weights from random-effects model*/
generate wR     = 1/(VlnES+tau2)
list wR

/*The total weight*/
egen tot_wR = total(wR)

/*The relative weight*/
generate rel_wR = wR/tot_wR
list rel_wR

/*Then the weighted mean from random-effects model*/
egen rlnES = total(lnES*rel_wR)
display rlnES

/*The variance for the weighted mean*/
drop var
generate var    = 1/tot_wR
display var

/*Transform back to the original scale*/
generate rRR   = exp(rlnES)
display rRR

/*The lower limits*/
generate rLL    = exp(rlnES-1.96*sqrt(var))
display rLL
```

```
/*The upper limits*/
generate rUL   = exp(rlnES+1.96*sqrt(var))
display rUL

/*The z-statistic*/
generate zR    = rlnES/sqrt(var)
display zR

/*The p-value*/
generate pval_R = 2*(1-normal(abs(zR)))
display pval_R

generate pval4Q =  chi2tail(df, Q)
display pval4Q

/*The H index*/
generate H = sqrt(Q/df)
display H

/*The SE for logH */
if Q > K {
 generate se_logH = 0.5*(log(Q)-log(K-1))/(sqrt(2*Q)-sqrt(2*K-3))
      }
else if Q <= K {
 generate se_logH = sqrt(1/(2*(K-2))*(1-1/(3*(K-2)^2)))
      }
display se_logH

/*The lower limit*/
generate LL_H  = max(1,exp(log(H)-1.96*se_logH))
display LL_H

/*The upper limit*/
generate UL_H  = exp(log(H) +1.96*se_logH)
display UL_H

/*The I-square*/
generate I2 = (Q-df)/Q*100
display I2

/*The lower limit for I-square*/
generate LL_I2 = max(0,(LL_H^2-1)/LL_H^2*100)
display LL_I2
```

```
/*The upper limit for I-square*/
generate UL_I2 = max(0,(UL_H^2-1)/UL_H^2*100)
display UL_I2
/*### Reproduce R Results in Section 6.3.4 ###*/
ssc install metan


/* These parts are specific to R, which utilize R metafor
   and rma. We utilize alternative Stata code to produce
   similar results. */

/* For the fixed model. */
meta esize evtrt strt evctrl sctrl, esize(lnrratio)
    fixed(mhenszel)
list name _meta_es _meta_se
meta summarize, fixed(mhenszel)

/* For the random model. */
meta esize evtrt strt evctrl sctrl, esize(lnrratio)
    random(dlaird)
meta summarize, random(dlaird)

/*### Reproduce R Results in Section 6.4.1 ###*/
/*Get the data path*/
import excel using dat4Meta.xls, sheet("Data_tubeless")
         firstrow clear

/*Call "read_excel" to read the Excel data in specific data
    sheet */
keep if Outcome=="duration"

/* The following parts are specific to R, which utilize metacont
   to produce meta-analysis results. We utilize some alternative
   Stata codes to produce similar results*/

/*### Reproduce R Results in Section 6.4.2 ###*/
/* For the fixed model. */
 metan nE MeanE SDE nC MeanC SDC, label(namevar=Study)
    fixed hedges

/* For the random model. */
metan nE MeanE SDE nC MeanC SDC, label(namevar=Study)
   random hedges

/*### Reproduce R Results in Section 6.4.3 ###*/
rename nE n_t
```

```
rename nC n_c
rename MeanE m_t
rename MeanC m_c
rename SDE sd_t
rename SDC sd_c

/* First get the pooled sd to calculate the SMD */
generate pooled_sd = sqrt(((n_t-1)*sd_t^2
        +(n_c-1)*sd_c^2)/(n_t+n_c-2))
list pooled_sd

/*Calculate the standardized mean difference(SMD)*/
generate g = (m_t-m_c)/pooled_sd
list g

/*Hedges' correction factor*/
generate N = n_t+n_c
generate J = 1- 3/(4*N-9)
list J

/*Now the Hedges's gstar*/
generate gstar = J*g
list gstar

/*Calculate the variance of Hedges's SMD*/
generate var_gstar = (n_t+n_c)/(n_t*n_c)
        + gstar^2/(2*(n_t+n_c-3.94))
list var_gstar

/*The lower limit*/
generat lowCI_gstar = gstar-1.96*sqrt(var_gstar)
list lowCI_gstar

/*The upper limit*/
generate upCI_gstar  = gstar+1.96*sqrt(var_gstar)
list upCI_gstar

/*Calculate the individual weight*/
generate w = 1/var_gstar
list w

/*The total weight*/
egen tot_w = total(w)
display tot_w
```

```
/*Then the relative weight*/
generate rel_w = w/tot_w
list rel_w

/*The meta-estimate*/
egen M = total(rel_w*g)
display M

/*  The variance of M */
generate var_M = 1/tot_w
display var_M

/*  The SE */
generate se_M = sqrt(var_M)
display se_M

/*  The 95% CI */
generate lowCI_M = M-1.96*se_M
display lowCI_M
generate upCI_M = M+1.96*se_M
display upCI_M

/* Compute z */
generate z = M/se_M
display z

/* Compute p-value */
generate pval = 2*(1-normal(abs(z)))
display pval

/*Calculate the heterogeneity Q statistic*/
egen Q1=total(w*gstar^2)
egen Q2=total(w*gstar)
generate Q = Q1-Q2^2/tot_w
display Q

/*The number of studies*/
generate K  =6

/*The degrees of freedom*/
generate df = K-1

/*The U quantity*/
egen U1=total(w^2)
```

```
generate U  = tot_w - U1/tot_w
display U

/*Now we can calculate the tau-square estimate*/
generate tau2 = (Q-df)/U
display tau2

/*Compute the weights in the random-effects model*/
generate wR = 1/(var_gstar+tau2)
list wR

/* The total weight */
egen tot_wR = total(wR)
display tot_wR

/* The relative weight */
generate rel_wR = wR/tot_wR
list rel_wR

/*The meta-estimate from the random-effects model*/
egen MR = total(rel_wR*gstar)
display MR

/*The var and SE of MR*/
generate var_MR = 1/tot_wR
display var_MR
generate se_MR = sqrt(var_MR)
display se_MR

/*The 95% CI*/
generate lowCI_MR = MR - 1.96*se_MR
display lowCI_MR
generate upCI_MR = MR + 1.96*se_MR
display upCI_MR

/* The z value */
generate zR = MR/se_MR
display zR

/* The p-value */
generate pval_R = 2*(1-normal(abs(zR)))
display pval_R

display Q
```

```stata
generate pval_HG = chi2tail(df, Q)
display pval_HG

/*Calculate the H index*/
generate H = sqrt(Q/df)
display H

/*The standard error of log(H)*/
if Q > K {
 generate se_logH = 0.5*(log(Q)-log(K-1))/(sqrt(2*Q)-sqrt(2*K-3))
      }
else if Q <= K {
 generate se_logH = sqrt(1/(2*(K-2))*(1-1/(3*(K-2)^2)))
      }
display se_logH

/*The lower limit of 95% CI*/
generate LL_H  = max(1,exp(log(H)-1.96*se_logH))
display LL_H

/*The upper limit of 95% CI*/
generate UL_H  = exp(log(H) +1.96*se_logH)
display UL_H

/*Calculate the heterogeneity I-square index*/
generate I2 = (Q-df)/Q*100
display I2

/*The lower limit of I-square index*/
generate LL_I2 = max(0,(LL_H^2-1)/LL_H^2*100)
display LL_I2

/*The upper limit of I-square index*/
generate UL_I2 = max(0,(UL_H^2-1)/UL_H^2*100)
display UL_I2

/*### Reproduce R Results in Section 6.4.4 ###*/
/* For the fixed model. */
 meta esize n_t m_t sd_t n_c m_c sd_c, fixed
list Study _meta_es _meta_se
meta summarize, fixed(invvariance)

/* For the random model. */
 meta esize n_t m_t sd_t n_c m_c sd_c, random(dlaird)
meta summarize, random(dlaird)
```

7

Meta-Regression

Continuing from Chapter 6 to explain heterogeneity in meta-analysis, we explore meta-regression in this chapter to explain extra heterogeneity (or the residual heterogeneity) using study-level moderators or study-level independent variables. With study-level moderators associated with the reported effect-sizes as the dependent variable and their variance as weights, typical weighted regression analysis methods can be utilized. From this point of view, meta-regression is merely typical multiple regression applied for study-level data and therefore the theory of regression can be directly applied for meta-regression.

From the practical side, meta-regression can be used to determine whether continuous or discrete study characteristics influence study effect-size by regressing effect-size (dependent variable) on study characteristics (independent variables). The estimated coefficients of study characteristics and the associated statistical tests can then be used to assess whether study characteristics influence study effects sizes in a statistically significant manner. Similar to meta-analysis, there are typically two types of meta-regression. The first is random-effects meta-regression where both within-study variation and between-study variation are taken into account. The second is fixed-effects meta-regression where only within-study variation is taken into account (between-study variation is assumed to be zero). As pointed out by Normand (1999) and van Houwelingen et al. (2002), fixed-effects meta-regression is more powerful, but is less reliable if the between-study variation is significant. Therefore, random-effects meta-regression is more commonly used in the analysis which can provide a test of between-study variation (i.e., the Q-statistic from heterogeneity) along with the estimates and tests of effects of study characteristics from regression.

However, whether fixed-effects or random-effects meta-regression should be performed should be based on a detailed review of all aspects of the individual studies (see Sections 2.3 and 2.4 of Chapter 2 and Section 3.4 of Chapter 3). Following this review if it is reasonable to believe "a priori" that each study would provide an estimate of the same (or common) treatment effect, then a fixed-effects meta-regression model should be used. Otherwise, use a random-effects meta-regression model.

The structure of this chapter is similar to that of previous chapters. We introduce three data sets appearing in the literature in Section 7.1 to be used to illustrate the methods and R implementation. The first data set contains summary information from 13 studies on the effectiveness of Bacillus Calmette-Guerin (BCG) vaccine against tuberculosis. The second data set contains summary information from 28 studies on ischemic heart disease (IHD) to assess the association between IHD risk reduction and reduction in serum cholesterol. Both data sets are widely used in meta-regression as examples. We recompiled a third data set from Huizenga et al. (2009) to assess whether the ability to inhibit motor responses is impaired for adolescents with attention-deficit hyperactivity disorder (ADHD). We then introduce meta-regression methods in Section 7.2 and use the first data set to illustrate these methods step-by-step. In Section 7.4, we illustrate meta-regression using the R library `metafor` for the other two data sets. We switch R library from `meta` and `rmeta` to `metafor` in this chapter since the libraries of `rmeta` and `meta` do not have the functionality of meta-regression. Some discussions are given in Section 7.6.

Note to the readers: you need to install R packages `readxl` to read in the excel data file and `metafor` for meta-analysis.

7.1 Data

7.1.1 BCG Vaccine Data

This is a data set from clinical trials conducted to assess the impact of a BCG vaccine in the prevention of tuberculosis (TB). The data set is widely used to illustrate meta-regression; for example, in the books authored by Everitt and Hothorn (2006) (see Table 12.2), Hartung et al. (2008) (see Table 18.8) and Borenstein et al. (2009) (see Table 20.1) as well as in the paper by van Houwelingen et al. (2002) and the R library `metafor` by Viechtbauer (2010). The source data set was reported in the original publication in Colditz et al. (1994) which included 13 clinical trials of BCG vaccine each investigating the effectiveness of BCG in the treatment of TB.

It should be noticed that the numbers reported in these references are different even though all of them referenced this data set as BCG with 13 studies from the same publications. The data tables reported from Everitt and Hothorn (2006), Borenstein et al. (2009), and Colditz et al. (1994) are the total number of cases in both BCG and control. However, the data set reported in the R `metafor` library and van Houwelingen et al. (2002) are the numbers of "negative cases." We will use this data structure in this chapter which is given in Table 7.1.

In this table, `author` denotes the authorship from the 13 studies, `year` is publication year of these 13 studies, `tpos` is the number of TB positive cases in the BCG vaccinated group, `tneg` is the number of TB negative cases in the BCG vaccinated group, `cpos` is the number of TB positive cases in the

TABLE 7.1
Data from Studies on Efficacy of BCG Vaccine for Preventing TB

Author	Year	tpos	tneg	cpos	cneg	ablat	alloc
Aronson	1948	4	119	11	128	44	Random
Ferguson & Simes	1949	6	300	29	274	55	Random
Rosenthal et al.	1960	3	228	11	209	42	Random
Hart & Sutherland	1977	62	13536	248	12619	52	Random
Frimodt-Moller et al.	1973	33	5036	47	5761	13	Alternate
Stein & Aronson	1953	180	1361	372	1079	44	Alternate
Vandiviere et al.	1973	8	2537	10	619	19	Random
TPT Madras	1980	505	87886	499	87892	13	Random
Coetzee & Berjak	1968	29	7470	45	7232	27	Random
Rosenthal et al.	1961	17	1699	65	1600	42	Systematic
Comstock et al.	1974	186	50448	141	27197	18	Systematic
Comstock & Webster	1969	5	2493	3	2338	33	Systematic
Comstock et al.	1976	27	16886	29	17825	33	Systematic

control group, `cneg` is the number of TB negative cases in the control group, `ablat` denotes the absolute latitude of the study location (in degrees), and `alloc` denotes the method of treatment allocation with three levels: random, alternate, or systematic assignment.

The purpose of the original meta-analysis was to quantify the preventative efficacy of the BCG vaccine against TB which was facilitated by a random-effects meta-analysis which concluded that the BCG vaccine significantly reduced the risk of TB− in the presence of significant heterogeneity. The heterogeneity was explained partially by geographical latitude. In this chapter, we use this data set to illustrate the application of R `metafor` library.

7.1.2 Ischemic Heart Disease

This is a data set from 28 randomized clinical trials of IHD conducted to assess the association between IHD risk reduction and the reduction in serum cholesterol – originally analyzed in Law et al. (1994). This data set was used by Thompson and Sharp (1999) to illustrate the increased benefit of IHD risk reduction in association with greater reduction in serum cholesterol and to explain heterogeneity in meta-analysis. The data are shown in Table 7.2 where `trial` denotes the study number from 1 to 28 with original trial reference and more detailed information listed in Law et al. (1994), `cpos` is the number of IHD events in the control group, `cneg` is the number of non-IHD event in the control group, `tpos` is the number of IHD events in the treated group, `tneg` is the number of non-IHD events in the treated group, and `chol` denotes the cholesterol reduction in unit mmol/l. In this chapter, we will illustrate the application of R to analyze this data set.

TABLE 7.2

Data on IHD Events from 28 Studies with Serum Cholesterol Reduction

Trial	cpos	cneg	tpos	tneg	chol
1.00	210.00	5086.00	173.00	5158.00	0.55
2.00	85.00	168.00	54.00	190.00	0.68
3.00	75.00	292.00	54.00	296.00	0.85
4.00	936.00	1853.00	676.00	1546.00	0.55
5.00	69.00	215.00	42.00	103.00	0.59
6.00	101.00	175.00	73.00	206.00	0.84
7.00	193.00	1707.00	157.00	1749.00	0.65
8.00	11.00	61.00	6.00	65.00	0.85
9.00	42.00	1087.00	36.00	1113.00	0.49
10.00	2.00	28.00	2.00	86.00	0.68
11.00	84.00	1946.00	54.00	1995.00	0.69
12.00	5.00	89.00	1.00	93.00	1.35
13.00	121.00	4395.00	131.00	4410.00	0.70
14.00	65.00	357.00	52.00	372.00	0.87
15.00	52.00	142.00	45.00	154.00	0.95
16.00	81.00	148.00	61.00	168.00	1.13
17.00	24.00	213.00	37.00	184.00	0.31
18.00	11.00	41.00	8.00	20.00	0.61
19.00	50.00	84.00	41.00	83.00	0.57
20.00	125.00	292.00	82.00	339.00	1.43
21.00	20.00	1643.00	62.00	6520.00	1.08
22.00	0.00	52.00	2.00	92.00	1.48
23.00	0.00	29.00	1.00	22.00	0.56
24.00	5.00	25.00	3.00	57.00	1.06
25.00	144.00	871.00	132.00	886.00	0.26
26.00	24.00	293.00	35.00	276.00	0.76
27.00	4.00	74.00	3.00	76.00	0.54
28.00	19.00	60.00	7.00	69.00	0.68

7.1.3 ADHD for Children and Adolescents

ADHD is one of the most common neurobehavioral disorders in children and adolescents. Typical symptoms of ADHD include difficulty staying focused and paying attention, very high levels of activity, and difficulty controlling behavior, etc. Among these symptoms, a key one is the inability to inhibit motor responses when asked to do so. There are many studies using the well-established stop-signal paradigm to measure this response in children with ADHD which typically showed a delayed stop-signal reaction time (SSRT) in comparison with healthy age-matched controls. To further study prolonged SSRT, Huizenga et al. (2009) performed a meta-analysis of 41 studies comparing SSRT in children or adolescents diagnosed with ADHD to normal control subjects. Since between-study variation in effect-sizes was large, a random-effects meta-regression analysis was conducted to investigate whether this variability could be explained by regression covariates from the between-study reaction time in "Go task" complexity. These covariates included a global index of Go task complexity measured as the mean reaction time in control subjects (RTc) and another more specific index measured as the spatial compatibility of the stimulus-response mapping.

It was found that the between-study variations were explained partially by the regression covariate RTc. There was a statistically significant relationship between the SSRT difference and RTc where the increased SSRT difference was positively associated with increasing RTc as well as in studies that employed a noncompatible mapping compared with studies that incorporated a spatially compatible stimulus-response mapping.

In this chapter, we use R `metefor` to analyze this data set. The data in original Tables 1 and 2 from Huizenga et al. (2009) are re-entered into the ExcelBook `dat4Meta` with data in Excel sheet `Data.adhd` and explanation in sheet `readme.adhd`. This data contain 41 studies and 26 variables, which would take up too much space to be included here as a table, and we will read it into the R later for illustration.

7.2   The Methods in Meta-Regression

As described in Section 3.2, the fundamental assumption for the fixed-effects model is that all studies share a common (true) overall effect-size δ. With this assumption, the true effect-size is the same (and therefore the name of fixed-effects) in all the studies with each observed effect-size δ_i varying around δ with a normal sampling error; i.e., ϵ_i distributed as $N(0, \hat{\sigma}_i^2)$ where $\hat{\sigma}_i^2$ are assumed to be known (directly or indirectly calculated from summary data).

This fundamental assumption may be impractical for some studies with substantially different effect-sizes. The random-effects model relaxes this fundamental assumption by assuming (1) that the effect-size $\hat{\delta}_{iR}$ from each study i is an estimate of its own underlying true effect-size δ_{iR} with sampling variance $\hat{\sigma}_i^2$ and (2) that the δ_{iR} from all studies follow an overall global distribution denoted by $N(\delta, \tau^2)$ with τ^2 as the between-study variance. If $\tau^2 = 0$, then $\delta_{1R} = \cdots = \delta_{KR} \equiv \delta$ which leads to homogeneity from all effects. In this sense, the random-effects model incorporates heterogeneity from the studies.

We have seen from Chapter 6 that even with the random-effects model, there can exist significant extra-heterogeneity. The meta-regression is then used to model this extra-heterogeneity with some study-level variables (or moderators) to account for the extra heterogeneity in the true effects. This meta-regression can be expressed as a mixed-effects model as follows:

$$\hat{\delta}_{iR} = \delta_{iR} + \epsilon_i \qquad (7.1)$$

and

$$\delta_{iR} = \beta_0 + \beta_1 x_{i1} + \cdots + \beta_p x_{ip} + \nu_i \tag{7.2}$$

where x_{ij} is the jth ($j = 1, \ldots, p$) moderator variable for the ith ($i = 1, \ldots, K$) study with associated regression parameter β_j, where β_0 is the global effect-size δ defined in Section 3.2 when all $\beta_1 = \cdots = \beta_p \equiv 0$. Note that ν_i is defined as $\nu_i \sim N(0, \tau^2)$ where τ^2 denotes the amount of residual heterogeneity that is not accounted for by the moderators in the meta-regression model. For this, the meta-regression is aimed to identify which moderators are significantly related to the study effects which can be used to account for the extra heterogeneity. Methodologically, the meta-regression is essentially a simple case of the general linear mixed-effects model with known heteroscedastic sampling variances provided from the study summary tables. Therefore, the parameter estimation and statistical inference can be easily provided from the mixed-effects model.

We have illustrated the details for fixed-effects and random-effects models in Chapters 3–5 using R packages `meta` and `rmeta`. These models are also implemented in R package `metafor`. Details about this package can be found in Viechtbauer (2010).

We are switching R library from `meta` and `rmeta` to `metafor` since this library includes the method of meta-regression. Readers can still use `meta` and `rmeta` for the meta-analysis following the procedures in Chapter 4 for categorical data and Chapter 5 for continuous data.

7.3   Meta-Analysis of BCG Data

7.3.1   Random-Effects Meta-Analysis

To use the R library, `metafor`, the original summary data from Table 7.1 have to be used to calculate the effect-sizes and their associated variances. To reproduce the results from Borenstein et al. (2009) and Viechtbauer (2010), we use the same log risk ratio to estimate effect-size. This effect-size is a measure of the log risk ratio between the treated (i.e., vaccinated) group and control group. Hence, a negative ES indicates that BCG is favored over the control in preventing TB infection. To further promote the `metafor` library, most of the R programs in this section are modified from Viechtbauer (2010). For practice, readers can simply change `measure` from `RR` for the log risk ratio to `OR` for log odds-ratio, `RD` for the risk difference, `AS` for the arcsine transformed risk difference, and `PETO` for the log odds-ratio estimated with Peto's method as discussed in Chapter 4 and re-run the analysis to verify.

To calculate the effect-sizes using log risk ratio, we call `escalc` as follows:

```
> # Calculate the ES using "escalc"
> dat  = escalc(measure="RR",ai=tpos,bi=tneg,ci=cpos,
```

```
            di = cneg, data = dat.bcg, append = TRUE)
> # print the numerical data (Delete columns 2,3,9 to
  save space)
> print(dat[,-c(2,3,9)], row.names = FALSE)
```

trial	tpos	tneg	cpos	cneg	ablat	yi	vi
1	4	119	11	128	44	-0.8893	0.3256
2	6	300	29	274	55	-1.5854	0.1946
3	3	228	11	209	42	-1.3481	0.4154
4	62	13536	248	12619	52	-1.4416	0.0200
5	33	5036	47	5761	13	-0.2175	0.0512
6	180	1361	372	1079	44	-0.7861	0.0069
7	8	2537	10	619	19	-1.6209	0.2230
8	505	87886	499	87892	13	0.0120	0.0040
9	29	7470	45	7232	27	-0.4694	0.0564
10	17	1699	65	1600	42	-1.3713	0.0730
11	186	50448	141	27197	18	-0.3394	0.0124
12	5	2493	3	2338	33	0.4459	0.5325
13	27	16886	29	17825	33	-0.0173	0.0714

It can be seen that two additional columns are appended (resulting from the option of append=TRUE) to the original dataframe. They are yi for the effect-size of log risk ratio with the corresponding (estimated) sampling variance denoted by vi. From this calculation, we can see that 11 out of 13 studies have a negative effect-size which indicates that BCG vaccination is favored over control in preventing TB infection; i.e., the TB infection risk is lower in the BCG treatment group than in the control group in 11 of 13 studies.

To perform the meta-analysis, the function rma in metafor is called with the option method to specify the choice of a fixed- or a random-effects model. For the fixed-effects model, we can easily specify method="FE". But for the random-effects model, there are several methods to be selected depending on which methods are to be used to estimate the between-study variance τ^2. We have extensively discussed and used the DerSimonian-Laird estimator in the previous chapter which is specified as method="DL" in function rma. Other methods implemented include:

1. method="HS" as the Hunter-Schmidt estimator discussed in Hunter and Schmidt (2004),

2. method="HE" as the Hedges estimator discussed in Hedges and Olkin (1985),

3. method="SJ" as the Sidik-Jonkman estimator discussed in Sidik and Jonkman (2005a) and Sidik and Jonkman (2005b),

4. method="EB" as the empirical Bayes estimator discussed in Morris (1983) and Berkey et al. (1995),

5. `method="ML"` and `method="REML"` as the maximum-likelihood estimator and the restricted maximum-likelihood estimator discussed in Viechtbauer (2005) with `REML` as the *default* method since `REML` is asymptotically unbiased and efficient.

The meta-analysis for the BCG data with `REML` is implemented in the following R code chunk:

```
> # Call `rma' to fit the BCG data
> meta.RE = rma(yi, vi, data = dat)
> # Print the summary
> meta.RE

Random-Effects Model (k = 13; tau^2 estimator: REML)

tau^2(estimated amount of total heterogeneity):0.3132(SE=0.1664)
tau(square root of estimated tau^2 value):      0.5597
I^2(total heterogeneity / total variability):   92.22%
H^2(total variability / sampling variability): 12.86


Test for Heterogeneity:
Q(df = 12) = 152.2330, p-val < .0001


Model Results:
estimate      se     zval     pval     ci.lb     ci.ub
 -0.7145  0.1798  -3.9744  <.0001   -1.0669  -0.3622  ***
---

Signif. codes: 0 *** 0.001 ** 0.01 * 0.05 . 0.1
```

From the summary, we can see that the overall effect-size from a random-effects model estimated by `REML` is statistically significant (estimate = -0.7145 and p-value < 0.0001). The estimated total amount of heterogeneity $\hat{\tau}^2$ is 0.3132(SE = 0.1664), the percentage of total variability due to heterogeneity is $\hat{I}^2 = 92.22\%$, and the ratio of the total variability to the sampling variability is $\hat{H}^2 = 12.86$. Furthermore, the `Test for Heterogeneity` is statistically significant since $\hat{Q} = 152.233$ with $df = 12$ and p-value < .0001. This meta-analysis can be simply summarized into the `forest` plot as shown in Figure 7.1.

7.3.2   Meta-Regression Analysis

To explain the extra-heterogeneity, we use all the moderators from the data which include `ablat`, `year`, and `alloc` and call the `rma` with default `REML` method with the following R code chunk:

```
> metaReg = rma(yi, vi, mods = ~ablat+year+alloc, data = dat)
> # Print the meta-regression results
> metaReg
```

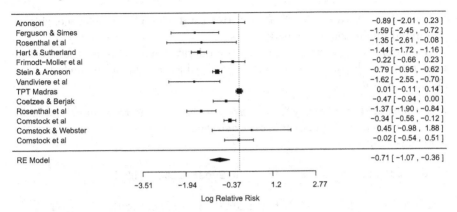

FIGURE 7.1
Forest plot from the random-effects model for BCG data.

```
Mixed-Effects Model (k = 13; tau^2 estimator: REML)

tau^2 (estimated amount of residual heterogeneity):  0.1796
                                                     (SE=0.1425)
tau(square root of estimated tau^2 value):           0.4238
I^2(residual heterogeneity/unaccounted variability):73.09%
H^2(unaccounted variability/sampling variability):   3.72
R^2(amount of heterogeneity accounted for):          42.67%

Test for Residual Heterogeneity:
QE(df = 8) = 26.2030, p-val = 0.0010

Test of Moderators (coefficients 2:5):
QM(df = 4) = 9.5254, p-val = 0.0492

Model Results:
                estimate       se     zval     pval     ci.lb    ci.ub
intrcpt         -14.4984  38.3943  -0.3776   0.7057  -89.7498  60.7531
ablat            -0.0236   0.0132  -1.7816   0.0748   -0.0495   0.0024  .
year              0.0075   0.0194   0.3849   0.7003   -0.0306   0.0456
allocrandom      -0.3421   0.4180  -0.8183   0.4132   -1.1613   0.4772
allocsystematic   0.0101   0.4467   0.0226   0.9820   -0.8654   0.8856
---

Signif. codes:  0 *** 0.001 ** 0.01 * 0.05 . 0.1
```

Although the Test for Residual Heterogeneity is still statistically significant ($Q_E = 26.2030$ with $df = 8$ and p-value $= 0.0010$) from this meta-regression, the estimated between-study variance dropped to 0.1796 from the previous meta-analysis of 0.3132 which indicates that

$(0.3132 - 0.1796)/0.3132 = 42.7\%$ of the total amount of heterogeneity is accounted for by the three moderators.

However, both `year` as a continuous moderator and `alloc` as a categorical moderator are highly insignificant. So we reduce the model to include only `ablat` as follows:

```
> metaReg.ablat = rma(yi, vi, mods = ~ablat, data = dat)
> # Print the meta-regression results
> metaReg.ablat
```

```
Mixed-Effects Model (k = 13; tau^2 estimator: REML)

tau^2 (estimated amount of residual heterogeneity):   0.0764
                                                       (SE=0.0591)
tau (square root of estimated tau^2 value):            0.2763
I^2(residual heterogeneity/unaccounted variability):68.39%
H^2 (unaccounted variability / sampling variability):3.16
R^2 (amount of heterogeneity accounted for):           75.62%


Test for Residual Heterogeneity:
QE(df = 11) = 30.7331, p-val = 0.0012


Test of Moderators (coefficient 2):
QM(df = 1) = 16.3571, p-val < .0001


Model Results:
          estimate      se     zval     pval    ci.lb   ci.ub
intrcpt     0.2515  0.2491   1.0095   0.3127  -0.2368  0.7397
ablat      -0.0291  0.0072  -4.0444   <.0001  -0.0432 -0.0150  ***
---
Signif. codes:  0 *** 0.001 ** 0.01 * 0.05 . 0.1
```

As can be seen from the output, with only `ablat`, the estimated residual heterogeneity $\hat{\tau}^2$ dropped to 0.0764 (SE = 0.0591) suggesting that there is confounding among `ablat`, `year`, and `alloc`. In addition, the `ablat` is more strongly statistically significant as seen from the p-value which dropped to $p < 0.0001$ as compared to $p = 0.0748$ in the previous meta-regression model.

In fact, the moderator `ablat` itself accounts for $(0.3132 - 0.0764)/0.3132 = 75.6\%$ of the total amount of heterogeneity and the absolute latitude is significantly related to the effectiveness of the BCG vaccine in preventing TB which can be quantified in the estimated meta-regression equation as follows:

$$log(RR) = 0.2515 - 0.0291 \times ablat \qquad (7.3)$$

This estimated equation and the entire meta-regression summary can be graphically displayed in Figure 7.2 using the following R code chunk:

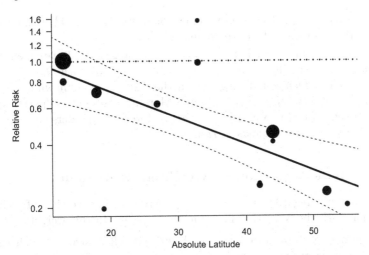

FIGURE 7.2
Plot for the meta-regression from the random-effects model for BCG data.

```
> # Create a new latitude vector
> newlat = 0:60
> # Using the meta-regression and calculate the predicted values
> preds  = predict(metaReg.ablat, newmods = newlat, transf = exp)
> # Use the inverse-variance to create a weighting for the data
> wi     = 1/sqrt(dat$vi)
> size   = 1 + 3 * (wi - min(wi))/(max(wi) - min(wi))
> # Plot the RR
> plot(dat$ablat, exp(dat$yi), pch = 19, cex = size,
  xlab = "Absolute Latitude", ylab = "Relative Risk",
  las = 1, bty = "1", log = "y")
> # Add a thicker line for the meta-regression
> lines(newlat, preds$pred, lwd=3)
> # Add the CIs
> lines(newlat, preds$ci.lb, lty = "dashed")
> lines(newlat, preds$ci.ub, lty = "dashed")
> # Add a dotted horizontal line for equal-effectiveness
> abline(h = 1, lwd=3,lty = "dotted")
```

It can be seen from this equation and the associated Figure 7.2 that the higher the absolute latitude, the more effective is the BCG vaccine. When the ablat is less than 20° and close to zero (i.e., study conducted closer to equator, the effect-size would be close to zero (as evidenced from the non-significant intercept parameter and Figure 7.2)) which means that the vaccination has no real effect on TB. As ablat increases, say to a latitude of 60°, the log RR as calculated from above equation is −1.49 which corresponds to a risk ratio of

0.224. In this latitude, the BCG vaccine would decrease the TB risk by 77.6% and effectively prevent the development of TB.

It should be emphasized that the Test for Residual Heterogeneity is still statistically significant as seen from $Q_E = 30.7331$ with $df = 11$ and p-value $= 0.0012$ which would suggest that there are more unknown moderators that impact effectiveness of the vaccine. More analyses can be performed on this data set as seen in Viechtbauer (2010). Interested readers can reanalyze this data using other methods in rma.

7.3.3   Meta-Regression vs Weighted Regression

It is commonly regarded that the meta-regression is a version of weighted regression with the weighting factor as $w_i = \frac{1}{\hat{\sigma}_i^2 + \hat{\tau}^2}$. In this weighting factor, $\hat{\sigma}_i^2$ is the observed variance associated with the effect-size $\hat{\delta}_i$ which can be calculated using escalc depending on data type and different measure specifications whereas $\hat{\tau}^2$ is the estimated residual variance which can be obtained from rma.

However, if we simply call lm incorporating this weighting factor, the standard errors and the associated inferences (i.e., p-values) can be wrong even though the parameter estimates are correct. For example, using the meta-regression *metaReg.ablat* in the previous section, we can use the following R code chunk for illustration:

```
> # Create the weighting factor
> wi = 1/(dat$vi+metaReg.ablat$tau2)
> # Call `lm' for weighted regression
> weightedReg = lm(yi~ablat, data=dat, weights=wi)
> # Print the summary
> summary(weightedReg)


Call: lm(formula = yi ~ ablat, data = dat, weights = wi)

Weighted Residuals:
   Min    1Q Median     3Q    Max
-2.412 -0.538 -0.225  0.490  1.799


Coefficients:
            Estimate Std. Error t value Pr(>|t|)
(Intercept)   0.2515     0.2839    0.89   0.3948
ablat        -0.0291     0.0082   -3.55   0.0046 **

Residual standard error: 1.14 on 11 degrees of freedom
Multiple R-squared:  0.534,       Adjusted R-squared:  0.491
F-statistic: 12.6 on 1 and 11 DF,  p-value: 0.00457
```

Comparing this output with the output from *metaReg.ablat* from the above subsection, we can see that the parameter estimates are the same as $\hat{\beta}_0$ for intercept $= 0.2515$ and $\hat{\beta}_1$ for ablat $= -0.0291$. However, the estimated standard errors and p-values are all different.

So, what is wrong? The key to making correct inferences is from the model specification. In meta-regression, the model is assumed to be

$$y_i = \beta_0 + \beta_1 x_{i1} + \cdots + \beta_p x_{pi} + e_i \qquad (7.4)$$

where $e_i \sim N(0, w_i)$ with known w_i. However in the weighted regression as illustrated in *weightedReg*, the model assumed seems to be the same as

$$y_i = \beta_0 + \beta_1 x_{i1} + \cdots + \beta_p x_{pi} + e_i \qquad (7.5)$$

However, the error distribution by default is $e_i \sim N(0, \sigma^2 \times w_i)$. lm will then estimate σ^2 which can be seen from the ANOVA table to be $\hat{\sigma} = 1.14$. With meta-regression, this σ^2 should set to 1.

Therefore, the correct procedure as implemented in rma would be to use matrix algebra to calculate the weighted hat matrix $H_w = (X'WX)^{-1}$, where X is the design matrix with the first column as 1s and the remaining p columns as $X = (x_{i1}, \ldots, x_{pi})$ and W is the weighting matrix with w_i as the diagonal elements. With this H_w, the parameter estimates would be $\hat{\beta} = H_w \times (X'Wy)$ which is the same from both the meta-regression in equation (7.4) and the weighted linear model as in equation (7.5).

With this notation, the correct standard error would be estimated as $se(\hat{\beta}) = \sqrt{H_w}$ for the meta-regression instead of the $se(\hat{\beta}) = \hat{\sigma} \times \sqrt{H_w}$ from the weighted linear model. From this correct standard error, appropriate inference can then be made. This procedure can be more explicitly illustrated by the following R code chunk:

```
> # Take the response vector
> y = dat$yi
> # Make the design matrix
> X = cbind(1,dat$ablat)
> # Make the weight matrix
> W = diag(wi)
> # Calculate the parameter estimate
> betahat = solve(t(X)%*%W%*%X)%*%t(X)%*%W%*%y
> # Calculate the estimated variance
> var.betahat =  diag(solve(t(X)%*%W%*%X))
> # Calculate the standard error
> se.betahat = sqrt(var.betahat)
> # Calculate z-value assuming asymptotic normal
> z = betahat/se.betahat
> # Calculate the p-value
> pval = 2*(1-pnorm(abs(z)))
```

```
> # Calculate the 95% CI
> ci.lb = betahat-1.96*se.betahat
> ci.ub = betahat+1.96*se.betahat
> # Make the output similar to metaReg.ablat
> Mod.Results = cbind(betahat, se.betahat,z,pval,ci.lb,ci.ub)
> colnames(Mod.Results) = c("estimate", "se","zval","pval",
                            "ci.lb","ci.ub")
> rownames(Mod.Results) = c("intrcpt", "ablat")
> # Print the result
> round(Mod.Results,4)

        estimate      se  zval    pval    ci.lb   ci.ub
intrcpt   0.2515  0.2491  1.01  0.3127  -0.2368   0.740
ablat    -0.0291  0.0072 -4.04  0.0001  -0.0432  -0.015
```

This reproduces the results from metaReg.ablat.

7.4 Meta-Analysis of IHD Data

7.4.1 IHD Data

The data in Table 7.2 were recompiled and typed into the excel data book with data sheet named as Data.IHD which can be loaded into R using following R code chunk:

```
> # Load the library
> require(readxl)
> # Get the data path
> datfile = "File path to the Excel Book 'dat4Meta.xls'"
> # Call "read_excel" to read the Excel data  with specific data
    sheet
> dat.IHD  = read_excel(datfile, sheet="Data.IHD")
```

It should be noted that there are two 0s in cpos for trials 22 and 23. In performing the meta-analysis and meta-regression, 0.5 is added to these two 0s.

7.4.2 Random-Effects Meta-Analysis

To reproduce the results from Thompson and Sharp (1999), we use the same log odds-ratios in this section as the measure for the effect-sizes. To calculate the effect-sizes using log odds-ratio, we can call escalc as follows:

```
> # Calculate the ES using "escalc"
> ES.IHD  = escalc(measure="OR",ai=tpos,bi=tneg,ci=cpos,
```

```
            di = cneg, data = dat.IHD, append = TRUE)
> # print the numerical data
> print(ES.IHD, row.names = FALSE)
```

trial	cpos	cneg	tpos	tneg	chol	yi	vi
1	210	5086	173	5158	0.55	-0.2079	0.0109
2	85	168	54	190	0.68	-0.5767	0.0415
3	75	292	54	296	0.85	-0.3421	0.0387
4	936	1853	676	1546	0.55	-0.1443	0.0037
5	69	215	42	103	0.59	0.2395	0.0527
6	101	175	73	206	0.84	-0.4878	0.0342
7	193	1707	157	1749	0.65	-0.2308	0.0127
8	11	61	6	65	0.85	-0.6696	0.2894
9	42	1087	36	1113	0.49	-0.1778	0.0534
10	2	28	2	86	0.68	-1.1221	1.0473
11	84	1946	54	1995	0.69	-0.4667	0.0314
12	5	89	1	93	1.35	-1.6534	1.2220
13	121	4395	131	4410	0.70	0.0760	0.0164
14	65	357	52	372	0.87	-0.2643	0.0401
15	52	142	45	154	0.95	-0.2257	0.0550
16	81	148	61	168	1.13	-0.4103	0.0414
17	24	213	37	184	0.31	0.5792	0.0788
18	11	41	8	20	0.61	0.3994	0.2903
19	50	84	41	83	0.57	-0.1865	0.0683
20	125	292	82	339	1.43	-0.5708	0.0266
21	20	1643	62	6520	1.08	-0.2469	0.0669
22	0	52	2	92	1.48	1.0430	2.4299
23	0	29	1	22	0.56	1.3695	2.7450
24	5	25	3	57	1.06	-1.3350	0.5909
25	144	871	132	886	0.26	-0.1041	0.0168
26	24	293	35	276	0.76	0.4371	0.0773
27	4	74	3	76	0.54	-0.3144	0.6100
28	19	60	7	69	0.68	-1.1383	0.2266

As explained previously, two additional columns are appended (resulting from the option `append=TRUE`) to the original dataframe where column `yi` is the effect-size for log odds-ratio with the corresponding (estimated) sampling variance denoted by column `vi`. Pay special attention to trial numbers 22 and 23 where 0.5 was added as control events in order to calculate the log odds-ratio and the variances, resulting in log odds-ratios of 1.043 and 1.369 with large variances of 2.4299 and 2.7450, respectively.

The meta-analysis with default `REML` is implemented in the following R code chunk:

```
> # Call `rma' to fit the BCG data
> meta.RE = rma(yi, vi, data = ES.IHD)
```

```
> # Print the summary
> meta.RE

Random-Effects Model (k = 28; tau^2 estimator: REML)

tau^2 (estimated amount of total heterogeneity):0.0321(SE=0.0207)
tau (square root of estimated tau^2 value):      0.1790
I^2 (total heterogeneity / total variability):  47.77%
H^2 (total variability / sampling variability): 1.91

Test for Heterogeneity:
Q(df = 27) = 49.9196, p-val = 0.0046

Model Results:
estimate      se     zval     pval     ci.lb     ci.ub
 -0.2193  0.0571  -3.8401   0.0001   -0.3312   -0.1074   ***
```

From the summary, we can see that the overall effect-size from a random-effects model estimated by REML is statistically significant (estimate $= -0.2193$ and p-value $= 0.0001$). The estimated total amount of heterogeneity $\hat{\tau}^2$ is 0.0321(SE $= 0.0207$), the percentage of total variability due to heterogeneity is $\hat{I}^2 = 47.77\%$, and the ratio of the total variability to the sampling variability is $\hat{H}^2 = 1.91$. Furthermore, the Test for Heterogeneity is statistically significant since $\hat{Q} = 49.9196$ with $df = 27$ and p-value $= 0.0046$.

7.4.3   Meta-Regression Analysis

To explain the extra-heterogeneity, we use the cholesterol reduction (chol) as a moderator and call the rma for a meta-regression analysis using the following R code chunk:

```
> metaReg.RE.REML = rma(yi, vi, mods = ~chol, data = ES.IHD)
> # Print the meta-regression results
> metaReg.RE.REML

Mixed-Effects Model (k = 28; tau^2 estimator: REML)

tau^2 (estimated amount of residual heterogeneity):  0.0107
                                                  (SE=0.0122)
tau (square root of estimated tau^2 value):          0.1035
I^2 (residual heterogeneity/unaccounted variability):22.84%
H^2 (unaccounted variability/sampling variability): 1.30
R^2 (amount of heterogeneity accounted for):         66.60%

Test for Residual Heterogeneity:
QE(df = 26) = 38.2448, p-val = 0.0575
```

```
Test of Moderators (coefficient 2):
QM(df = 1) = 8.9621, p-val = 0.0028

Model Results:
         estimate      se    zval    pval   ci.lb   ci.ub
intrcpt    0.1389  0.1258  1.1037  0.2697 -0.1078  0.3855
chol      -0.5013  0.1675 -2.9937  0.0028 -0.8295 -0.1731  **
```

It can be seen from this meta-regression that the `Test for Residual Heterogeneity` is no longer statistically significant at the 5%-level ($Q_E = 38.2448$ with $df = 26$ and p-value $= 0.0575$), the estimated between-study variance dropped to 0.0107 from the previous meta-analysis of 0.0321 which indicates that $(0.0321 - 0.0107)/0.0321 = 66.7\%$ of the total amount of heterogeneity is accounted for by the cholesterol reduction with estimated meta-regression equation as:

$$log(OR) = 0.1389 - 0.5013 \times chol \qquad (7.6)$$

This estimated equation and the entire meta-regression summary are graphically displayed in Figure 7.3 using the following R code chunk:

```
> # Create a new cholesterol reduction vector
> newx    = seq(0,1.5, length=100)
> # Using the meta-regression and calculate the predicted values
> preds   = predict(metaReg.RE.REML, newmods = newx, transf=exp)
> # Use the inverse-variance to create a weighting for the data
> wi      = 1/sqrt(ES.IHD$vi+metaReg.RE.REML$tau2)
```

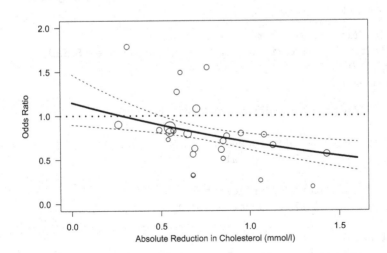

FIGURE 7.3
Plot for the meta-regression from the random-effects model for IHD data.

```
> size   =  1 + 2*(wi - min(wi))/(max(wi) - min(wi))
> # Plot the OR
> plot(ES.IHD$chol, exp(ES.IHD$yi),pch = 1,cex = size,
  xlim=c(0, 1.6), ylim=c(0,2), las = 1, bty = "l",
  ylab = "Odds Ratio", xlab = "Absolute Reduction in Cholesterol
  (mmol/l)")
> # Add a thicker line for the meta-regression
> lines(newx, preds$pred, lwd=3)
> # Add the CIs
> lines(newx, preds$ci.lb, lty = "dashed")
> lines(newx, preds$ci.ub, lty = "dashed")
> # Add a dotted horizontal line for equal-effectiveness
> abline(h = 1, lwd=3,lty = "dotted")
```

7.4.4   Comparison of Different Fitting Methods

As pointed in Section 7.3.1, there are several methods in `rma` for fitting a fixed- or a random-effects model. The `method="FE"` is for fixed-effects models. For random-effects models, there are choices to estimate the variance τ^2; i.e., the DerSimonian-Laird estimator specified as `method="DL"`, the Hunter-Schmidt estimator specified as `method="HS"`, the Hedges estimator specified as `method="HE"`, the Sidik-Jonkman estimator specified as `method="SJ"`, the empirical Bayes estimator specified as `method="EB"`, the maximum-likelihood estimator specified as `method="ML"` and the restricted maximum-likelihood estimator specified as `method="REML"`. Different methods to estimate τ^2 will impact outcomes from the meta-regression. We are illustrating this impact using the ICH data which can be easily implemented as in the following R code chunk:

```
> # The fixed-effects meta-regression
> metaReg.FE = rma(yi, vi, mods = ~chol, data = ES.IHD,
  method="FE")
> metaReg.FE

Fixed-Effects with Moderators Model (k = 28)

Test for Residual Heterogeneity:
QE(df = 26) = 38.2448, p-val = 0.0575

Test of Moderators (coefficient 2):
QM(df = 1) = 11.6748, p-val = 0.0006

Model Results:
          estimate      se     zval    pval    ci.lb    ci.ub
intrcpt     0.1153  0.0972   1.1861  0.2356  -0.0752   0.3059
chol       -0.4723  0.1382  -3.4168  0.0006  -0.7432  -0.2014  ***
```

```
---
Signif. codes:  0 *** 0.001 ** 0.01 * 0.05 . 0.1

> # The random-effects meta-regression with "DL"
> metaReg.RE.DL = rma(yi, vi, mods = ~chol, data = ES.IHD,
    method="DL")
> metaReg.RE.DL

Mixed-Effects Model (k = 28; tau^2 estimator: DL)

tau^2(estimated amount of residual heterogeneity):   0.0170
                                                     (SE = 0.0162)
tau(square root of estimated tau^2 value):           0.1305
I^2(residual heterogeneity/unaccounted variability):32.02%
H^2(unaccounted variability/sampling variability):   1.47
R^2(amount of heterogeneity accounted for):          42.75%


Test for Residual Heterogeneity:
QE(df = 26) = 38.2448, p-val = 0.0575

Test of Moderators (coefficient 2):
QM(df = 1) = 8.0471, p-val = 0.0046

Model Results:
          estimate      se     zval    pval    ci.lb    ci.ub
intrcpt     0.1491  0.1378   1.0826  0.2790  -0.1209   0.4192
chol       -0.5137  0.1811  -2.8367  0.0046  -0.8686  -0.1588  **
---
Signif. codes:  0 *** 0.001 ** 0.01 * 0.05 . 0.1

> # The random-effects meta-regression with "HS"
> metaReg.RE.HS = rma(yi, vi, mods = ~chol, data = ES.IHD,
    method="HS")
> metaReg.RE.HS

Mixed-Effects Model (k = 28; tau^2 estimator: HS)

tau^2(estimated amount of residual heterogeneity):    0.0116
                                                      (SE=0.0114)
tau(square root of estimated tau^2 value):            0.1076
I^2(residual heterogeneity/unaccounted variability):  24.25%
H^2(unaccounted variability / sampling variability):  1.32
R^2(amount of heterogeneity accounted for):           53.26%


Test for Residual Heterogeneity:
QE(df = 26) = 38.2448, p-val = 0.0575
```

```
Test of Moderators (coefficient 2):
QM(df = 1) = 8.8185, p-val = 0.0030


Model Results:
          estimate      se     zval    pval    ci.lb    ci.ub
intrcpt     0.1404  0.1276   1.1005  0.2711  -0.1097   0.3905
chol       -0.5032  0.1694  -2.9696  0.0030  -0.8353  -0.1711  **
---
Signif. codes: 0 *** 0.001 ** 0.01 * 0.05 . 0.1

> # The random-effects meta-regression with "HE"
> metaReg.RE.HE = rma(yi, vi, mods = ~chol, data = ES.IHD,
  method="HE")
> metaReg.RE.HE


Mixed-Effects Model (k = 28; tau^2 estimator: HE)


tau^2(estimated amount of residual heterogeneity):   0.0618
                                                  (SE=0.2090)
tau (square root of estimated tau^2 value):          0.2486
I^2 (residual heterogeneity/unaccounted variability): 63.08%
H^2 (unaccounted variability/sampling variability): 2.71
R^2 (amount of heterogeneity accounted for):         0.00%


Test for Residual Heterogeneity:
QE(df = 26) = 38.2448, p-val = 0.0575


Test of Moderators (coefficient 2):
QM(df = 1) = 5.0345, p-val = 0.0248


Model Results:
          estimate      se     zval    pval    ci.lb    ci.ub
intrcpt     0.1895  0.1962   0.9661  0.3340  -0.1950   0.5741
chol       -0.5647  0.2517  -2.2438  0.0248  -1.0579  -0.0714  *
---
Signif. codes:  0 *** 0.001 ** 0.01 * 0.05 . 0.1

> # The random-effects meta-regression with "SJ"
> metaReg.RE.SJ = rma(yi, vi, mods = ~chol, data = ES.IHD,
  method="SJ")
> metaReg.RE.SJ


Mixed-Effects Model (k = 28; tau^2 estimator: SJ)


tau^2 (estimated amount of residual heterogeneity):  0.1389
                                                  (SE=0.0618)
```

```
tau (square root of estimated tau^2 value):          0.3727
I^2 (residual heterogeneity/unaccounted variability): 79.34%
H^2 (unaccounted variability/sampling variability): 4.84
R^2 (amount of heterogeneity accounted for):         12.50%


Test for Residual Heterogeneity:
QE(df = 26) = 38.2448, p-val = 0.0575


Test of Moderators (coefficient 2):
QM(df = 1) = 3.3004, p-val = 0.0693


Model Results:
          estimate      se     zval    pval    ci.lb    ci.ub
intrcpt     0.2169  0.2619   0.8279  0.4077  -0.2966   0.7303
chol       -0.6053  0.3332  -1.8167  0.0693  -1.2584   0.0477  .
---
Signif. codes:  0 *** 0.001 ** 0.01 * 0.05 . 0.1

> # The random-effects meta-regression with "ML"
> metaReg.RE.ML = rma(yi, vi, mods = ~chol, data = ES.IHD,
    method="ML")
> metaReg.RE.ML

Mixed-Effects Model (k = 28; tau^2 estimator: ML)

tau^2 (estimated amount of residual heterogeneity):   0.0000
                                                   (SE=0.0045)
tau (square root of estimated tau^2 value):          0.0022
I^2 (residual heterogeneity/unaccounted variability): 0.01%
H^2 (unaccounted variability / sampling variability): 1.00
R^2 (amount of heterogeneity accounted for):         99.98%


Test for Residual Heterogeneity:
QE(df = 26) = 38.2448, p-val = 0.0575


Test of Moderators (coefficient 2):
QM(df = 1) = 11.6726, p-val = 0.0006


Model Results:
          estimate      se     zval    pval    ci.lb    ci.ub
intrcpt     0.1153  0.0972   1.1860  0.2356  -0.0753   0.3059
chol       -0.4723  0.1382  -3.4165  0.0006  -0.7432  -0.2013  ***
---
Signif. codes: 0 *** 0.001 ** 0.01 * 0.05 . 0.1

> # The random-effects meta-regression with "EB"
```

```
> metaReg.RE.EB = rma(yi, vi, mods = ~chol, data = ES.IHD,
    method="EB")
> metaReg.RE.EB

Mixed-Effects Model (k = 28; tau^2 estimator: EB)

tau^2 (estimated amount of residual heterogeneity):   0.0299
                                                     (SE=0.0244)
tau (square root of estimated tau^2 value):           0.1730
I^2 (residual heterogeneity/unaccounted variability): 45.28%
H^2 (unaccounted variability / sampling variability): 1.83
R^2 (amount of heterogeneity accounted for):          45.35%


Test for Residual Heterogeneity:
QE(df = 26) = 38.2448, p-val = 0.0575


Test of Moderators (coefficient 2):
QM(df = 1) = 6.7671, p-val = 0.0093


Model Results:
          estimate      se     zval    pval    ci.lb    ci.ub
intrcpt     0.1651  0.1579   1.0454  0.2958  -0.1444   0.4746
chol       -0.5331  0.2049  -2.6014  0.0093  -0.9348  -0.1314  **

---
Signif. codes:  0 *** 0.001 ** 0.01 * 0.05 . 0.1
```

We summarize the results from this series of model fittings along with the meta-analysis in Section 7.4.2 and the meta-regression in Section 7.4.3 in Table 7.3.

In this table, the column "Method" denotes the fitting method with the first "Meta" for meta-analysis in Section 7.4.2, "FE" for fixed-effects meta-regression, and the next 7 for random-effects regression analyses (prefixed

TABLE 7.3
Summary of Model Fittings

Method	Intercept(SE)	Slope(SE)	$\hat{\tau}^2$	$\hat{Q}$	p-value
Meta	−0.219(0.057)	NA	0.032	49.920	0.005
FE	0.115(0.097)	−0.472(0.138)	0.000	38.245	0.057
RE.DL	0.149(0.138)	−0.514(0.181)	0.017	38.245	0.057
RE.HS	0.140(0.128)	−0.503(0.169)	0.012	38.245	0.057
RE.HE	0.190(0.196)	−0.565(0.252)	0.062	38.245	0.057
RE.SJ	0.217(0.262)	−0.605(0.333)	0.139	38.245	0.057
RE.ML	0.115(0.097)	−0.472(0.138)	0.000	38.245	0.057
RE.EB	0.165(0.158)	−0.533(0.205)	0.030	38.245	0.057
RE.REML	0.139(0.126)	−0.501(0.167)	0.011	38.245	0.057

with "RE"). The second and third columns are the estimated intercept and slope along with their standard errors from the meta-regression. Notice that for meta-analysis (i.e., the first row), there is no estimated slope parameter which is denoted by "NA." The column labeled $\hat{\tau}^2$ is the estimated between (residual)-variance where $\hat{\tau}^2 = 0$ is for fixed-effects (i.e., "FE") meta-regression. The last two columns are for the estimated heterogeneity (Q) quantity and its associated p-value from the χ^2-test and they are the same for all meta-regressions since $\hat{Q}$ is independent of the $\hat{\tau}^2$. From this table, we can see that the estimates for the parameters and between-study variance are slightly different. However, the fundamental conclusion is the same; i.e., there is a statistically significant relationship between the serum cholesterol reduction and IHD risk reduction.

Similar analyses can be performed by using different measures of study effects. For this data, we used log odds-ratio. Other possible choices are Peto's log odds-ratio, log relative risk, risk difference, and the arcsine transformed risk difference. Analyses can be performed with the library `metafor`, using the function `escalc` to specify `measure=PETO` for Peto's log odds-ratio, `measure=RR` for log relative risk, `measure=RD` for risk difference, and `measure=AS` for the arcsine-transformed risk difference. We leave these as exercises for interested readers.

7.5 Meta-Analysis of ADHD Data

7.5.1 Data and Variables

The data can be loaded into R using library `gdata` as follows:

```
> # Load the library
> require(readxl)
> # Get the data path
> datfile = "File path to ExcelBook 'dat4Meta.xls'"
> # Call "read_excel" to read the Excel data in specific data
    sheet
> dat.ADHD = read_excel(datfile, sheet="Data.adhd", na = "NA")
> # Print the dimmension of the dataframe
> dim(dat.ADHD)
```

```
[1] 41 26
```

We do not intend to print the whole data set since it contains a large number of rows and columns. Readers can print the data set and compare it with the values from Tables 1 and 2 from the paper. It can be seen that there are 41 rows (i.e., 41 studies) and 26 columns (i.e., 26 variables associated with each study).

The dependent variable was chosen as the SSRT difference between ADHD and control subjects with the associated variance (named as `ssrt12ssrtc` and `var.ssrta2ssrtc` in the dataframe). Two variables were chosen to be the independent variables for the meta-regression. One is the reaction time in the control (i.e., `crt`) which is a global index indicator of Go task complexity and it is continuous. The other independent variable is the spatial compatibility (named as `cmp` which is a more specific index of stimulus-response mapping in the Go task and is nominal variable with "−1" as "spatially noncompatible" and "1" as "spatially compatible."

7.5.2 Meta-Analysis

We first look into the SSRT difference between ADHD and control subjects which can be implemented into `metafor` as meta-regression without independent variables. The R code chunk is as follows:

```
> # Call `rma' from metafor for default random-effect MA
> metareg.No = rma(ssrta2ssrtc,var.ssrta2ssrtc, data = dat.ADHD)
> # Print the summary
> metareg.No
```

```
Random-Effects Model (k = 41; tau^2 estimator: REML)

tau^2 (estimated amount of total heterogeneity):349.0573
                                                (SE=239.2865)
tau (square root of estimated tau^2 value):      18.6831
I^2 (total heterogeneity/total variability):     32.87%
H^2 (total variability/sampling variability): 1.49


Test for Heterogeneity:
Q(df = 40) = 63.4688, p-val = 0.0105


Model Results:
estimate       se     zval     pval     ci.lb     ci.ub
 67.3725   5.4115  12.4499   <.0001   56.7662   77.9789  ***
---
Signif. codes:  0 *** 0.001 ** 0.01 * 0.05 . 0.1
```

From the summary, we can see that the average SSRT difference between ADHD and control is 67.37 which is statistically significantly different from zero (p-value < 0.001). Furthermore, a statistically significant variation between studies was found as indicated by the heterogeneity statistic $Q=63.4688$ with df of 40 and p-value $= 0.0105$.

Readers can use R library `rmeta` or `meta` to reproduce these results and we leave this as practice for interested readers.

7.5.3   Meta-Regression Analysis

To identify the sources of heterogeneity, a meta-regression between SSRT difference and task complexity as assessed by RTc can be conducted to explain the extra-heterogeneity. The R implementation can be done using the R code chunk as follows:

```
> # Meta-regression to RTc
> metareg.crt <- rma(ssrta2ssrtc,var.ssrta2ssrtc, mods =~crt,
                                           data = dat.ADHD)
> # Print the summary
> metareg.crt

Mixed-Effects Model (k = 35; tau^2 estimator: REML)
tau^2 (estimated amount of residual heterogeneity):   218.9710
                                                    (SE=230.0648)
tau (square root of estimated tau^2 value):           14.7977
I^2 (residual heterogeneity/unaccounted variability): 22.26%
H^2 (unaccounted variability / sampling variability): 1.29
R^2 (amount of heterogeneity accounted for):          31.12%


Test for Residual Heterogeneity:
QE(df = 33) = 44.8954, p-val = 0.0811


Test of Moderators (coefficient 2):
QM(df = 1) = 3.4841, p-val = 0.0620


Model Results:
          estimate       se    zval    pval     ci.lb     ci.ub
intrcpt    16.8440  24.4404  0.6892  0.4907  -31.0583   64.7463
crt         0.0779   0.0417  1.8666  0.0620   -0.0039    0.1597
```

A great feature for this **metafor** library is the plotting functionality and can be used to display the typical forest plot, residual funnel plot, and other residual plots by simply calling the **plot** command as follows to produce Figure 7.4:

```
> # Plot all from this meta-regression
> plot(metareg.crt)
```

We can see from these figures again that the SSRT difference between ADHD and control is statistically significantly larger than zero. The funnel plot and the two other residual plots indicate symmetry and no systematic deviations. From the summary of the meta-regression, we can conclude that there is a positive regression ($\hat{\beta} = 0.0779$ with p-value $= 0.0620$) between the SSRT difference and the task complexity as measured by RTc. With this

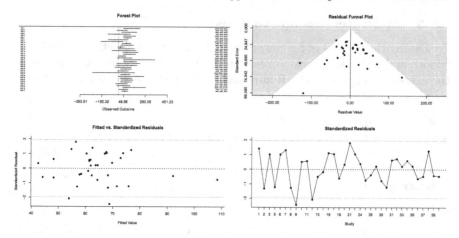

FIGURE 7.4
All plots from the meta-regression.

meta-regression, the heterogeneity statistic is now reduced to $Q = 44.8954$ which is now statistically nonsignificant (p-value $= 0.0811$). This relationship can be graphically illustrated in Figure 7.5.
which is produced using the following R code chunk:

```
> # Figure 1 from the paper
> plot(ssrta2ssrtc~crt, las=1, xlab="RTc", ylab="SSRTa-SSRTc",
                                        data = dat.ADHD)
> # Add the meta-regression line to the plot
> abline(metareg.crt$b, lwd=2)
> # Fill `spatilly compatible"
> points(ssrta2ssrtc~crt,data=dat.ADHD[dat.ADHD$cmp==1,], pch=16)
```

From this figure, a positive relationship between the SSRT difference and RTc can be seen graphically which is consistent with the meta-regression summary from the above analysis. In addition, it can be seen from this figure that small SSRT differences are associated with spatially compatible responses as denoted by the filled circles and large SSRT differences with noncompatible responses as denoted by the open circles.

This observation can be statistically tested by meta-regression using the following R code chunk:

```
> # Meta-regression to spatially compatible response
> metareg.cmp = rma(ssrta2ssrtc,var.ssrta2ssrtc, mods =~cmp,
                                        data = dat.ADHD)
> # Print the summary
> metareg.cmp
```

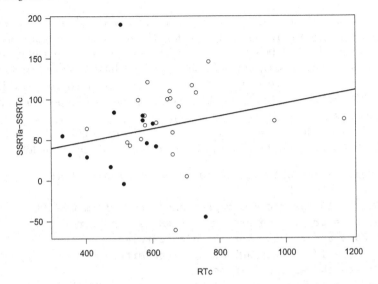

FIGURE 7.5
Reproduction of Figure 1 in the original paper for SSRT differences between subjects with ADHD and control subjects as a function of RTc for studies with spatially compatible (filled circles) versus a noncompatible mapping (open circles).

```
Mixed-Effects Model (k = 41; tau^2 estimator: REML)

tau^2 (estimated amount of residual heterogeneity):   210.4249
                                                     (SE=202.7994)
tau (square root of estimated tau^2 value):            14.5060
I^2 (residual heterogeneity/unaccounted variability): 22.36%
H^2 (unaccounted variability/sampling variability): 1.29
R^2 (amount of heterogeneity accounted for):           39.72%


Test for Residual Heterogeneity:
QE(df = 39) = 51.3191, p-val = 0.0895

Test of Moderators (coefficient 2):
QM(df = 1) = 6.8837, p-val = 0.0087

Model Results:
          estimate      se     zval    pval    ci.lb    ci.ub
intrcpt    63.9132  5.0850  12.5691  <.0001  53.9469  73.8795  ***
cmp       -13.3413  5.0850  -2.6237  0.0087 -23.3076  -3.3750  **
---
Signif. codes:  0 *** 0.001 ** 0.01 * 0.05 . 0.1
```

It can be seen from the summary that there was indeed a statistically significant relationship with spatial compatibility (slope estimate of $\hat{\beta} = 13.34$ and p-value $= 0.0087$). Incorporating this spatial compatibility effect into meta-regression as an independent variable reduced between-study variation; the heterogeneity statistic $Q = 51.32$ as compared to the original Q of 63.4688. With this independent variable, the test of heterogeneity is statistically significant (p-value $= 0.0087$).

To include all the meta-regression results into Figure 7.5, a better presentation can be produced with the following R code chunk as follows:

```
> # Create a new data series to cover the range of RTc
> new.crt = 300:1200
> # Calculate the predict values and the CI from the MR
> preds   = predict(metareg.crt, newmods = new.crt)
> # Create the weights for the size circles
> wi      = 1/sqrt(dat.ADHD$var.ssrta2ssrtc)
> # Create the size of circles
> size    = 1+2*(wi - min(wi))/(max(wi) - min(wi))
> # Make the plot
> plot(ssrta2ssrtc~crt, las=1, xlab="RTc", cex=size,
                    ylab="SSRTa-SSRTc",data = dat.ADHD)
> # Add the regression line
> abline(metareg.crt$b, lwd=2)
> # Use filled circles for `spatially compatibility
> points(ssrta2ssrtc~crt,data=dat.ADHD[dat.ADHD$cmp==1,],
    cex=size,pch=16)
> # Add CIs
> lines(new.crt, preds$ci.lb, lty = "dashed")
> lines(new.crt, preds$ci.ub, lty = "dashed")
> # Add the significant line
> abline(h = 1, lty = "dotted", lwd=3)
```

This produces a better presentation as seen in Figure 7.6.

7.5.4   Summary of ADHD Meta-Analysis

Readers can see that we have reproduced the results from Huizenga et al. (2009) that SSRT for ADHD subjects was significantly higher than for normal control subjects, and task complexity was significantly related to SSRT differences and explained part of the heterogeneity. In practice, these differences could be related to other variables as seen from the data. Huizenga et al. (2009) discussed further tests for potential confounders and we leave this further analysis to interested readers as practice.

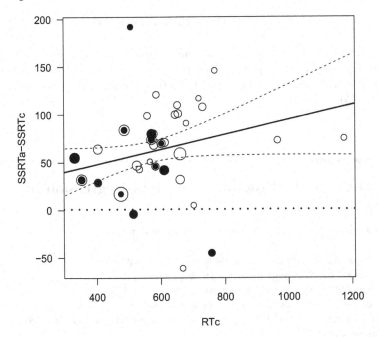

FIGURE 7.6
The summary plot for the data and the meta-regression.

7.6 Discussion

In this chapter, we discussed meta-regression to use study-level moderators to account for extra-heterogeneity in meta-analysis. The methods for meta-regression are essentially a special case of regression with weightings obtained from within-study and between-study which can be fixed-effects and random-effects models. With meta-regression models, we can quantify the relationship between study effect-sizes and extra study moderators and test their statistical significance.

We illustrated the models used in meta-regression with three data sets from the literature using the R library `metafor`. We showed how straightforward it is to use this library for any kind of meta-regression as well as meta-analysis.

There are many references and books discussing methods and applications in meta-regression. The utility of this chapter is to illustrate these developed methodologies and their step-by-step implementation in R. Interested readers can follow the steps and reuse the R for their own research and meta-regression analysis.

We have referred to some books and publications in this chapter. We further recommend the paper by Thompson and Higgins (2002) and the books by Roberts and Stanley (2005), Petitti (2000), Pigott (2012), and Schwarzer et al. (2015) to readers.

Appendix: Stata Programs for Meta-Regression by Manyun Liu

The Stata program below corresponds to the R program.

```
/*### Reproduce R Results in Section 7.1.1 ###*/
/* Because the dat.bcg data is in R metafor,
   we created a new Excel document sheet Data_bcg
   for dat4Meta.xls to provide the data. */
/* You can use the following command to load the excel file */
/*Changes the wd*/
cd "File path to the ExcelBook"
import excel using dat4Meta.xls, sheet("Data_bcg") firstrow clear

/* present the data */
browse

/* Or we can use list command to present the data */
list

/*### Reproduce R Results in Section 7.1.2 ###*/
/* You can use the following command to load the excel file */
import excel using dat4Meta.xls, sheet("Data.IHD") firstrow clear
list

/*### Reproduce R Results in Section 7.3.1 ###*/
/* This part is specific to R, which utilizes R metafor.
We utilize alternative Stata code to produce similar results*/

import excel using dat4Meta.xls, sheet("Data_bcg") firstrow clear
meta esize tpos tneg cpos cneg, esize(lnrratio) fixed(mhaenszel)
generate yi= _meta_es
generate vi= _meta_se^2
list trial tpos tneg cpos cneg ablat yi vi

/* Call `meta' to fit the BCG data */
meta esize tpos tneg cpos cneg, esize(lnrratio)
```

```
/* Print the summary */
meta summarize, random(reml)

meta forestplot, random(reml)

/*### Reproduce R Results in Section 7.3.2 ###*/
/* alloc as a categorical moderator is not allowed in Stata meta*/

meta regress ablat year

meta regress ablat

/*This graphic part is unique to R, we produce a bubble plot instead*/
estat bubbleplot, xtitle("Absolute Latitude")
  lineopts(color(black)lwidth(medthick))
  color(black) ciopts(lpattern(dash))


/*### Reproduce R Results in Section 7.3.3 ###*/
/* Create the weighting factor
      metaReg.ablat$tau2=0.07635469 */
generate wi = 1/(vi+0.07635469)

/* weighted regression */
regress yi ablat [aweight=wi]

/* Take the response vector */
mkmat yi
matrix y = yi

/* Make the design matrix */
mkmat ablat
matrix X=(1\1\1\1\1\1\1\1\1\1\1\1\1),ablat

/* Make the weight matrix */
mkmat wi
matrix W = diag(wi)

/* Calculate the parameter estimate */
matrix betahat = inv(X'*W*X)*X'*W*y

/* Calculate the estimated variance */
matrix betahat_temp=inv(X'*W*X)
matrix var_betahat = vecdiag(betahat_temp)

/* Calculate the standard error */
ssc install matmap
matmap var_betahat se_betahat, map(sqrt(@))
```

```
/* Calculate z-value assuming asymptotic normal */
matrix z = J(2,1,0)
matrix se_betahat = se_betahat'
forvalues i = 1/2  {
matrix z[`i',1]= betahat[`i',1]/se_betahat[`i',1]
}

/* Calculate the p-value */
matrix pval = J(2,1,0)
forvalues i = 1/2  {
matrix pval[`i',1]= 2*(1-normal(abs(z[`i',1])))
}

/* Calculate the 95% CI */
matrix ci_lb = J(2,1,0)
forvalues i = 1/2  {
matrix ci_lb[`i',1]= betahat[`i',1]-1.96*se_betahat[`i',1]
}
matrix ci_ub = J(2,1,0)
forvalues i = 1/2  {
matrix ci_ub[`i',1]= betahat[`i',1]+1.96*se_betahat[`i',1]
}

/* Make the output similar to metaReg.ablat */
matrix Mod_Results = betahat,se_betahat,z,pval,ci_lb,ci_ub
matrix rownames Mod_Results = intrcpt ablat
matrix colnames Mod_Results = betahat se_betahat z pval ci_lb ci_ub
matmap Mod_Results Mod_Results, map(round(@,0.0001))

/* Print the result */
matrix list Mod_Results

/*### Reproduce R Results in Section 7.4.1 ###*/
/* Load the Excel data  with specific data sheet */
import excel using dat4Meta.xls, sheet("Data.IHD") firstrow clear

/*### Reproduce R Results in Section 7.4.2 ###*/
meta esize tpos tneg cpos cneg
generate yi= _meta_es
generate vi= _meta_se^2
list trial cpos cneg tpos tneg chol yi vi

/* Call `meta' to fit the BCG data */
meta esize tpos tneg cpos cneg

/* Print the summary */
meta summarize, random(reml)

/*### Reproduce R Results in Section 7.4.2.1 ###*/
```

```
meta regress chol

estat bubbleplot, xtitle("Absolute Reduction in
        Cholesterol (mmol/l)")
lineopts(color(black)lwidth(medthick)) color(black)
        ciopts(lpattern(dash))

/*### Reproduce R Results in Section 7.4.3 ###*/
/* The fixed-effects meta-regression */
meta regress chol, fixed

/* The random-effects meta-regression with "DL" */
meta regress chol, random(dlaird)

/* The random-effects meta-regression with "HS" */
meta regress chol, random(hschmidt)

/* The random-effects meta-regression with "HE" */
meta regress chol, random(hedges)

/* The random-effects meta-regression with "SJ" */
meta regress chol, random(sjonkman)

/* The random-effects meta-regression with "ML" */
meta regress chol, random(mle)

/* The random-effects meta-regression with "EB" */
meta regress chol, random(ebayes)

/*### Reproduce R Results in Section 7.5.1 ###*/
/* Load the Excel data  with specific data sheet */
import excel using dat4Meta.xls, sheet("Data.adhd") firstrow clear

/* Describe the dataframe */
describe

/*### Reproduce R Results in Section 7.5.2 ###*/
generate sessrta2ssrtc=sqrt(varssrta2ssrtc)
metareg ssrta2ssrtc, wsse(sessrta2ssrtc) bsest(reml)

/*### Reproduce R Results in Section 7.5.3 ###*/
/* Meta-regression to RTc */
destring crt, replace ignore(NA)
metareg ssrta2ssrtc crt, wsse(sessrta2ssrtc) bsest(reml)

/* metareg of Stata only offers bubble plot */
metareg ssrta2ssrtc crt, wsse(sessrta2ssrtc) bsest(reml) graph

/* similar Figure 1 from the paper */
```

```
metareg ssrta2ssrtc crt, wsse(sessrta2ssrtc) graph

/* Meta-regression to spatially compatible response */
metareg ssrta2ssrtc cmp, wsse(sessrta2ssrtc) bsest(reml)

/* similar Figure 7.5 */
metareg ssrta2ssrtc crt, wsse(sessrta2ssrtc) bsest(reml)
predict fit
predict stdp, stdp
predict stdf, stdf
gen t = invttail(e(df_r)-1, 0.025)
gen confl = fit - t*stdp
gen confu = fit + t*stdp
sort crt
gen wi = 1/sqrt(varssrta2ssrtc)
egen min=min(wi)
egen max=max(wi)
gen size = 1+2*(wi - min)/(max - min)
gen byte compatibility1 = cmp > 0
gen compatibility=compatibility1*crt
mvdecode compatibility, mv(0=.)
twoway rarea confl confu crt,lpattern(dash) lcolor(black) ||
line fit crt,lcolor(black)|| ,
yline(1,lpattern(dot) lcolor(black))||
scatter ssrta2ssrtc crt[aw=size], msymbol(Oh)||
scatter ssrta2ssrtc compatibility[aw=size],mfcolor(black)|| ,
xtitle("RTc") ytitle("SSRTa-SSRTc")
```

8

Multivariate Meta-Analysis

It is not uncommon for studies to have multiple outcome measures which lead to statistical multivariate analysis. For example, the data set lui in Section 15.3 contains two correlation coefficients between land use intensity and response diversity (variable named as r.FDis) or functional redundancy (variable named as r.nbsp) along with the total observations (variable named as n) across 18 land use intensity gradients from nine countries and five biomes. There are more examples in multivariate meta-analysis literature (Bujkiewicz et al., 2013; Jackson et al., 2011; Riley, 2009). For example, in medical research, we often compare multiple outcomes at multiple time points between different intervention groups as seen in Ishak et al. (2007).

The results of studies with multiple outcomes and/or endpoints are typically synthesized via conventional univariate meta-analysis (UMA) on each outcome separately, ignoring the correlations between the outcomes. For example, in the field of orthopedic surgery, when the effect of an antifibrinolytic agent on two outcomes of operative blood loss and blood transfusions is of interest, two univariate meta-analyses were utilized for pooling each effect size and for estimating their related precision. A joint synthesis of the amounts of blood loss and blood transfusions would, however, be more meaningful as the two outcomes are clearly correlated (higher amount of blood loss needing higher number of blood transfusions). The impact of ignoring the within-study correlation has been explored extensively in the statistical literature, with issues including overestimated variance of the pooled effect size and biased estimates, which in turn may influence statistical inferences. In this case, multivariate meta-analysis should be used to synthesize multiple outcomes while taking into account their correlations, often resulting in superior parameter estimation. The goal of this chapter is therefore to increase the awareness of the advantages of multivariate meta-analysis and promote its use.

Methodologically, multivariate meta-analysis is an extension of the UMA with multiple outcome measures where the correlations among the multiple outcomes are taken into account. With study-level moderators or predictors, multivariate meta-regression can also be developed in parallel with multivariate regression techniques.

In this chapter, we introduce multivariate meta-analysis using the R package mvmeta as detailed in Gasparrini and Kenward (2012). This package includes a collection of functions to perform fixed- and random-effects multivariate meta-analysis along with UMA as well as meta-regression. We further illustrate the R package `metafor` for comparison.

8.1   The Model and the Package of `mvmeta`

Suppose there are M outcomes $\mathbf{y_i} = (y_{1i}, y_{2i}, \ldots, y_{Mi})$ reported from K studies where $\mathbf{y_i}$ is the vector of M outcomes of y_{mi} from the mth $(m = 1, \ldots, M)$ outcome and ith study $(i = 1, \ldots, K)$. For p-study level moderators or predictors, the general multivariate meta-regression model is formulated as follows:

$$\mathbf{y_i} \sim N_M(\mathbf{X_i}\beta, \mathbf{S_i} + \Psi) \tag{8.1}$$

where $\mathbf{y_i}$ is distributed as multivariate normal with mean $\mathbf{X_i}\beta$ and variance-covariance matrix of $\mathbf{S_i} + \Psi$. In this formulation, $\mathbf{X_i}$ is a $K \times Kp$ design matrix and β is the vector of fixed-effects coefficients. $\mathbf{S_i}$ is the within-covariance matrix from the M outcomes which is assumed known. Ψ is the so-called between-study covariance matrix which is assumed to be zero for fixed-effects meta-models, but estimated from the data in random-effects meta-models.

It is easily seen that when $p=1$, the general multivariate meta-regression model (8.1) becomes the multivariate meta-analysis model where $\mathbf{X_i}$ reduces to an identity matrix and β reduces to the intercepts. When $M = 1$, this model reduces to the corresponding univariate meta-regression or meta-analysis model.

Therefore, the purpose is to estimate and make statistical inference for the coefficients β and, for random-effects models, estimate the between-study covariance matrix Ψ as seen in equation (8.1). The R package `mvmeta` was developed for this purpose.

This R package is accessed from http://cran.r-project.org/web/packages/mvmeta/index.html. The reference manual is in the pdf file `mvmeta.pdf`. With this package installed in R, the reader can access its help manual using `library(help=mvmeta)`. We use some examples from this package in this chapter to further promote and illustrate its functionalities.

8.2   Bivariate Meta-Data from Five Clinical Trials on Periodontal Disease

There are several examples on multivariate meta-data in the `mvmeta` package. We illustrate multivariate meta-analysis using data `berkey98` which includes five published clinical trials on periodontal disease as reported in Berkey et al. (1998, 1995).

When the package is installed in R, it can be accessed by calling the library as follows:

```
> library(mvmeta)
```

This `berkey98` meta-data is loaded into R as follows:

```
> # Load the Data
> data(berkey98)
> # Print the data
> berkey98
```

```
           pubyear npat   PD    AL var_PD cov_PD_AL var_AL
Pihlstrom     1983   14 0.47 -0.32 0.0075    0.0030 0.0077
Lindhe        1982   15 0.20 -0.60 0.0057    0.0009 0.0008
Knowles       1979   78 0.40 -0.12 0.0021    0.0007 0.0014
Ramfjord      1987   89 0.26 -0.31 0.0029    0.0009 0.0015
Becker        1988   16 0.56 -0.39 0.0148    0.0072 0.0304
```

It is seen that this data set includes five published studies that compare surgical and nonsurgical treatments for medium-severity periodontal disease. The two outcome measures are average improvement (surgical minus non-surgical, in mm) in probing depth (PD) and attachment level (AL). In this dataframe, seven variables are reported with **pubyear** as the publication year of the trial, **npat** as the number of patients in each trial, PD as the estimated improvement from surgical to nonsurgical treatment in PD (mm), AL as the estimated improvement from surgical to nonsurgical treatment in AL (mm), var_PD as the variance for PD, cov_PD_AL as the covariance between PD and AL and var_AL as the variance for AL.

8.3   Meta-Analysis with R Package mvmeta

8.3.1   Fixed-Effects Meta-Analysis

The fixed-effects meta-analysis is implemented using `method="fixed"` as follows:

```
> # Call mvmeta with fixed-effects
> berkey.mvmeta.fixed = mvmeta(cbind(PD,AL),
          S=berkey98[,c("var_PD","cov_PD_AL","var_AL")],
          method="fixed",data=berkey98)
> # Print the summary
> summary(berkey.mvmeta.fixed)
```

```
Call:  mvmeta(formula = cbind(PD, AL) ~ 1, S = berkey98[,
         c("var_PD", "cov_PD_AL", "var_AL")], data = berkey98,
         method = "fixed")
```

```
Multivariate fixed-effects meta-analysis
Dimension: 2
```

```
Fixed-effects coefficients
      Estimate  Std. Error        z Pr(>|z|)  95%ci.lb  95%ci.ub
PD      0.3072      0.0286  10.7513   0.0000    0.2512   0.3632***
AL     -0.3944      0.0186 -21.1471   0.0000   -0.4309  -0.3578***
```

```
Multivariate Cochran Q-test for heterogeneity:
Q = 128.2267 (df = 8), p-value = 0.0000
I-square statistic = 93.8%
```

```
5 studies,10 observations,2 fixed and 0 random-effects parameters
   logLik      AIC        BIC
-45.4416   94.8833   95.4884
```

From the output, we note that both PD and AL are statistically significant with estimates of effects of 0.3072 and -0.3944 for PD and AL, respectively. And there is statistically significant heterogeneity as reported by the Multivariate Cochran Q-test for heterogeneity with $Q = 128.2267$ ($df = 8$) which gives a p-value $= 0.0000$.

8.3.2   Random-Effects Meta-Analysis

The random-effects meta-model with default method of "REML" is illustrated as follows:

```
> berkey.mvmeta.REML = mvmeta(cbind(PD,AL), method="reml",
    S=berkey98[,c("var_PD","cov_PD_AL","var_AL")],data=berkey98)
> #Print the summary
> summary(berkey.mvmeta.REML)
```

```
Call:  mvmeta(formula = cbind(PD, AL) ~ 1, S = berkey98[,
         c("var_PD","cov_PD_AL", "var_AL")], data = berkey98,
         method = "reml")
```

```
Multivariate random-effects meta-analysis
Dimension: 2
Estimation method: REML
```

```
Fixed-effects coefficients
      Estimate Std. Error        z  Pr(>|z|)  95%ci.lb  95%ci.ub
```

```
PD     0.3534     0.0588  6.0057     0.0000     0.2381  0.4688 ***
AL    -0.3392     0.0879 -3.8589     0.0001    -0.5115 -0.1669 ***
```

```
Between-study random-effects (co)variance components
Structure: General positive-definite
     Std. Dev   Corr
PD     0.1083     PD
AL     0.1807  0.6088
```

```
Multivariate Cochran Q-test for heterogeneity:
Q = 128.2267 (df = 8), p-value = 0.0000
I-square statistic = 93.8%
```

```
5 studies, 10 observations, 2 fixed, and 3 random-effects
    parameters
logLik    AIC     BIC
2.0823  5.8353  6.2325
```

Again both PD and AL are statistically significant with estimates of effects of 0.3534 and -0.3392 for PD and AL, respectively, with the same conclusion for the test of heterogeneity. For the random-effects meta-model, the estimated between-studies standard deviations are $\hat{\tau}_{PD} = 0.1083$ and $\hat{\tau}_{AL} = 0.1807$ with estimated correlation of 0.6088.

Slightly different estimates (but the same statistical conclusions) will result if the maximum likelihood method is used as seen from the following R code chunk:

```
> berkey.mvmeta.ML = mvmeta(cbind(PD,AL),
    S=berkey98[,c("var_PD","cov_PD_AL","var_AL")],
    method="ml",data=berkey98)
> summary(berkey.mvmeta.ML)
```

```
Call:  mvmeta(formula = cbind(PD, AL) ~ 1, S = berkey98[,
    c("var_PD","cov_PD_AL", "var_AL")], data = berkey98,
    method = "ml")
```

```
Multivariate random-effects meta-analysis
Dimension: 2
Estimation method: ML
```

```
Fixed-effects coefficients
     Estimate Std. Error     z Pr(>|z|) 95%ci.lb  95%ci.ub
PD     0.3448     0.0495  6.9714  0.0000   0.2479   0.4418 ***
AL    -0.3379     0.0798 -4.2365  0.0000  -0.4943  -0.1816 ***
```

```
Between-study random-effects (co)variance components
```

```
Structure: General positive-definite
     Std. Dev    Corr
PD    0.0837      PD
AL    0.1617   0.6992


Multivariate Cochran Q-test for heterogeneity:
Q = 128.2267 (df = 8), p-value = 0.0000
I-square statistic = 93.8%


5 studies,10 observations, 2 fixed and 3 random-effects parameters
  logLik      AIC        BIC
  5.8407   -1.6813   -0.1684
```

8.3.3 Meta-Regression

To account for between-study heterogeneity, we use the study-level moderator, which in this data set is the year of the clinical trial as studyyear. The implementation is straightforward and we only show the random-effects meta-regression with "REML." Interested readers can experiment using the method="fixed" and method="ml".

The R code chunk is as follows:

```
> # meta-reg to study year
> berkey.mvmetareg.REML = mvmeta(cbind(PD,AL)~pubyear,
     S=berkey98[,c("var_PD","cov_PD_AL","var_AL")],data=berkey98)
> # Print the result
> summary(berkey.mvmetareg.REML)

Call:  mvmeta(formula = cbind(PD, AL) ~ pubyear, S = berkey98[,
          c("var_PD","cov_PD_AL", "var_AL")], data = berkey98)

Multivariate random-effects meta-regression
Dimension: 2
Estimation method: REML


Fixed-effects coefficients
PD :
              Estimate Std. Error       z Pr(>|z|) 95%ci.lb 95%ci.ub
(Intercept)    -9.2816    43.3419 -0.2141   0.8304 -94.2302  75.6670
pubyear         0.0049     0.0219  0.2225   0.8239  -0.0380   0.0477


AL :
              Estimate Std. Error       z Pr(>|z|) 95%ci.lb 95%ci.ub
(Intercept)    22.5415    59.4308  0.3793   0.7045 -93.9408 139.0237
pubyear        -0.0115     0.0300 -0.3850   0.7002  -0.0703   0.0472


Between-study random-effects (co)variance components
```

```
Structure: General positive-definite
     Std. Dev   Corr
PD    0.1430     PD
AL    0.2021   0.5614
```

```
Multivariate Cochran Q-test for residual heterogeneity:
Q = 125.7557 (df = 6), p-value = 0.0000
I-square statistic = 95.2%
```

```
5 studies, 10 observations, 4 fixed, and 3 random-effects
    parameters
 logLik      AIC      BIC
-3.5400  21.0799  19.6222
```

It is seen from the summary that the moderator is not statistically significant for any PD (p-value $= 0.8239$) and AL (p-value $= 0.7002$). Because of this nonsignificance, the Cochran heterogeneity statistic Q changed slightly from 128.2267 in the meta-model to 125.7557 in the meta-regression.

8.4 Meta-Analysis with R Package metafor

8.4.1 Rearrange the Data Format

In order to use the metafor package for multivariate meta-analysis, meta-data should be rearranged accordingly. We load the metafor package first:

```
> # Load the package
> library(help=metafor)
```

For example, the data berkey98 are first rearranged by the two outcomes with each outcome as a separate row within the study as follows:

```
> dat.berkey1998
```

	trial	author	year	ni	outcome	yi	vi
1	1	Pihlstrom et al.	1983	14	PD	0.4700	0.0075
2	1	Pihlstrom et al.	1983	14	AL	-0.3200	0.0077
3	2	Lindhe et al.	1982	15	PD	0.2000	0.0057
4	2	Lindhe et al.	1982	15	AL	-0.6000	0.0008
5	3	Knowles et al.	1979	78	PD	0.4000	0.0021
6	3	Knowles et al.	1979	78	AL	-0.1200	0.0014
7	4	Ramfjord et al.	1987	89	PD	0.2600	0.0029
8	4	Ramfjord et al.	1987	89	AL	-0.3100	0.0015
9	5	Becker et al.	1988	16	PD	0.5600	0.0148
10	5	Becker et al.	1988	16	AL	-0.3900	0.0304

```
      v1i    v2i
1   0.0075 0.0030
2   0.0030 0.0077
3   0.0057 0.0009
4   0.0009 0.0008
5   0.0021 0.0007
6   0.0007 0.0014
7   0.0029 0.0009
8   0.0009 0.0015
9   0.0148 0.0072
10  0.0072 0.0304
```

Interested readers can compare this rearranged data with the original data format as follows:

```
> berkey98
```

	pubyear	npat	PD	AL	var_PD	cov_PD_AL	var_AL
Pihlstrom	1983	14	0.47	-0.32	0.0075	0.0030	0.0077
Lindhe	1982	15	0.20	-0.60	0.0057	0.0009	0.0008
Knowles	1979	78	0.40	-0.12	0.0021	0.0007	0.0014
Ramfjord	1987	89	0.26	-0.31	0.0029	0.0009	0.0015
Becker	1988	16	0.56	-0.39	0.0148	0.0072	0.0304

With this rearranged data format, we then construct a list of the variance-covariance matrices of the observed outcomes for the five studies to create a block diagonal matrix, V, for `metafor`:

```
> # Rearrange the variance-covariance matrices for each study
> V = lapply(split(dat.berkey1998[,c("v1i", "v2i")],
                    dat.berkey1998$trial), as.matrix)
> # Print the V
> # Construct block diagonal matrix
> V <- bldiag(V)
> # Print V for metafor
> V
```

```
        [,1]   [,2]   [,3]   [,4]  [,5]   [,6]   [,7]
[1,]  0.0075 0.0030 0.0000 0e+00 0.0000 0.0000 0.0000
[2,]  0.0030 0.0077 0.0000 0e+00 0.0000 0.0000 0.0000
[3,]  0.0000 0.0000 0.0057 9e-04 0.0000 0.0000 0.0000
[4,]  0.0000 0.0000 0.0009 8e-04 0.0000 0.0000 0.0000
[5,]  0.0000 0.0000 0.0000 0e+00 0.0021 0.0007 0.0000
[6,]  0.0000 0.0000 0.0000 0e+00 0.0007 0.0014 0.0000
[7,]  0.0000 0.0000 0.0000 0e+00 0.0000 0.0000 0.0029
[8,]  0.0000 0.0000 0.0000 0e+00 0.0000 0.0000 0.0009
```

```
[9,]  0.0000 0.0000 0.0000 0e+00 0.0000 0.0000 0.0000
[10,] 0.0000 0.0000 0.0000 0e+00 0.0000 0.0000 0.0000

        [,8]    [,9]   [,10]
[1,]  0.0000 0.0000 0.0000
[2,]  0.0000 0.0000 0.0000
[3,]  0.0000 0.0000 0.0000
[4,]  0.0000 0.0000 0.0000
[5,]  0.0000 0.0000 0.0000
[6,]  0.0000 0.0000 0.0000
[7,]  0.0009 0.0000 0.0000
[8,]  0.0015 0.0000 0.0000
[9,]  0.0000 0.0148 0.0072
[10,] 0.0000 0.0072 0.0304
```

8.4.2   Fixed-Effects Meta-Analysis

With the rearranged data and variance-covariance matrix, V, we now fit
the fixed-effects meta-analysis model using metafor with the option of
method="FE" as follows:

```
> # Call "rma.mv" to fit fixed-effects
> berkey.metafor.FE = rma.mv(yi,V, mods=~outcome-1,
        random=~outcome|trial, struct="UN",method="FE",
        data=dat.berkey1998)
> print(berkey.metafor.FE, digits=4)

Multivariate Meta-Analysis Model (k = 10; method: FE)

Test for Residual Heterogeneity: QE(df=8)=128.2267, p-val< .0001
Test of Moderators (coefficients 1:2):QM(df=2)=871.3189,
    p-val<.0001

Model Results:
            estimate      se     zval    pval   ci.lb   ci.ub
outcomeAL   -0.3944  0.0186 -21.1471 <.0001 -0.4309 -0.3578 ***
outcomePD    0.3072  0.0286  10.7513 <.0001  0.2512  0.3632 ***
```

We note that the fixed-effects model results in Section 8.3.1 are reproduced.

8.4.3   Random-Effects Meta-Analysis

To fit the random-effects multivariate meta-analysis model using the metafor
package, we simply change the option to method="REML" (as default setting)
as follows:

```
> # Call "rma.mv" to fit fixed-effects
> berkey.metafor.RE = rma.mv(yi,V, mods=~outcome-1,
      random=~outcome|trial, struct="UN",method="REML",
      data=dat.berkey1998)
> # Print the model fit
> print(berkey.metafor.RE, digits=4)


Multivariate Meta-Analysis Model (k = 10; method: REML)

Variance Components:
outer factor: trial(nlvls = 5); inner factor:outcome(nlvls = 2)

            estim    sqrt  k.lvl  fixed  level
tau^2.1    0.0327  0.1807      5     no     AL
tau^2.2    0.0117  0.1083      5     no     PD

      rho.AL  rho.PD    AL  PD
AL         1  0.6088     -  no
PD    0.6088       1     5   -


Test for Residual Heterogeneity:
QE(df = 8) = 128.2267, p-val < .0001
Test of Moderators (coefficients 1:2):
QM(df = 2) = 108.8616, p-val < .0001

Model Results:
            estimate      se     zval    pval    ci.lb    ci.ub
outcomeAL    -0.3392  0.0879  -3.8589  0.0001  -0.5115  -0.1669***
outcomePD     0.3534  0.0588   6.0057  <.0001   0.2381   0.4688***
```

We note that this reproduces the results in Section 8.3.2.

With this random-effects model, we can also test the difference between the two outcomes with the following R code:

```
> anova(berkey.metafor.RE, L=c(1,-1))


Hypothesis:
1: outcomeAL - outcomePD = 0

Results:
    estimate      se     zval    pval
1:   -0.6926  0.0744  -9.3120  <.0001

Test of Hypothesis:
QM(df = 1) = 86.7139, p-val < .0001
```

This tests the null hypothesis $H_0: outcomeAL - outcomePD = 0$. As seen from the output, the estimated difference is -0.6926, standard error is 0.0744, and z-value is -9.3120. The associated p-value is <0.0001, which indicates that these two outcomes are statistically significantly different. That is to say that the estimated improvement from surgical to nonsurgical treatment in PD (i.e., PD) is statistically significantly larger than the estimated improvement from surgical to nonsurgical treatment in AL (i.e., AL).

8.4.4 Meta-Regression

Similarly, we perform meta-regression including publication year as moderator for both outcomes as follows:

```
> berkey.metafor.Reg = rma.mv(yi, V, mods = ~ outcome
                        + outcome:year - 1,
            random = ~ outcome | trial, struct="UN",
            data=dat.berkey1998, method="REML")
> print(berkey.metafor.Reg, digits=4)

Multivariate Meta-Analysis Model (k = 10; method: REML)

Variance Components:
outer factor: trial   (nlvls = 5)
inner factor: outcome (nlvls = 2)

            estim   sqrt  k.lvl  fixed  level
tau^2.1    0.0409  0.2021     5     no     AL
tau^2.2    0.0204  0.1430     5     no     PD

      rho.AL  rho.PD   AL  PD
AL         1  0.5614    -  no
PD    0.5614       1    5   -


Test for Residual Heterogeneity:
QE(df = 6) = 125.7557, p-val < .0001
Test of Moderators (coefficients 1:4):
QM(df = 4) = 76.7102, p-val < .0001

Model Results:
                estimate       se     zval    pval     ci.lb     ci.ub
outcomeAL        22.5415  59.4308   0.3793  0.7045  -93.9407  139.0237
outcomePD        -9.2815  43.3417  -0.2141  0.8304  -94.2296   75.6667
outcomeAL:year   -0.0115   0.0300  -0.3850  0.7002   -0.0703    0.0472
outcomePD:year    0.0049   0.0219   0.2225  0.8239   -0.0380    0.0477
```

As seen from the output, this reproduces the results in Section 8.3.3.

8.5   Discussions

In this chapter, we illustrated features of the package mvmeta for multivariate meta-analysis along with the R package metafor. This package can also be used for meta-regression to incorporate study-level moderators and predictors. To promote application of the package, we illustrated its use with an example for both fixed-effects and random-effects models.

There are more packages that can be used for multivariate meta-analysis. We illustrated the R package metafor, used in the previous chapters for UMA, can also be used for multivariate meta-analysis as demonstrated in Section 8.4.

In addition, mvtmeta is another R package for multivariate meta-analysis developed by Chen et al. (2012). It can be accessed from http://cran.r-project.org/web/packages/mvtmeta/index.html. This package contains two functions mvtmeta_fe for fixed-effects multivariate meta-analysis and mvtmeta_re for random-effects multivariate meta-analysis which are easy to implement. This package implemented the method in Chen et al. (2012). In this paper, they developed a noniterative method of moments estimator for the between-study covariance matrix in the random-effects multivariate meta-analysis which is a multivariate extension of the DerSimonian and Laird's univariate method of moments estimator, and invariant to linear transformations.

Another function that can be used for multivariate meta-analysis is from the genetic analysis package, i.e., gap which can be accessed at http://cran.r-project.org/web/packages/gap/. This package is in fact designed to be an integrated package for genetic data analysis of both population and family data. The function mvmeta can be used for multivariate meta-analysis based on generalized least squares (GLS). This function can input a data matrix of parameter estimates (denoted by b) and their variance-covariance matrix from individual studies (denoted by V) and output a GLS estimate and heterogeneity statistic. The usage is mvmeta(b,V). An example is given in the package for readers to follow.

For a Bayesian approach to multivariate meta-analysis, DPpackage is a good reference and can be obtained from http://cran.r-project.org/web/packages/DPpackage/. This package contains functions to provide inference via simulation from the posterior distributions for Bayesian nonparametric and semiparametric models which is motivated by the Dirichlet Process prior so named as DPpackage. In this package, the function DPmultmeta is used for Bayesian analysis in semiparametric random-effects multivariate meta-analysis model.

Appendix: Stata Programs for Multivariate Meta-Analysis by Manyun Liu

The Stata program below corresponds to the R program.

```
/*### Reproduce R Results in Section 8.2 ###*/
ssc install mvmeta

/* Because the berkey98 data is in R library, we created a new
 Excel sheet berkey98 for dat4Meta.xls to provide the data.*/
/* You can use the following command to load the excel file */
/*Changes the wd*/
cd "C:\Users\"
import excel using dat4Meta.xls, sheet("berkey98") firstrow clear

/* present the data */
browse

/* Or we can use list command to present the data */
list

/*### Reproduce R Results in Section 8.3.1 ###*/
# Call mvmeta with fixed-effects
rename PD y1
rename AL y2
rename var_PD V11
rename var_AL V22
rename cov_PD_AL V12

ssc install heterogi
mvmeta y V ,fixed i2

/*### Reproduce R Results in Section 8.3.2 ###*/
# Call mvmeta with random-effects
mvmeta y V ,reml i2

# Call mvmeta with method ml
mvmeta y V ,ml i2

/*### Reproduce R Results in Section 8.3.3 ###*/
# meta-reg to study year
mvmeta y V pubyear ,reml i2
```

9

Publication Bias in Meta-Analysis

Hani Samawi

9.1 Introduction

In a meta-analysis, publication bias or selection bias is the term in which the research that appears in the literature is unrepresentative of the population of completed studies. In a meta-analysis, the studies selected and included are vital to draw a correct conclusion. When only positive studies (those that demonstrate statistical significance or if not statistically significant do not reflect qualitative interaction) of a drug are included in a meta-analysis, publication bias may occur.

On the other hand, although meta-analysis provides a mathematically accurate synthesis of summary measures of the studies included in the analysis, if the studies are a biased sample of all relevant studies, the mean effect computed by the meta-analysis may reflect this bias. Customarily, studies that report relatively large or statistically significant effect sizes are more likely to be published than studies that report smaller or negative effect sizes. Consequently, a sample of these published studies included in a meta-analysis may reflect publication bias. Although the problem of publication bias is not unique to systematic reviews, it received more attention from systematic reviews and meta-analyses.

Begg's funnel plot or Egger's plot is used to display graphically the existence of publication bias. Statistical tests for publication bias are usually based on the fact that clinical studies with small sample sizes (and therefore large variances) may be more prone to publication bias than large clinical studies. Thus, when estimates from all studies plotted against their variances (sample size), a symmetrical funnel should be seen when there is no publication bias, while a skewed asymmetrical funnel is a signal of potential publication bias. We illustrate this funnel plot and testing procedure for publication bias using the R and Stata system in the following sections.

In this chapter, we discuss meta-analysis publication bias and the attendant reasons. We discuss some of the methods that have been developed to assess the likely impact of bias in any given meta-analysis study. Finally, we introduce some testing procedures and provide illustrative examples using R and STAT system.

9.2   Reasons for Publication Bias in Systematic Review

In planning a systematic review, it is customary for researchers to develop inclusion criteria to guide the types of studies that are included. In perfect hypothetical situations, researchers may be able to locate all reviews that meet their criteria. However, in reality, this is not always possible. Moreover, not including some studies may result in loss of information when the missing studies are a random subset of all relevant studies. This loss of data may impact inferential results, including wider confidence intervals, and less powerful tests, but should have no systematic impact on the effect size. However, if the missing studies are not missing at random, or are otherwise preferentially not included, then the sample of chosen studies will be biased. In the literature, the concern is that studies with a relatively large or statistically significant effect size for a specific question are more likely to be published than studies with smaller or negative effect sizes. This bias in the published literature will be carried over to a meta-analysis using that literature.

To this end, Borenstein et al. (2009) explained in their book, chapter two, that Dickersin in 2005 reviewed several investigations and established that studies with statistically significant results are more likely to be published than those with statistically insignificant results. He argued that if the effect size is large enough for given sample size, the result has a greater chance of being statistically significant. Consequently, the groups of studies focused on the magnitude of a relationship and the observed effects distributed over a range of values. Those studies with effects in the direction of the higher end of that range have a higher likelihood of being statistically significant and published. As Hedges (1984, 1989) indicated, this trend would result in substantial biases in the relationships' magnitude, especially when those studies have relatively small sample sizes.

Furthermore, Clarke and Clarke (2000) investigated the list of references from healthcare protocols and reviews published in The Cochrane Library in 1999. They found that about 92% of the references included in those studies were journal articles. However, for the remaining 8%, about 4% were from conference proceedings, about 2% were unpublished material, and slightly over 1% were from books or book chapters. Similarly, Mallet et al. (2002) investigated sources of the unpublished literature included in the first 1000 Cochrane systematic reviews. They found that nearly half of them did not include any data from unpublished sources.

Moreover, Easterbrook et al. (1991), Dickersin et al. (1992), and Dickersin and Min (1993) conducted investigations to identify groups of studies when they were initiated, followed them over time, and recorded which were published and which were not. They found that nonstatistically significant studies were less likely to be published than statistically significant studies. In addition, they found that even the statistically significant ones, when released, could be subject to long delays before publication. For example, Rothstein (2006) indicated that in 95 meta-analytic reviews published studies in Psychological Bulletin, between 1995 and 2005, 23 out of the 95 did not include any unpublished data. However, some researchers argued that it is legitimate to exclude studies that have not been published in peer-reviewed journals due to their low quality (see Weisz et al., 1995). On the other hand, other reasons may lead to an upward bias in effect size and manifest as publication bias, including duplication bias (Tramer et al., 1997); language bias (Egger et al., 1997; Jüni et al., 2002); availability bias; cost bias; familiarity bias; and citation bias (Götzsche, 1987; Ravnskov, 1992).

9.3 Dealing with Publication Bias

In a meta-analysis, when the available research results are different from those of all research conducted in an area, reviewers are at risk of reaching the wrong conclusions about what that body of research shows. This could, in some cases, cause dramatic concerns, especially in clinical trials and drug development. For example, including studies in a meta-analysis of an ineffective or dangerous treatment falsely viewed as safe and effective may overestimate the actual effect sizes (efficacy and safety). Some approaches in dealing with these concerns appear in the literature. However, as indicated by Borenstein et al. (2009), the only actual test for publication bias is to compare effects in the formal published studies with effects in the unpublished studies. Therefore, the best approach is for the researcher to perform an accurate, comprehensive search of the literature, hoping to minimize bias. For example, Cochrane reviews one of the approaches which tend to include more studies with smaller effect sizes than those found in similar reviews published in medical journals. Similar to Cochrane reviews, serious efforts to find unpublished, and difficult to find studies, are recommended to reduce publication bias.

More resources are needed to locate and retrieve information and studies from sources other than published journal articles, such as dissertations, theses, conference papers, government, and technical reports. However, it is not generally acceptable to conduct a synthesis that unconditionally excludes these types of research reports (Borenstein et al., 2009). Borenstein et al. (2009) suggested that it could be beneficial when searches are balanced between published articles and other sources of data. Additional guidance in the process of literature searching and information retrieval can found in Reed and Baxter (2009) and Rothstein and Hopewell (2009), among others.

To investigate and understand the impact of publication bias, Borenstein et al. (2009) proposed the following model that identifies which studies are likely to be missing by making the following assumptions: "(1) Large studies are likely to be published regardless of statistical significance because these involve substantial commitments of time and resources. (2) Moderately sized studies are at risk of being lost, but with a moderate sample size, even modest effects will be important, and so only some studies may be lost. (3) Small studies are at the highest risk of being lost. Because of the small sample size, only the most substantial effects are likely to be significant, with studies of low and moderate effects possibly not published."

Borenstein et al. (2009) indicated that using their model, they expect the bias to increase as the sample size decreases. The methods described below are based on Borenstein et al.'s model. They argued that more sophisticated techniques found in the literature to estimate the number of missing studies and/or to adjust the observed effect to account for bias are rarely used in actual research due to the difference between sample size and effect size. Thus if such a relationship is found, it will be considered that some studies are missing.

9.4   Assessing the Potential of the Publication Bias

The first step in assessing potential publication bias is to thoroughly understand the data. Rearranging forest plot size in ascending (or descending) order, so that larger studies appear toward the bottom and smaller studies appear toward the top (or vice versa), has no impact on the summary effect, allowing researchers to see the relationship between sample size and effect size. This approach is the first data articulation to get some sense about the data and check for potential publication bias. Table 9.1 contains the classical and famous data from the Cochrane Collaboration logo reviews. Those reviews resulted from a systematic review of the pre-1980 clinical study literature on corticosteroid therapy of premature labor and its effect on neonatal death. The meta-analysis figure is part of the logo of the Cochrane Collaboration (http://www.cochrane.org). We present meta-analyses of this data set using the R and Stata systems. The response measure in this data set is binary (death or alive).

Figures 9.1 and 9.2 are forest and funnel plots, respectively, of the studies in Table 9.1 using the Stata system. Since this study is about corticosteroid therapy in premature labor and its effect on neonatal death, a decrease in risk is indicated by a risk ratio of less than 1.0. Only two studies showed an increase of risk of death, while the majority of studies show decreased risks of death when corticosteroid therapy in premature labor was used. On the other hand, the last rows show the summary data for the random-effects model. The overall risk ratio is 0.49, and the 95% confidence interval is (0.34, 0.70). The test of heterogeneity yields $T^2 = 0.31$, $I^2 = 92.22\%$, $H^2 = 12.86$, $Q(12) = 152.23$ (p-value < 0.0001).

Figure 9.1 shows that the smallest study weight (%) has the largest risk ratio. However, the study is not statistically significant. Additionally, as we

TABLE 9.1

Data from Cochrane Collaboration Logo: Use y as the Log Relative Risk (Log-RR) and v is the Variance of the Log Relative Risk

Trial	Author	Treatment Yes	Treatment No	Control Yes	Control No	Log-RR y	Sample Variance v
1	Aronson	4	119	11	128	−0.8893	0.3256
2	Ferguson & Simes	6	300	29	274	−1.5854	0.1946
3	Rosenthal et al.	3	228	11	209	−1.3481	0.4154
4	Hart & Sutherland	62	13,536	248	12,619	−1.4416	0.02
5	Frimodt-Moller et al.	33	5,036	47	5,761	−0.2175	0.0512
6	Stein & Aronson	180	1,361	372	1,079	−0.7861	0.0069
7	Vandiviere et al.	8	2,537	10	619	−1.6209	0.223
8	TPT Madras	505	87,886	499	87,892	0.012	0.004
9	Coetzee & Berjak	29	7,470	45	7,232	−0.4694	0.0564
10	Rosenthal et al.	17	1,699	65	1,600	−1.3713	0.073
11	Comstock et al.	186	50,448	141	27,197	−0.3394	0.0124
12	Comstock & Webster	5	2,493	3	2,338	0.4459	0.5325
13	Comstock et al.	27	16,886	29	17,825	−0.0173	0.0714

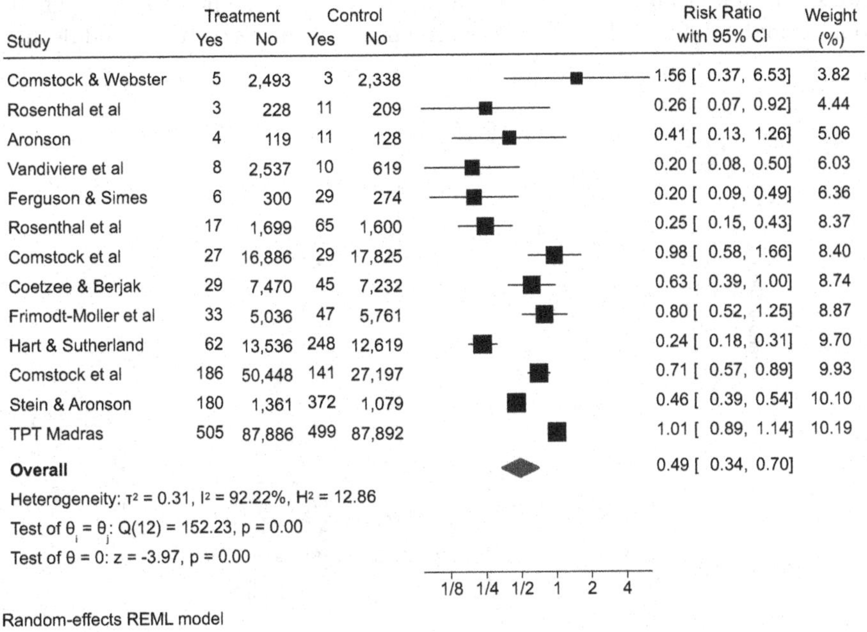

Study	Treatment Yes	No	Control Yes	No	Risk Ratio with 95% CI	Weight (%)
Comstock & Webster	5	2,493	3	2,338	1.56 [0.37, 6.53]	3.82
Rosenthal et al	3	228	11	209	0.26 [0.07, 0.92]	4.44
Aronson	4	119	11	128	0.41 [0.13, 1.26]	5.06
Vandiviere et al	8	2,537	10	619	0.20 [0.08, 0.50]	6.03
Ferguson & Simes	6	300	29	274	0.20 [0.09, 0.49]	6.36
Rosenthal et al	17	1,699	65	1,600	0.25 [0.15, 0.43]	8.37
Comstock et al	27	16,886	29	17,825	0.98 [0.58, 1.66]	8.40
Coetzee & Berjak	29	7,470	45	7,232	0.63 [0.39, 1.00]	8.74
Frimodt-Moller et al	33	5,036	47	5,761	0.80 [0.52, 1.25]	8.87
Hart & Sutherland	62	13,536	248	12,619	0.24 [0.18, 0.31]	9.70
Comstock et al	186	50,448	141	27,197	0.71 [0.57, 0.89]	9.93
Stein & Aronson	180	1,361	372	1,079	0.46 [0.39, 0.54]	10.10
TPT Madras	505	87,886	499	87,892	1.01 [0.89, 1.14]	10.19
Overall					0.49 [0.34, 0.70]	

Heterogeneity: $\tau^2 = 0.31$, $I^2 = 92.22\%$, $H^2 = 12.86$

Test of $\theta_i = \theta_j$: Q(12) = 152.23, p = 0.00

Test of $\theta = 0$: z = -3.97, p = 0.00

1/8 1/4 1/2 1 2 4

Random-effects REML model

FIGURE 9.1

Corticosteroid therapy in premature labor and its effect on neonatal death-forest-plot.

move from the lowest to the largest study, the plot of most effects shifts toward the right. This behavior may predict bias is present. As suggested by Borenstein et al. (2009), when meta-analysis includes some studies from different resources, the plot could also be grouped by source, which may help to observe if other studies tend to have smaller effects than the others.

The funnel plot is another way to display the relationship between study size and effect size. At first, the funnel plotted with effect size on the X-axis and the sample size (or variance) on the Y-axis. Therefore, large studies appear toward the top of the graph, and in general, they cluster around the mean effect size. However, smaller studies appear toward the bottom of the chart and tend to spread across a broader range of values (Light and Pillemer, 1984; Light et al., 1994).

Borenstein et al. (2009) argued that using the standard error instead of using the sample size or variance on the Y-axis could spread out the points on the bottom half of the scale, where the smaller studies are plotted. There-fore, it is expected, in the absence of publication bias, that the studies will be distributed symmetrically about the mean effect size due to the random-ness of the sampling error. However, in the presence of publication bias, the distribution of studies shows symmetry at the top, a few studies missing in the middle, and more studies missing near the bottom. Consequently, when the effect direction is to the right, near the bottom of the plot, where the nonsignificant studies are located, we expect a gap in the plot to the right. In our example, Figure 9.2 supports the presence of asymmetry. In the middle and

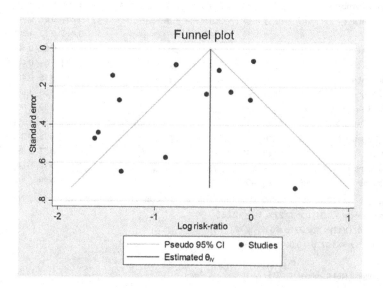

FIGURE 9.2
Corticosteroid therapy in premature labor and its effect on neonatal death (funnel-plot).

the bottom of the funnel plot, most studies appear toward the left (indicating more risk), which could suggest that some studies are missing from the right.

9.4.1   R Codes

```
# Get the R data
library("metafor")
data("dat.bcg", package = "metafor")
###############################
# Calculate the ES using "escalc"
dat = escalc(measure="RR",ai=tpos,bi=tneg,ci=cpos,
             di = cneg, data = dat.bcg, append = TRUE)
# print the numerical data (Delete columns 2,3,9 to save space)
print(dat, row.names = FALSE)
###################################################
# Call `rma' to fit the BCG data
meta.RE = rma(yi, vi, data = dat)
# Print the summary
meta.RE
plot(meta.RE)
funnel(meta.RE)
######################
```

9.4.2   Stata Codes

```
. import spss using "c:\..."

. meta esize tpos tneg cpos cneg, esize(lnrratio)
. meta forestplot, random(reml)
```

9.5   Statistical Tests for Funnel-Plot Asymmetry

Although forest and funnel plots are used as visual diagnostic tools for small-study effects in meta-analysis, asymmetry of these plots, especially the funnel plot, could indicate a potential small-study effects that could be interpreted as publication bias. However, the interpretation of a funnel plot is profoundly subjective, and there are other possible causes of funnel plot asymmetry. Those causes are presented in Rothstein et al. (2005) (Table 5.2), which are listed first in Egger et al. (1997). Therefore, there is a need for a less subjective interpretation of the evidence for funnel plot asymmetry. This need led investigators to develop several tests in the literature and use them to examine the relationship between effect size and sample size. Using similar notation as in Rothstein et al. (2005), we will denote the study effect estimate (standardized mean difference or log odds ratio) from the ith study by θ_i and its corresponding variance and standard error as v_i and s_i, respectively.

9.5.1 Begg and Mazumdar's Rank Correlation Method

Begg and Mazumdar's rank correlation test, proposed by Begg and Mazumdar (1994), is an adjusted rank correlation approach, which examines the association between the effect estimates and their sampling variances. They suggested to first stabilize the variances by deriving standardized effect sizes $\{\theta_i^*\}$, where

$$\theta_i^* = \frac{(\theta_i - \overline{\theta})}{\sqrt{v_i^*}}$$

where $\overline{\theta} = \sum \theta_i v_i^{-1} / \sum v_i^{-1}$, and $v_i^* = v_i - \left(\sum v_i^{-1}\right)^{-1}$ is the variance of $(\theta_i - \overline{\theta})$.

The test is based on deriving Kendall's rank correlation between θ_i^* and v_i^*, which is based on comparing the ranks of the two quantities (Begg and Mazumdar, 1994). Then the test is given by

$$z = \frac{x - y}{\sqrt{k\left(k - 1\right)\left(2k + 5\right)/18}},$$

where k is the number of available studies, x is the concordant ranks, and y is the discordant ranks. Note that for lager k, $z \sim N\left(0, 1\right)$.

9.5.2 Egger's Linear Regression Test

A linear regression method is introduced by Egger et al. (1997) by regressing $z_i = \theta_i / s_i$ on its precision $prec_i = 1/s_i$:

$$E(z_i) = \beta_0 + \beta_1 prec_i..$$

The suggested test is of the null hypothesis that $\beta_0 = 0$ (no funnel plot asymmetry) which can be derived directly from the usual regression output. This test is two-sided. Egger's test is widely used as a test for funnel plot asymmetry. For more discussions about Egger's test, including the weighted and the unweighted versions of the test and its extension, we refer the reader to Rothstein et al. (2005) (Chapter 6).

The validity and power of the regression test and the rank correlation test are of concern. Begg and Mazumdar (1994) and Sterne et al. (2000) conducted simulations studies, and both reach to the same conclusion that the power of the regression tests is low if the number of studies used in the analysis is 10 or fewer, or the bias is not severe. However, the regression test for funnel plot asymmetry has higher power than the rank correlation test.

And that would give an advantage to the regression method over the rank correlation test when the power of the test is at best moderate. However, the regression test is only appropriate when the use of meta-analysis makes sense.

Finally, as discussed above, there are possible reasons for funnel plot asymmetry other than publication bias. Therefore, the funnel plot asymmetry tests discussed so far should not be viewed as tests for detecting publication bias, but rather as tests for "small-study effects" in a meta-analysis (see, Rothstein et al., 2005).

9.5.3   Illustration with R and Stata System

9.5.3.1   Using Data from Cochrane Collaboration Logo (Table 9.1)

As described earlier, this study includes 13 pre-1980 clinical studies from the literature of corticosteroid therapy in premature labor and its effect on neonatal death. Figure 9.2 indicated asymmetry of the funnel plot.

R-codes

```
# test for symmetry
ranktest(meta.RE) \# rank test
regtest(meta.RE) \# regression test
########################### Stata-Codes
. meta bias, egger
. meta bias, begg
```

Table 9.2 shows results from the rank correlation and regression tests of funnel plot asymmetry for Cochrane Collaboration logo data. Both tests failed to show any significant evidence to indicate funnel plot asymmetry. However, the p-value of the regression test is smaller than that of the rank correlation test.

9.5.3.2   Using the Effect of Streptokinase After a Myocardial Infarction (strepto.dta) Data

This illustration uses data extracted from Stata 16 manual (2019). This meta-analysis study, conducted by Lau et al. (1992), included 33 studies conducted between 1959 and 1988 to assess the effect of streptokinase medication to break down clots of heart attack patients. The patients in this experiment were randomly treated with streptokinase or a placebo. Note that breaking down clots

TABLE 9.2

Tests of Symmetry of the Funnel Plot

Test Name	Test Size	p-value
Regression-based Egger test for small-study effects	−0.80	0.4218
Rank Correlation test (Kendall's score)	0.06	0.9514

reduces damage to the heart muscle in myocardial infarction (heart attack) patients. Lau et al. (1992) used meta-analysis to investigate when the effect of streptokinase became statistically significant (Table 9.3 and Figure 9.3).

In this illustration, we present Stata system codes and analysis. There was no statistical evidence study heterogeneity (see Table 9.3 and Figure 9.4). Figure 9.5 shows a shift of the smaller studies toward the right, which indicates small studies effect and funnel plot asymmetry. However, both the regression test and the rank correlation test showed p-values larger than 0.05. Therefore, Table 9.4 shows no statistical evidence of funnel plot asymmetry. However, again the p-value using the regression method (0.1372) is smaller than from the rank correlation method (0.1410). Note that these tests make sense if there is a reasonable amount of dispersion in the sample sizes and the number of studies included in the meta-analysis. Also, both tests have low power as indicated by Borenstein et al. (2009).

TABLE 9.3

Summary of the Effect of Streptokinase after a Myocardial Infarction Data

```
Effect-size label:   Log Odds-Ratio
      Effect size:   _meta_es
        Std. Err.:   _meta_se
      Study label:   study
```

Meta-analysis summary		Number of studies =	33
Random-effects model		Heterogeneity:	
Method: REML		tau2 =	0.0003
		I2 (%) =	0.52
		H2 =	1.01

Study	Log Odds-Ratio	[95% Conf. Interval]		% Weight
Fletcher	1.838	-0.549	4.226	0.08
Dewar	0.754	-0.664	2.171	0.22
European 1	-0.379	-1.130	0.373	0.79
European 2	0.454	0.102	0.806	3.60
Heikinheimo	-0.222	-0.885	0.442	1.02
Italian	-0.012	-0.697	0.674	0.95
Australian 1	0.282	-0.267	0.831	1.49
Franfurt 2	0.973	0.251	1.696	0.86
NHLBI SMIT	-0.950	-2.360	0.460	0.23
Frank	0.042	-1.159	1.242	0.31
Valere	-0.060	-1.056	0.937	0.45
Klein	-1.163	-3.544	1.217	0.08
UK-Collab	0.094	-0.382	0.570	1.97
Austrian	0.576	0.143	1.009	2.38
Australian 2	0.469	-0.137	1.075	1.22
Lasierra	1.504	-0.929	3.938	0.08
N Ger Collab	-0.195	-0.617	0.227	2.51
Witchitz	0.251	-1.113	1.616	0.24
European 3	0.578	-0.053	1.210	1.12
ISAM	0.137	-0.239	0.513	3.15
GISSI-1	0.215	0.102	0.327	32.81
Olson	0.898	-1.568	3.364	0.07
Baroffio	2.751	-0.175	5.677	0.05
Schreiber	1.216	-1.145	3.578	0.08
Cribier	-0.095	-2.932	2.742	0.06
Sainsous	0.761	-0.686	2.208	0.21
Durand	0.535	-1.051	2.120	0.18
White	1.841	0.319	3.362	0.19
Bassand	0.560	-0.732	1.852	0.27
Vlay	0.875	-1.667	3.418	0.07
Kennedy	0.461	-0.309	1.230	0.76
ISIS-2	0.294	0.196	0.392	42.35
Wisenberg	1.584	-0.142	3.310	0.15
theta	0.264	0.197	0.331	

```
Test of theta = 0: z = 7.73                    Prob > |z| = 0.0000
Test of homogeneity: Q = chi2(32) = 39.48      Prob > Q = 0.1703
```

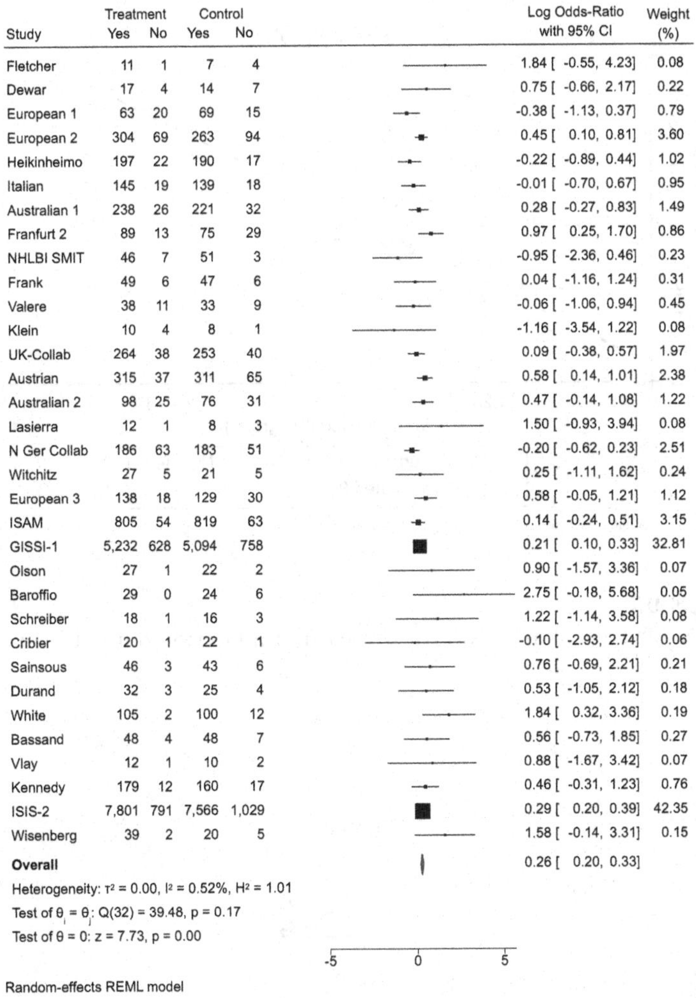

Study	Treatment Yes	Treatment No	Control Yes	Control No		Log Odds-Ratio with 95% CI	Weight (%)
Fletcher	11	1	7	4		1.84 [-0.55, 4.23]	0.08
Dewar	17	4	14	7		0.75 [-0.66, 2.17]	0.22
European 1	63	20	69	15		-0.38 [-1.13, 0.37]	0.79
European 2	304	69	263	94		0.45 [0.10, 0.81]	3.60
Heikinheimo	197	22	190	17		-0.22 [-0.89, 0.44]	1.02
Italian	145	19	139	18		-0.01 [-0.70, 0.67]	0.95
Australian 1	238	26	221	32		0.28 [-0.27, 0.83]	1.49
Franfurt 2	89	13	75	29		0.97 [0.25, 1.70]	0.86
NHLBI SMIT	46	7	51	3		-0.95 [-2.36, 0.46]	0.23
Frank	49	6	47	6		0.04 [-1.16, 1.24]	0.31
Valere	38	11	33	9		-0.06 [-1.06, 0.94]	0.45
Klein	10	4	8	1		-1.16 [-3.54, 1.22]	0.08
UK-Collab	264	38	253	40		0.09 [-0.38, 0.57]	1.97
Austrian	315	37	311	65		0.58 [0.14, 1.01]	2.38
Australian 2	98	25	76	31		0.47 [-0.14, 1.08]	1.22
Lasierra	12	1	8	3		1.50 [-0.93, 3.94]	0.08
N Ger Collab	186	63	183	51		-0.20 [-0.62, 0.23]	2.51
Witchitz	27	5	21	5		0.25 [-1.11, 1.62]	0.24
European 3	138	18	129	30		0.58 [-0.05, 1.21]	1.12
ISAM	805	54	819	63		0.14 [-0.24, 0.51]	3.15
GISSI-1	5,232	628	5,094	758		0.21 [0.10, 0.33]	32.81
Olson	27	1	22	2		0.90 [-1.57, 3.36]	0.07
Baroffio	29	0	24	6		2.75 [-0.18, 5.68]	0.05
Schreiber	18	1	16	3		1.22 [-1.14, 3.58]	0.08
Cribier	20	1	22	1		-0.10 [-2.93, 2.74]	0.06
Sainsous	46	3	43	6		0.76 [-0.69, 2.21]	0.21
Durand	32	3	25	4		0.53 [-1.05, 2.12]	0.18
White	105	2	100	12		1.84 [0.32, 3.36]	0.19
Bassand	48	4	48	7		0.56 [-0.73, 1.85]	0.27
Vlay	12	1	10	2		0.88 [-1.67, 3.42]	0.07
Kennedy	179	12	160	17		0.46 [-0.31, 1.23]	0.76
ISIS-2	7,801	791	7,566	1,029		0.29 [0.20, 0.39]	42.35
Wisenberg	39	2	20	5		1.58 [-0.14, 3.31]	0.15
Overall						0.26 [0.20, 0.33]	

Heterogeneity: $\tau^2 = 0.00$, $I^2 = 0.52\%$, $H^2 = 1.01$

Test of $\theta_i = \theta_j$: Q(32) = 39.48, p = 0.17

Test of $\theta = 0$: z = 7.73, p = 0.00

-5   0   5

Random-effects REML model

FIGURE 9.3

The effect of streptokinase after a myocardial infarction data (forest-plot).

Stata-Codes and Meta-Analysis Results

```
. use https://www.stata-press.com/data/r16/strepto
(Effect of streptokinase after a myocardial infarction)
. meta esize nsurvt ndeadt nsurvc ndeadc
```

```
Meta-analysis setting information
 Study information
   No. of studies: 33
```

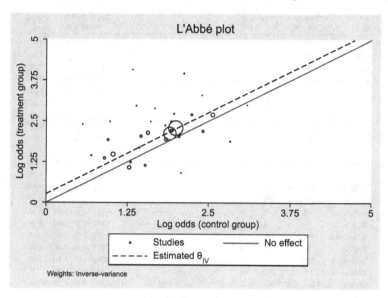

FIGURE 9.4
The effect of streptokinase after a myocardial infarction data (L'Anne'-plot).

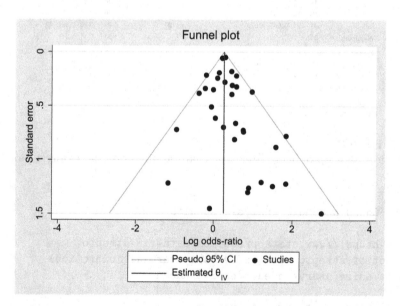

FIGURE 9.5
The effect of streptokinase after a myocardial infarction data (funnel-plot).

TABLE 9.4
Tests of Symmetry of the Funnel Plot

Test Name	Test Size	*p*-value
Regression-based Egger test for small-study effects	1.49	0.1372
Rank Correlation test (Kendall's score)	1.47	0.1410

```
          Study label: Generic
          Study size: _meta_studysize
        Summary data: nsurvt ndeadt nsurvc ndeadc
         Effect size
                Type: lnoratio
               Label: Log Odds-Ratio
            Variable: _meta_es
    Zero-cells adj.: 0.5, only0
           Precision
          Std. Err.: _meta_se
                  CI: [_meta_cil, _meta_ciu]
            CI level: 95\%
   Model and method
               Model: Random-effects
              Method: REML
```

```
Contains data from https://www.stata-press.com/data/r16/strepto.dta
  obs:          33                    Effect of streptokinase after a myocardial infarction
  vars:          7                    14 May 2019 18:24
                                      (_dta has notes)

               storage   display    value
variable name   type     format     label    variable label

study           str12    %12s                Study name
year            int      %10.0g              Publication year
ndeadt          int      %10.0g              Number of deaths in treatment group
nsurvt          int      %9.0g               Number of survivors in treatment group
ndeadc          int      %10.0g              Number of deaths in control group
nsurvc          int      %9.0g               Number of survivors in control group
studyplus       str13    %13s                Study label for cumulative MA
```

```
. meta summarize
. meta forestplot

Effect-size label: Log Odds-Ratio
     Effect size: _meta_es
       Std. Err.: _meta_se


.meta labbeplot

Effect-size label: Log Odds-Ratio
       Effect size: _meta_es
```

```
        Std. Err.: _meta_se
   Summary data: nsurvt ndeadt nsurvc ndeadc
          Model: Common-effect
         Method: Inverse-variance
```

. meta funnelplot

```
Effect-size label: Log Odds-Ratio
      Effect size: _meta_es
        Std. Err.: _meta_se
            Model: Common-effect
           Method: Inverse-variance
```

. meta bias, egger

. meta bias, beg

Moreover, as discussed by Rothstein et al. (2005), the funnel plot's interpretation is profoundly subjective, and there are other possible causes of funnel plot asymmetry. Those causes are presented in Rothstein et al. (2005) (Table 5.2), which are listed first in Egger et al. (1997). Among those causes are selection biases (i.e., publication bias, location biases, language bias, citation bias, multiple publication bias), true heterogeneity, data irregularities, artifact, and chance. Therefore, it is essential to ask if there is evidence of any bias, and if we are confident that the effect is not an artifact of bias?

9.6   Other Issues of Publication Bias and Remedies

Rosenthal's (1979) Fail-safe N is an approach for dealing with publication bias. This approach concern is that the studies with smaller effects are missing. If the missing studies were retrieved and included in the analysis, the *p*-value for the summary effect would no longer be significant. Therefore, Rosenthal's Fail-safe N approach computes how many missing studies would be needed to be retrieved and incorporated in the analysis before the *p*-value became insignificant. Although Rosenthal's Fail-safe N approach is essential for publication bias, this approach focuses on statistical significance rather than practical significance. This approach did not focus on how many hidden studies are required to reduce the effect to the point that it is not of practical importance. Also, the approach assumes that the mean effect size of the studies not included is zero when it could be negative. Moreover, the Fail-safe N approach is based on significance tests that combine *p*-values across studies. Hence, this approach is not generally appropriate for analyses that focus on effect sizes.

To address the shortcomings of Rosenthal's Fail-safe N approach, Orwin and Boruch (1983) proposed a variant on the Rosenthal formula. Orwin's method allows us to determine how many missing studies would affect a specified level other than zero. Therefore, the researcher may select a value that represents the smallest effect, which is deemed to be of practical importance, and ask how many missing studies would be required to bring the summary effect below this point. Also, it allows the researcher to specify the mean effect in the absent studies as some value other than zero.

On the hand, a third approach, named "Trim and Fill" by Duval and Tweedie (2000a, b), is introduced. The Trim and Fill approach tries to estimate how much impact the bias had and to estimate the effect size that would have been in the absence of bias. Trim and Fill's approach is based on an iterative algorithm that tends to remove the extremely small studies from the positive side of the funnel plot and re-calculate the effect size at each iteration until the funnel plot becomes symmetric about the (new) effect size found.

Duval and Tweedie (2000a, b) indicated that, in theory, this would yield an unbiased estimate of the effect size. However, as this trimming generates the adjusted effect size, it also reduces the variance of the effects. Hence we will have narrower confidence intervals. This algorithm will then add the original studies back into the analysis and introduce a mirror image for each. This imputation method has no impact on the point estimate but corrects the variance.

This approach is used to address an essential question in mate-analysis, which is, what is our best estimate of the unbiased effect size? This approach lends itself to an intuitive visual display. The software that incorporates Trim and Fill method can also create a funnel plot that includes both the observed and the imputed studies, so the researcher can see how the effect size shifts when the imputed studies are included in the plot. When the change in the funnel plot is minor, one could be more confident that the reported effect is valid. A problem with this method is that it depends strongly on the assumptions of the model for why studies are missing. One or two aberrant studies can influence the algorithm for detecting asymmetry.

Using Stata software and the data presented in Section 9.5.3.2, we have the following Stata codes and output.

```
. meta trimfill, funnel

 Effect-size label: Log Odds-Ratio
       Effect size: _meta_es
         Std. Err.: _meta_se
Nonparametric trim-and-fill analysis of publication bias
Linear estimator, imputing on the left
 Iteration              Number of studies = 39
   Model: Random-effects          observed = 33
   Method: REML                     imputed = 6
```

```
Pooling
  Model: Random-effects
  Method: REML
```

Table 9.5 shows the results of the trim-and-fill analysis of publication bias using data of the effect of streptokinase after a myocardial infarction. There were six missing studies estimated by the trim-and-fill approach and replaced symmetrically in Figure 9.5 to generate Figure 9.6. The replaced missing studies are orange colored circles in Figure 9.6. Moreover, Table 9.5 presents the overall estimate of the odds ratio of 0.254 with 95% confidence interval (0.186, 0.323). There is a reduction in the estimated odds ratio of the original data 0.264 with 95% confidence interval (0.197, 0.331).

TABLE 9.5

Nonparametric Trim-and-Fill Analysis of Publication Bias Results of the Effect of Streptokinase after a Myocardial Infarction Data

Studies	Log Odds-Ratio	[95% Conf. Interval]	
Observed	0.264	0.197	0.331
Observed + Imputed	0.254	0.186	0.323

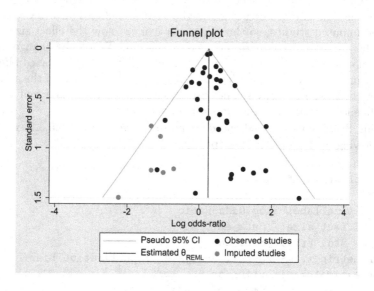

FIGURE 9.6

A filed funnel plot with imputed missing studies.

10

Strategies to Handle Missing Data in Meta-Analysis

Haresh Rochani and Mario Keko

10.1 Introduction

Meta-analysis is the process of integration of the results from multiple studies with the goal of estimating the true effect of an intervention on a particular effect size (ES) of interest. Meta-analysis and systematic review are very similar in terms of narrative summary; however, meta-analyst usually pools summary estimates numerically from individual published studies which are often insufficiently powered to draw definitive results of a particular research question. In individual published studies, complete data are rarely available, especially when a requirement of the study is to collect information on a large number of individuals or large number of variables or simply because the individual study did not collect the outcome and/or moderator which is required to pool the summary estimates.

In almost all meta-analysis research, the issue of missing data is relatively common and can have a significant effect on the conclusions that can be drawn from the data (Graham, 2009). In general, presence of missing data can reduce the representativeness of the samples and may complicate the analysis. Meta-analyses or any statistical analyses that improperly treat missing data can lead to biased summary estimates and ultimately lead to loss of efficiency. This may limit the generalization of results to a wider population and can diminish our ability to understand true underlying phenomena. There may be many potential sources of missing data in meta-analysis. For example, whole study may be missing from the review because it was never published which is commonly known as publication bias in meta-analysis. An outcome or ESs may be missing from individual studies under review or predictors may be missing for the models of ES variation. There may be missing summary data from individual studies due to incomplete reporting.

For investigators, it is very crucial to understand the reasons for missing data for their studies in order to accurately estimate the parameters of interest. In practice, it is difficult to verify the reasons for missing data unless researchers have the ability to go back and collect the data which were missing.

Currently available missing data methods work under the assumptions which are based on the reasons for missingness in given observed data. Rubin (1976) defined the taxonomy of missing data mechanisms based on how the probability of a missing value relates to the data both missing and observed. In general, missing data mechanisms represent the statistical relationship between observed data and probability of missing. This taxonomy has been widely adopted in the statistical literature. There are mainly three types of missing data mechanisms:

Missing Completely at Random (MCAR)

Data are said to be MCAR when we assume that the probability of missingness in the variable of interest does not depend on the values of that variable that are either missing or observed. In other words, probability of being missing is the same for all the cases and observed data are considered to be a random sample of original data . In meta-analysis, primary authors may differ in reporting practices. This may result in missing outcome or predictors where it is reasonable to assume that data are MCAR. Let us denote the data as D and M as the missing indicator matrix, which has values 1 if the variable is observed and 0 if the variable is not observed. For MCAR, missingness in D is independent of the data being observed or missing, or equivalently $p(M|D, \theta) = p(M|\theta)$, where θ are the unknown parameters.

Missing at Random (MAR)

Data are said to be MAR when we assume that the probability of missingness in the variable of interest is associated only with components of observed variables and not with the components that are missing. In other words, probability of being missing is the same only within groups defined by the observed data which is not a random sample of original data. As applied to meta-analysis, some studies may report the subject-level systolic blood pressure (SBP) as a function of age groups, while others report SBP as the average reported by their clinicians. So missing values for a particular measure of SBP in a particular study is not necessarily related to the value of SBP itself but to the choices of the primary author and constraint to the published version of the study. In mathematical terms, MAR mechanism can be written as $p(M|D, \theta) = p(M|D_{obs}, \theta)$.

Missing Not at Random (MNAR)

If neither MCAR or MAR assumptions are reasonable for given data, then data can be assumed as MNAR. In this case, the probability of missing depends on the unobserved data. Participants may dropout for the reasons that are associated with an outcome. For example, participants in longitudinal randomized clinical trials focusing on quality of life outcomes in terminally ill patients may dropout significantly because of their declining quality of life outcomes over time. It is very reasonable to assume that in this type of studies, participants may be dropping out of the study because of their low quality of life outcomes. As applied to meta-analysis, publication bias can be considered as MNAR data. Finally, MNAR assumption allows missingness in the variable of interest to depend on the unobserved values in the data set. In terms of notation, it can be written as $p(M|D, \theta) = p(M|D_{miss}, \theta)$. In missing data literature, MCAR or MAR mechanisms are more often referred as ignorable missing mechanisms while MNAR mechanism is termed as nonignorable missing mechanism.

In this chapter, we will review the most widely used and powerful missing data methods available for meta-analysis. We also will discuss the strategies and approaches to apply each missing data methods in practice. In general, this chapter explores application of missing data methods on missing outcomes or missing predictors from the published studies. One common cause of missing data in meta-analysis is publication bias when search strategies are only focused on published research. Publication bias has been discussed extensively in Chapter 8 of this book. Finally, real data examples will be provided to demonstrate the application of one of the missing data methods.

10.2 Strategies to Handle Missing Data in Meta-Analysis

It is extremely common to have missing data in many areas of research which can have a significant effect on the conclusions that can be drawn from the data. Meta-analyst faces unique challenges pooling the summary estimates from the studies with missing data. It is very important to understand the extend of missing data in each study included for analysis. For example, standard process of data extraction from clinical trial studies includes the number of individuals analyzed in each arm with summary statistics. However, each study should be reviewed carefully to pull out the important information such as the number of participants with missing data in each arm. Many studies also provide the information about the possible reasons for missing participants in the study. Reviewing this information gives a good amount of confidence about making reasonable assumptions for missing data mechanisms (Mavridis and White, 2020).

In practice, it is crucial to understand how missing data were handled at each published study. Only 34% of the studies published in PubMed reported handling missing data by year 2000 while by 2013, almost 100% of the trials published in major medical journals reported handling of missing data (Chan and Altman, 2005; Bell et al., 2014). It is possible that different studies under review assumed different missing mechanisms for their analysis. The distribution of reasons for missing data may be used to impute missing values or information can certainly be used to do sensitivity analysis for combining the estimates from the studies.

In recent years, many methods have been developed to handle the missing data under various missing mechanism assumptions. Most widely used missing data methods can be divided in three main categories: (1) deletion methods (list-wise deletion, pair-wise deletion); (2) single imputation methods (mean imputation, regression imputation, last observation carry forward, hot deck imputations); and (3) model-based methods (maximum likelihood (ML), multiple imputation (MI) methods). In this section, we will discuss the overview of these methods along with practical implications for meta-analysis data.

10.2.1   Deletion Methods

Deletion methods are the simplest and most convenient way to address the issue of missing observations in given data sets. These methods give valid inferences only if missing data mechanism is assumed to be MCAR (Schafer, 1999). There are two main ways of using deletion methods: list-wise deletion (complete case analysis) and pair-wise deletion (available case analysis).

10.2.1.1   List-Wise Deletion (Complete Case Analysis)

In list-wise deletion, researchers use only those cases with all variables fully observed by dropping partially observed cases. Complete case analysis assumes that complete cases are a random sample of the original targeted sample which implies that the data are MCAR. This procedure is a default procedure in many widely used statistical softwares such as SAS, Stata, and R. When the data set has few missing observations, assumption of MCAR is more likely to apply. However, when large number of missing observations are present in the data set then it is difficult to justify MCAR assumption for given data. The main advantage of using complete case analysis is the ease of implementation as researchers can estimate the parameter of interest by using standard statistical methods. One of the disadvantages of using this method is that the researcher can lose many observations even though they were observed for some of the variables but not for all the variables in the data set. This leads to decrease in power of the analysis and ignore the information in incomplete cases (Kim and Curry, 1997; Little and Rubin, 2019). Meta-analysis using published studies with all observed variables can produce biased pooled estimates if the assumption of MCAR does not hold. In some regression analysis, complete case analysis may produce unbiased estimates of regression coefficients; however, the standard errors do not accurately reflect the fact that variables have missing observations (White and Carlin, 2010). This concept can also be translated in fixed-effects and random-effects models in meta-analysis.

10.2.1.2 Pair-Wise Deletion (Available Case Analysis)

Pair-wise deletion or available case analysis uses as much as of available data to estimate the parameters. For example, descriptive statistics such as means and standard deviations of a variable with missing observations can be estimated from available data which might be different and more powerful than complete case analysis as discussed in previous section. However, the potential problems increase when interest is focused on bivariate or multivariable analysis. For example, in estimating the correlation between five variables with 10% ,20%,30%,40%, and 50% missing values, respectively, variance-covariance matrix estimate using available cases could be based on different subsets of the original data set. While Kim and Curry (1997) argue that estimates can be improved by using available cases instead of complete cases, others (Anderson et al., 1983; Haitovsky, 1968; Little and Rubin, 2019) have demonstrated the problems with this procedure. If the data are MCAR, then variance-covariance matrix estimation may provide unbiased estimates because each of the subsets is a representative sample of original data. However, if data are MAR, then each of the subset is not a representative of the original data and may produce biased estimates.

10.2.2 Single Imputation Methods

In single imputation methods, missing values are replaced with single values assuming the replaced values are true values that would have been observed if the data would have been complete. Single imputation methods do not take into account the uncertainty about prediction of those imputed missing values. When the data are missing, we can never be completely certain about the imputed values.

Mean imputation is the method where a missing value on a certain variable is replaced by the mean of the available cases. This method tends to underestimate the variance and also decreases the magnitude of the covariance and correlation which can lead to biased estimate irrespective of underlying missing mechanisms (Enders, 2010; Eekhout et al., 2012).

Single regression imputation is also one of the single imputation methods where the missing values are replaced with predicted values from a regression equation coming from complete observations. This method assumes that the imputed values fall directly on a regression line with nonzero slope which implies the perfect correlation between the predictors and missing outcome variables. In contrast to single regression imputation, stochastic regression imputation error is added to the predicted value from the regression equation which is drawn from a normal distribution. This method can produce unbiased estimates with MAR data; however, the standard error may be underestimated because the uncertainty about the imputed values is not included. This ultimately leads to higher probability of Type I error (Enders, 2010).

In general, single imputation methods are very easy to apply to a data set; however, they have many pitfalls in terms of obtaining valid inferences. There are many missing data methods which are available in widely used statistical packages such as SAS, STATA, and R which are based on solid statistical theory and modeling. In next section, we will focus on these model-based methods to handle missing data in meta-analysis.

10.2.3   Model-Based Methods For Missing Data

ML and MI methods are very popular and widely used statistical methods to handle missing data based on model approach. These two methods generally provide unbiased estimates given that the underlying missing mechanism assumption is true. Both methods have very similar statistical properties and are more superior than ad hoc methods described in previous section of this chapter.

10.2.3.1   Maximum Likelihood Method

ML is one of the alternative methods to handle the missing data for statistical analysis including meta-analysis (Little and Rubin, 2019). Parameter estimates of interest can be estimated based on full likelihood function without any missing data. In presence of missing data, researchers have access to only observed data likelihood. Inferences based on observed data likelihood may be biased. Hence, the general idea of ML method for missing data is to obtain the full data likelihood based on observed data likelihood and underlying missing data mechanism assumption. Furthermore, the inferences can be drawn from this full data likelihood.

10.2.3.2   Multiple Imputations

MI is one of the widely used model-based statistical methods to address the issue of missing data. It is a very powerful technique developed by Rubin in 1970 based on Monte Carlo simulation method (Little and Rubin, 2019). As discussed in previous section, single imputation methods mainly have two disadvantages: (1) they do not incorporate uncertainty around the true value and (2) single imputation methods tend to increase Type I error in majority of analyses. One of the common misconceptions with MI is that imputed values should represent "real" values. Instead, the purpose of MI is to correctly reproduce variance-covariance matrix we would have observed if we had our data without any missing (Bruin, 2011). In general, there are three stages of MI techniques.

In the first stage, missing values in observed data are replaced with imputed values based on the specified imputation model. This process is repeated m times which result into m number of complete data sets. The imputed values in each data set are sampled from their predictive distribution based on the observed data under specified imputed missing data model. Therefore, this stage of MI is based on Bayesian approach. It is very important to specify the imputation model thoughtfully for improving the performance of MIs. This step requires to include variables in imputation model under the most plausible missing data mechanism assumption for given data. All the variables of primary interest of any statistical analysis such as the outcome variables, predictor variables, and covariates should be included in the imputation model. It is also important to have an imputation model which fits the distribution assumptions of the data. For example, if missing data are all continuous then multivariate normal distribution may be used for imputation. However, when data are not continuous or not normally distributed then other imputation algorithms can be used. In second stage, standard statistical methods are used to analyze the m imputed data sets generated in first stage. Estimated associations and ESs in each of the imputed data set will differ because of the variation introduced in the imputation of missing values. In third stage, the parameter estimates and standard errors obtained from each analyzed data set are then combined by using Rubin's rule for inference (Rubin, 1987). Rubin's rule of combining inferences from imputed data sets take account of the variability in estimates between imputed data sets.

Over the years, many MI methods have been developed in literature and it is the most recommended technique for handling missing data in any statistical analysis, including meta-analysis (Kleinke et al., 2020). One of the most widely and general parametric MI method uses Markov Chain Monte Carlo procedures. This method of MI assumes that all the variables in the imputation model have joint multivariate normal distribution. The assumption of multivariate normality may not hold for many data sets; however, simulation studies have shown that reliable results still can be produced given the sufficient sample size (Demirtas et al., 2008; Lee and Carlin, 2010). One of the MI methods developed by Van Buuren (2007) does not assume joint multivariate normal distribution. This approach of MI is commonly known as multiple imputation by chained equations (MICE). It uses separate conditional distribution for each variable in imputation model. If the variable only takes binary values or variable only takes positive integer values for count data, then MICE will impute these values accordingly. Currently, MICE is the most general method available for MI and has been adopted by many commonly used statistical softwares such as STATA, SAS, and R.

MI may give different results every time when the analysis is being conducted. This is because the first stage of MI uses random draws from the predictive distribution. This variability can be reduced by imputing a large number of data sets. However, ML produces deterministic results. Unlike the MI, ML method has no problem of incompatibility between analytic model and imputation model because it only uses one model. In contrast to some disadvantages of using MI compared to ML, it has many advantages as well. The major limitation of using ML method is that sometime full data likelihood function after assuming missing data mechanism is intractable and it becomes very difficult to maximize parameter estimates. Expectation-maximization algorithm is a very powerful method to handle these scenarios; however, obtaining the consistent estimates of standard error is the biggest obstacle of using these algorithms. Overall, ML and MI are very powerful model-based methods to handle missing data in meta-analysis which can produce unbiased estimates under ignorable as well as nonignorable missing mechanism assumptions. In practice, it is not possible to test the assumption of missing mechanism based on the observed data alone. Hence, sensitivity analysis should be performed to quantify the departure from the assumed missing mechanism for given data. Both ML and MI can be used to perform sensitivity analysis to explore the uncertainty due to missing data in meta-analysis.

10.3   Sensitivity Analysis by Informative Missingness Approach

Informative missingness (IM) approach is a unique way to handle missing observations in meta-analysis especially in aggregate (summary) data from published studies. When aggregate data in meta-analysis are MNAR but they are analyzed under the assumption of MAR or MCAR then nonresponse bias can occur. White et al. (2008) proposed the method of IM for binary outcomes with aggregate data by quantifying the ratio of the odds of the outcome among subjects with unobserved outcome to the odds of the outcome among observed subjects. They referred this quantity as informative missingness odds ratios (IMORs). Mavridis et al. (2015) extended the IM approach to meta-analyses with continuous outcomes by defining informative missingness parameters (IMPs) that relate the mean of the outcome between the missing and the observed participants. IMPs are like sensitivity parameters which measure the departure from MAR assumption (Kenward et al., 2001). Many statistical softwares such as STATA can perform sensitivity analysis for aggregate data (Chaimani et al., 2018). In our next section, we will show how to use IMORs to analyze binary outcome data for meta-analyses.

10.4   Application

In this section, we will show the application of missing data methods to meta-analysis with missing data especially missing binary outcome and missing predictors.

10.4.1 Meta-Analysis of Studies with Missing Outcome

When it comes to missing data in meta-analysis, it is often the case where the outcome variable is missing. In this section, we are demonstrating the approaches that can be used for dealing with missing binary outcomes by taking the example of Haloperidol vs Placebo in schizophrenia studies.

The published studies for Haloperidol meta-analysis data came from 17 clinical trials that compared the effectiveness of Haloperidol with Placebo in treating Schizophrenia (Irving et al., 2006). The outcome is binary and corresponds to the fact whether there was a success or failure in treating Schizophrenia for each study. Relative Risk (RR) was used to compare the treatments and an RR greater than 1 suggests that Haloperidol works better than Placebo in treating Schizophrenia. The outcome for some of the enrolled patients was missing in many studies. Depending on the most probable assumptions about these missing data, there are different approaches which can be used as explained below.

Available Case Analysis: Under the assumption of MCAR for the outcome, one of the possible approaches is to use the available case analysis. In this case, only the subjects for whom the outcome is known are used. Figure 10.1 shows the output from available case analysis. The test for ES =1 has a z score of 4.37 and the calculated ES is 1.567 from our available case analysis. This demonstrates that Haloperidol is significantly more effective than Placebo.

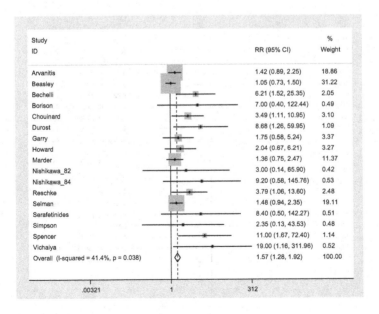

FIGURE 10.1
Available case analysis for Haloperidol vs Placebo data set.

Best Case Scenario: In this approach, the assumption being made is that all the subjects that have missing values in the Haloperidol group have a good outcome (considering them as success) and the missing values in the Placebo group have a bad outcome (considering them as failure). In missing data mechanism, this can be considered as MNAR assumption. Figure 10.2 shows the results for the Best-Case Scenario for the Haloperidol vs Placebo data set. The pooled ES is 2.416 and test of ES = 1 has a z score of 8.0, which corresponds to a p value of 0.000. Hence, under this assumption, Haloperidol is significantly more effective than Placebo.

Worst Case Scenario: In this approach, the assumption being made is that all the subjects who have missing outcome values in Haloperidol group have a bad outcome (considering them as failure) and that the subjects that have missing outcome in Placebo group have a good outcome (considering them as success). Figure 10.3 shows the forest plot of results from the worst-case analysis. The pooled ES is 0.994 and the Z test for ES = 1 has a value of 0.64 (p value = 0.52). This draws to the conclusion that using the worst-case scenario, there is no significant difference in the effectiveness in treating Schizophrenia between Haloperidol and Placebo.

IMOR: Association of the outcome between missing and observed data can be described by logarithm of IMOR. In Haloperidol group, if we assume that there are systematic differences between outcomes in missing and observed participants in positive direction, then we can give logIMOR a distribution with mean = 1 and SD = 1. Furthermore, in Placebo group, if we assume that

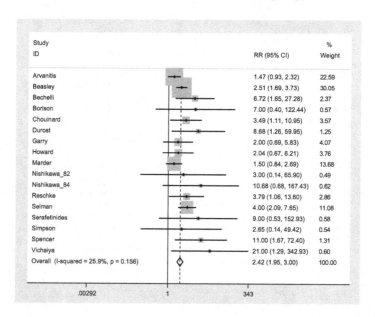

FIGURE 10.2
Best case analysis for Haloperidol vs Placebo data set.

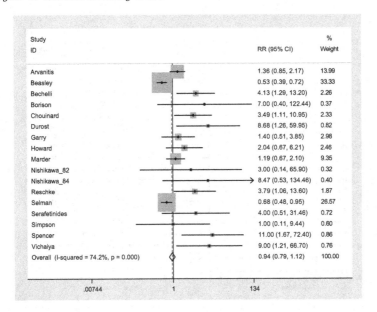

FIGURE 10.3
Worst-case scenario for Haloperidol vs Placebo data set.

response in missing participants is worse than observed participants then we can give the logIMOR a distribution with mean $= -1$ and SD $= 1$. In STATA statistical software, metamiss2 command can be used to perform this analysis (Chaimani et al., 2018). Figure 10.4 gives the forest plot from the output of IMOR approach under one of the MNAR assumption described above. The pooled ES is 2.22; the z score for the test ES $= 1$ is 5.08; and the corresponding value is p-value is 0.000. Hence, under one of the MNAR assumption using the IMOR approach, it can be concluded that Haloperidol is significantly more effective than Placebo in treating Schizophrenia. If we assume that the outcome in the missing participants is on average the same as the outcome in observed participants then that is equivalent to assuming MAR assumption. In general, based on expert opinion or any prior information available from existing literature, sensitivity analysis which measures the departure from MAR assumption can be performed by assuming various distributions on log IMOR.

10.4.2 Meta-Analysis of Studies with Missing Predictors

In this section, we will focus on the aggregated data with missing predictors. The data set was taken from Eagly et al. (2003) who examine the differences in transformational, transactional, and laissez-faire leadership styles by gender. The ES corresponds to the difference between the leadership style of the male and female leaders, divided by the pooled standard deviation. A positive ES indicates that men had a higher transformational leadership score

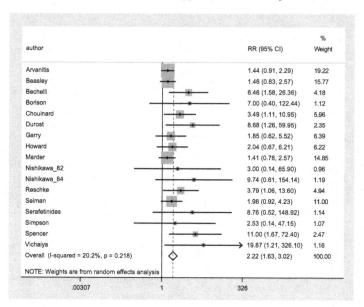

FIGURE 10.4
Informative missingness OR for Haloperidol vs Placebo data set.

than women, and a negative ES indicates that women had a higher score. The variables used to predict ES were the average age of the study participants, percentage of males in leadership roles, if the first author of the study was female (1 = Female, 0 = Male), size of organization which was subject of the study (taking values of 0 = Small, 1 = mixed and 2 = large) and whether random selection methods were utilized for the study (taking values of 0 = random, 1 = unsuccessful random, and 2 = nonrandom). As the last 3 variables were categorical, dummy variables were created according to their response levels and the reference category was set at the level equal to 0. In this data set, the average age of participants and percentage of male leaders was missing (not reported) in many studies.

The method used to measure the effect of each of the predictors on the reported ES was meta-regression. In this data set, only 22 out of 44 studies have reported all the moderators of interest. Table 10.1 demonstrates the estimates of effect of each predictor on ES by conducting a meta-regression analysis under MCAR assumption using available case analysis. By default, this type of analysis can be conducted on almost any statistical package with default options, as it excludes automatically the cases that have missing values in any of the variables of interest. Table 10.1 shows that age, male leaders percentage, female first author, and mixed organization size have a significant effect on reported ES (p value < 0.05).

In order to include the studies that have missing values in some of the variables of interest in the leadership example, we can utilize MI procedure.

TABLE 10.1

Available Case Analysis for Leadership Data

Variable	Coefficient	SE	Z	P value	Lower 95% CI	Upper 95% CI
Intercept	1.3361	0.3735	3.5773	0.0003	0.6040	2.0681
Age	−0.0323	0.0068	−4.7811	0.0000	−0.0456	−0.0191
Male leaders pct	0.0077	0.0024	3.2724	0.0011	0.0031	0.0124
Female first author	−0.2553	0.1170	−2.1814	0.0292	−0.4846	−0.0259
Size Org 1[a]	−0.4982	0.2422	−2.0575	0.0396	−0.9729	−0.0236
Size Org 2[a]	−0.3164	0.2062	−1.5348	0.1248	−0.7205	0.0877
Random selection 1[b]	−0.1038	0.1098	−0.9451	0.3446	−0.3189	0.1114
Random selection 2[b]	0.1182	0.1311	0.9015	0.3673	−0.1388	0.3752

[a] Reference category is Small.
[b] Reference category is Random.

Under the assumption of MAR and due to the presence of categorical variables in our model, we will use MIs with chained equations. The missing values were imputed for 30 times to generate 30 data sets with complete observations. Then meta-regression was used to estimate the effect of each predictor on ES for each data set. Finally, the estimated parameters were pooled together to have a final estimate of effect for each predictor by Rubin's rule.

TABLE 10.2

Multiple Imputation under MAR Assumption for Leadership Data

Variable	Coefficient	SE	Z	P value	Lower 95% CI	Upper 95% CI
Intercept	0.5333	0.3544	1.5000	0.1500	−0.2125	1.2790
Age	−0.0113	0.0071	−1.5900	0.1380	−0.0268	0.0042
Male leaders pct	0.0035	0.0025	1.3900	0.1900	−0.0020	0.0091
Female first author	−0.0444	0.0923	−0.4800	0.6360	−0.2382	0.1493
Size Org 1[a]	−0.2131	0.2002	−1.0600	0.2970	−0.6247	0.1985
Size Org 2[a]	−0.2050	0.1938	−1.0600	0.3000	−0.6030	0.1930
Random Selection 1[b]	−0.2501	0.1219	−2.0500	0.0510	−0.5016	0.0014
Random Selection 2[b]	−0.1037	0.1410	−0.7400	0.4710	−0.3995	0.1921

[a] Reference category is Small.
[a] Reference category is Random.

Table 10.2 represents the final estimates of effect of each predictor on ES produced from MI procedure. Furthermore, based on expert opinion or based on existing literature, MI can be performed under any specific MNAR model.

10.5 Conclusion

In this chapter, we have reviewed available missing data methods to conduct meta-analysis with major focus on missing outcome and missing predictors. It is well known that the observed data are not sufficient to identify the underlying missing mechanism. Therefore, sensitivity analyses should be performed over various plausible models for the nonresponse mechanism (Little and Rubin, 2019). In general, the stability of conclusions (inferences) over the plausible models gives an indication of their robustness to unverifiable assumptions about the mechanism underlying missingness. Available case analysis and single imputation methods are very convenient ways to address the issue of missing data in aggregate data or individual participant data (if available for each study). However, these methods require the assumption of MCAR which very rarely holds in practice. Currently, MI and ML methods are very widely used methods under ignorable or nonignorable missing mechanisms. Finally, it is not possible to verify the missing mechanism based on observed data; hence, it is highly recommended to evaluate the departure from the assumed missing mechanism by doing sensitivity analysis.

11

Meta-Analysis for Evaluating Diagnostic Accuracy

Jingjing Yin and Jing Kersey

The meta-analysis (MA) of this chapter is to summarize and synergize the results of a group of diagnostic test accuracy (DTA) studies that evaluate the performance of diagnostic tests of the same disease. One single study of a diagnostic test is usually limited due to the small sample size and restricted population. Therefore, MA is needed to combine common results and investigates the differences between DTA studies in order to give better conclusions of the performance of the diagnostic tests. This chapter focuses on the statistical analysis basics of the MA of diagnostic studies for evaluating and comparing the diagnostic accuracy of tests. The methods discussed in this chapter are based primarily on sensitivity and specificity, as most studies report only the sensitivity and specificity. Additionally, analysis based on the summary ROC (SROC) curve will be discussed. Relevant R and Stata programming code for the methods discussed in this chapter will be given.

11.1 Introduction

In this chapter, we introduce the basics of the statistical analysis for evaluating the diagnosing performance of diagnostic tests/biomarkers and the MA for a group of DTA studies of the same disease. Such MA studies are generally referred to as Diagnostic Meta-Analysis.

The objective of the MA of DTA studies is to synergize the accuracy results from different studies and investigate the differences between studies in order to give better conclusions of the performance of the diagnostic tests. In addition, a MA of diagnostic studies can determine the sample size and research scope for each of the diagnostic studies considered; it can study the association of diagnostic accuracy with patient and clinical settings; it can help identify potential design mistakes and provide insights for future diagnostic studies; finally, it can increase the power of test when pooling similar studies together. One important consideration that is common to all MA studies is to determine the scope of analysis, such as which disease and which test(s) are of interest and the targeting population of patient and the reference/gold standard for evaluation in general before performing the MA for diagnostic studies. Then the scope of analysis will determine the inclusion/exclusion criteria of literature reviews.

The MA of DTA studies depends on summary diagnostic measures, such as sensitivity and specificity, diagnostic odds ratio (DOR), likelihood ratios, ROC indices such as the area under the ROC curve or predictive values. When the reported sensitivity or specificity estimates are similar for all DTA studies of interest, usually a summary measure of sensitivity and specificity is reported in a MA, which is generally referred to as the "summary point" approach. On the other hand, sensitivity or specificity estimates can be very different across DTA studies, particularly when the test measures are continuous, and different DTA studies have a very different threshold. In those cases, the SROC curve approach is more appropriate. The SROC curve approach demonstrates different values of sensitivity and specificity in a scatter plot and fits a smooth "summary curve" along the reported scatter points. The "summary curve" approach shows how the average sensitivity changes with the average specificity across all possible threshold choices through regression models. In addition, sensitivity and specificity are inherently correlated, so the MA of medical tests reporting both sensitivity and specificity becomes a bivariate problem, and bivariate analysis considering the correlation should be used. This chapter focuses on the statistical analysis basics of the MA of diagnostic studies using the sensitivity (i.e., true positive (TP) rate) and/or specificity (1-false positive (FP) rate) for evaluating the diagnostic accuracy of tests. This chapter summarizes and illustrates the most common approaches that either reporting "summary point" or "summary curve." This chapter also presents methods handling potential heterogeneity between diagnostic accuracy studies and the inherent correlation between sensitivity and specificity. A MA of diagnostic measures other than sensitivity and specificity can be derived from the MA summaries of the sensitivity, specificity-pairs by the given formulas listed in this chapter.

The organization of the chapter is as follows: Section 11.2 gives an overview of medical diagnostic accuracy studies and the basics of statistical methods, including ROC analysis for such studies. Section 11.3 presents MA methods for reporting a single value of sensitivity or specificity. However, it is not the best approach as usually sensitivity and specificity are reported together, and their estimates are naturally correlated. Therefore, the later sections focus on the joint inference approach of both sensitivity and specificity. Section 11.4 presents a bivariate model resulting in an estimated "summary point" in a MA of DTA when the reported sensitivity and specificity values do not vary significantly between studies. Section 11.5 presents the SROC curve analysis, including the random intercept model, bivariate model, and hierarchical summary ROC (HSROC) model, which all give a fitted "summary curve" when the reported sensitivity and specificity values vary significantly between DTA studies. Sections 11.6 and 11.7 gives step-by-step R and Stata programming demonstrations for the methods discussed in previous sections. Finally, Section 11.8 introduces other software in addition to R and Stata that can be used for MA of DTA studies.

11.2 Medical Diagnostic Tests Accuracy Studies

DTA studies aim to assess the diagnostic performance of a test/biomarker for differentiating between individuals with the disease status of interest and those without. The diagnostic test of interest does not always give the correct results, so we compare it with the reference standard or gold standard to determine the true disease status. The DTA generally describes four key components: the disease condition of interest; the diagnostic test(s) of interest; the reference standard (usually the existing best method that is commonly used in clinical practice for assessing the disease of interest); and the targeting patient population and clinical setting. A perfect diagnostic test would identify all truly diseased individuals as disease positive and nondiseased individuals as disease negative, so if the test results do not overlap for different disease status. While if the test results do not differ between different disease statuses, the test performs no better than random chance, thus is useless. Most diagnostic studies fall between. If the diagnostic test is binary, that is, the results are either positive or negative, and the disease conditions are also binary (i.e., nondiseased versus diseased), then we can form a two-by-two table in Table 11.1 that cross-classifies the test results with the true disease condition given by the reference standard. There are two types of diagnostic errors: false negative (FN) means incorrectly classifying a diseased individual as disease negative and FP is incorrectly classifying a nondiseased individual as disease positive. The corresponding correct cases are referred to as TP and true negative (TN). The proportion/rate of TPs is referred to as sensitivity, while the proportion/rate of TNs is referred to as specificity. Likewise, the FP rate is 1− specificity, and the FN rate is 1− sensitivity.

TABLE 11.1

Two-by-Two Table of Diagnostic Tests
Against True Disease Condition

	Test Results	
True condition	positive	negative
Present	TP	FN
Absent	FP	TN

From Table 11.1, the positive results for individuals with the disease condition are referred to as TPs, and the negative results for individuals without the disease condition are referred to as TNs. We can see these correct diagnosis results fall on the diagonal. The results lying off diagonals of Table 11.1 are FNs for those with a negative diagnosis but with the disease and FPs for those with a positive diagnosis but without the disease condition. The two most popular diagnostic measures are sensitivity and specificity, which are the proportion of TP over all of the disease samples and the proportion of TN over all of the nondisease samples.

In other situations where the diagnostic test is based on continuous biomarker measurements, a cut-off value c is needed to classify subjects into two groups (positive or negative diagnosis). Without loss of generality, assuming all the test measurements are higher in the disease group, the diagnosis is positive (T^+) if the measurement is greater than c and negative (T^-) if less than or equal to c. Different choices of diagnostic cut-off will result in different diagnosis for an individual. Thus for the targeting population, the proportions of positive and negative results depend on the cut-off c. Figure 11.1 gives the graphical representation of sensitivity and specificity under numeric diagnostic tests.

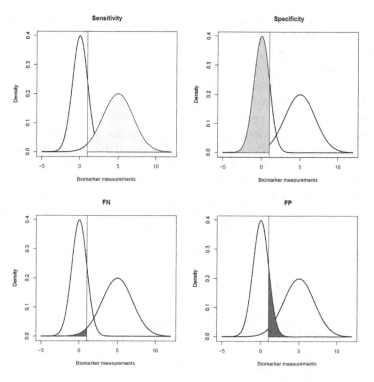

FIGURE 11.1
The plots of sensitivity, specificity, FN rate (FNR), and FP rate (FPR).

The figure gives the density plots of diagnostic test/biomarker measurements from two populations with and without the disease condition of interest. Moreover, the disease population on the right has larger measurements in general with larger variability. The sensitivity is defined as the area under the disease density that larger than the threshold c, and specificity is defined as the area under the nondisease density that less than the c. The incorrect diagnosis rates were the FN rate (FNR) under the non-disease density (1-sensitivity) and FP rate (FPR) under the disease density (1-specificity).

Mathematically, we can express sensitivity as $P(D+ > c|D+)$ for continuous test measures or $P(T + |D+)$ for binary test measures, and specificity as $P(D- \leq c|D-)$ or $P(T - |D-)$. The test accuracy is often described using complementary measures of sensitivity and specificity and reports them in pairs. For a continuous diagnostic test measure, there is a trade-off phenomenon between sensitivity and specificity that as threshold value c increases, sensitivity decreases while specificity increases (Yin and Tian 2014a). Figure 11.2 demonstrates such trade-off, and the sensitivity (in grey) decreases while specificity (in black) increases when the threshold value c increases. This trade-off phenomenon can potentially result in vastly different values of sensitivity and specificity estimates for the same diagnostic test in different DTA studies. Clinicians choose different values of c and can weigh sensitivity and specificity differently depending on the comparative cost of whether having an FN or FP result. If the cost of FP is higher, for instance,

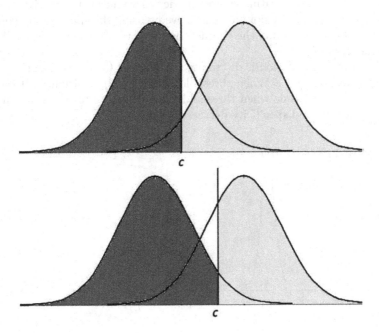

FIGURE 11.2
Trade-off between sensitivity and specificity when the threshold value changes.

if a positive diagnosis triggers an invasive procedure, e.g., Breast cancer, then we would prefer a high specificity. On the other hand, if the cost of FN is higher, such as for a life-threatening disease that has an inexpensive and effective diagnosis and treatment, e.g., cervical cancer, we should weigh sensitivity more heavily in this type of situations.

In some circumstances, for example, a certain test requires a minimally acceptable value for the specificity. Thus, the objective would be to make inferences on the range of sensitivity of the test at this given level of specificity. Likewise, sometimes clinicians may want to control for sensitivity, i.e., by giving a fixed minimally acceptable value of sensitivity, and thus make inference on the range of specificity. In other cases, when a diagnostic threshold for the test is known, an objective could be obtaining the range of sensitivity and/or specificity of the test corresponding to a given cut-off value. And you can balance the sensitivity and specificity by using the Youden index, which gives the threshold value with the largest sum of the two proportions (Yin and Tian 2014a).

Additionally, a popular graphical method for evaluating diagnostic accuracy is by the receiver operating characteristic (ROC) curve, which is the graph of a series values of sensitivity against 1-specificity as the cut-off value c runs through all possible values (Yin and Tian 2016). Hence the corresponding ROC curve and the ROC indices (Yin and Tian 2014b) can summarize sensitivity and specificity across all possible diagnostic thresholds (Figure 11.3). The name "receiver operating characteristic" curve means the receivers of the curve can operate at any point on the curve by using the appropriate diagnostic threshold to determine the characteristics of the test (Zhou et al. 2009). There are some ROCs.

The disease population is distributed as Normal (3, 1) and healthy population as Normal (0, 1). When threshold value $c = 2$, sensitivity = 0.84 and specificity = 0.98; while when threshold value decreases to $c = 1$, sensitivity increases to 0.98 and specificity decreases to 0.84.

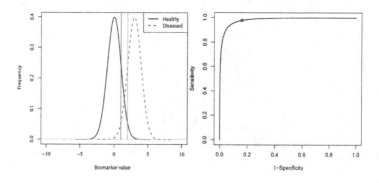

FIGURE 11.3
The construction of ROC curve from pairs of sensitivity and specificity.

If the diagnostic test of interest is inherently binary, we will apply the two most common measures of diagnostic accuracy: the sensitivity, i.e., the proportion of test-positive out of all diseased ($D+$) subjects or the specificity, i.e., the proportion of test-negative out of all nondisease ($D-$) subjects. A MA of DTA studies generally gives a summary of the sensitivity and specificity as they are the most common and primary measures to report for evaluating medical diagnostic tests in DTA studies. Moreover, unlike positive predictive value (PPV) and negative predictive value (NPV)that depend on disease prevalence, sensitivity and specificity are pretest diagnostic accuracy measures, which is independent of the disease prevalence. Prevalence is valid only if it is estimated from a cohort study. Since most DTA studies are with case-control design in order to obtain enough sample size in the case group, the prevalence cannot be estimated directly from the current DTA study. In addition, sensitivity and specificity always range from 0 to 1, which is easy to understand and compare across literature, while other measures may not have the restrictive range such as the diagnostic likelihood ratios (DLRs) or DOR ranges from zero to infinity (Huang et al. 2018). Moreover, the DOR and DLR values rise steeply when one of the pair (sensitivity, specificity) becomes nearly perfect, while the other one of the pair may stay unsatisfactory (Yin and Vogel 2017). Furthermore, if readers prefer to report other diagnostic measures of interest, the expressions of predictive values (PPV and NPV) and DLRs (LR+ and LR−) or DOR as functions of sensitivity and specificity are given below. You can calculate the overall predictive values (for a prespecified value of prevalence rate (pre) of the disease) and other diagnostic accuracy measures using the MA summaries of sensitivity (Se) and specificity (Sp) (Zhou et al. 2009):

$$PPV = \frac{Se \times Pre}{Se \times Pre + (1 - Sp) \times (1 - Pre)} \tag{11.1}$$

$$NPV = \frac{Sp \times (1 - Pre)}{(1 - Se) \times Pre + Sp \times (1 - Pre)} \tag{11.2}$$

$$LR(+) = \frac{P(T=1|D=1)}{P(T=1|D=0)} = \frac{P(T=1|D=1)}{1 - P(T=0|D=0)} = \frac{Se}{1 - Sp} \tag{11.3}$$

$$LR(-) = \frac{P(T=0|D=1)}{P(T=0|D=0)} = \frac{1 - P(T=1|D=1)}{P(T=0|D=0)} = \frac{1 - Se}{Sp} \tag{11.4}$$

$$DOR = \frac{TP/FN}{FP/TN} = \frac{Se/(1-Se)}{(1-Sp)/Sp} = \frac{Se \times Sp}{(1-Se) \times (1-Sp)} = \frac{Se \times Sp}{FPR \times FNR} \tag{11.5}$$

In this chapter, we will demonstrate how to do DTA MA with both R and Stata. The data set ChildrenUS is used in the demonstration. This data set

TABLE 11.2

ChildrenUS Data

Authors	FP	FN	TP	TN
Ang	13	14	145	102
Cha	1	0	3	7
Chang	2	4	26	18
Crady	4	4	22	68
Davidson	9	8	62	174
Hahn	97	50	444	3268
Han	1	0	13	79
Hayden	1	1	53	75
Kaiser	20	48	196	336
Karakas	9	9	26	138
Lessin	3	4	28	64
Lowe	7	0	20	51
Pena	6	28	22	83
Quillin	5	5	34	56
Ramachandran	6	5	55	206
Rice	7	5	36	55
Ronco	8	8	104	188
Rubin	5	5	40	60
Siegel	0	7	31	140
Sivit-92	5	6	46	123
Sivit-00	17	18	65	215
Vignault	4	2	31	33
Wong ML	1	4	25	61

(shown in Table 11.2) includes 23 studies on the ultrasonography test in diagnosing appendicitis in Children (Doria et al. 2006). The average numbers of children with and without appendicitis are 77 and 254, respectively. Each study provides the author of the study and the counts of TP, FP, TN, and FN.

We can see the reported sensitivity and specificity values along with the respective 95% confidence intervals from each DTA study in a forest plot, as in Figure 11.4.

11.3 Meta-Analysis Pooling a Single Value of the Sensitivity or the Specificity

There are two situations for MA of DTA studies: (1) the reported sensitivity and specificity estimates from different DTA studies are similar; (2) the sensitivity and specificity are significantly different. Generally, MA will give a "summary" point for the first case. This could happen in meta-analyses if the

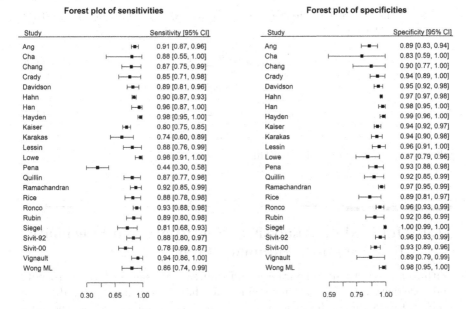

FIGURE 11.4
Forest plot for sensitivity and specificity of the ChildrenUS data.

diagnostic test of interest is continuous, and all DTA studies have the same or similar diagnostic threshold. This also applies to binary diagnostic tests if the sensitivity (or specificity) does not differ vastly between DTA studies. For the first situation, if only one proportion (either sensitivity or specificity) is of interest, general MA methods where the (weighted) average value of the statistic of interest (usually a single statistic) from different studies are reported. Such examples include the average proportion presented in the previous sections of the single sensitivity or specificity, the average relative risk in epidemiology studies, and the average standardized mean difference between the treatment and control groups in clinical studies. If both proportions are of interest, then we need to consider the correlation between the two proportions and apply the bivariate approach and report the summary values as a pair jointly. This section and the following Section 11.4 will focus on the "summary point" approach, and the later Section 11.5 will present methods for the "summary curve" for sensitivity and specificity pairs across different DTA studies.

For the binary test or the continuous test with the same threshold across DTA studies, if only one measure, either the sensitivity or the specificity is of interest, then we do not need to worry about the correlation between the two proportions. Therefore, the inference of MA using only the sensitivity, or the specificity marginally is the same as the general MA for a single statistic (i.e., a proportion), which is the weighted average with the weight to be the inverse of the variance of the reported proportions (θ_i) from each DTA study Zhou et al. (2009):

$$\widehat{\theta} = \frac{\sum_{i=1}^{G} \widehat{\theta}_i / \widehat{\sigma}_i^2}{\sum_{i=1}^{G} 1 / \widehat{\sigma}_i^2} \tag{11.6}$$

$$Var\left(\widehat{\theta}\right) = \frac{1}{\sum_{i=1}^{G} 1 / \widehat{\sigma}_i^2} \tag{11.7}$$

where σ_i^2 is the variance of the estimate of θ_i.

11.4 Joint Meta-Analysis of Sensitivity and Specificity Resulting in a Summary Point

Within each study, only when the cut-off values are prespecified, the sensitivity and specificity estimates are independent as they are estimated from different groups of individuals. However, if the cut-off value is estimated from the data, such as using the Youden index or other threshold optimization method, then the estimated sensitivity and specificity are correlated. Furthermore, due to the trade-off phenomena between the sensitivity and specificity when using different threshold values, the estimated study-specific values are likely negatively correlated, and such observation is referred to as the "threshold effect." Therefore, it is necessary to consider summarizing both sensitivity and specificity jointly in the MA for continuous diagnostic tests when reporting the MA summaries of both the sensitivity and specificity. In addition, even for binary tests, if both the sensitivity and the specificity are of interest, then we need to consider the correlation between the two proportions. However, the traditional MA analysis using the weighted average ignores the correlation between sensitivity and specificity. When both measures are in consideration, the weighted average approach in Section 11.4 will underestimate the summary sensitivity and specificity.

In addition, the weighted average approach assumes homogeneity between studies that variations between the reported sensitivity (specificity) values from the selected diagnostic studies are purely due to a random error; however, in reality, due to different clinical settings, tests operators and evaluators, or different patient characteristics, the diagnostic accuracy measures can be truly different between studies. Such a situation is referred to as between-study heterogeneity. The previous chapter in this book discussed measures to test if heterogeneity exists in a MA, and we can apply here to check if heterogeneity exists between DTA studies. A common way of accounting for between-study heterogeneity and correlation between sensitivity and specificity pairs is using the bivariate MA approach, which models the sensitivity (or true-positive rate (TPR)) and specificity (or false-positive rate (FPR)) directly and jointly. The bivariate model in a MA for DTA studies has two levels of modeling. At the first level, it models the variability of TPR (sensitivity) and FPR (1-specificity) within each DTA study, respectively, and assumes normal distributions for each. At the second level, the correlation between TPR and FPR is accounted directly by assuming a bivariate normal distribution, and the between-study heterogeneity was accounted for by using the average sensitivity and specificity Reitsma et al. (2005). Let $\xi_i = logit(FPR_i)$ and $\eta_i = logit(TPR_i)$ be the true population parameters for each study. A bivariate normal model for (ξ_i, η_i) is

$$(\xi_i, \eta_i) \sim N\left(\begin{pmatrix} \xi \\ \eta \end{pmatrix}, \begin{pmatrix} \sigma_\xi^2 & \sigma_{\xi\eta} \\ \sigma_{\xi\eta} & \sigma_\eta^2 \end{pmatrix} \right) \tag{11.8}$$

$$\widehat{\xi}_i | \xi \sim N\left(\xi_i, \frac{1}{r_{1i}} + \frac{1}{r_{0i}} \right), \tag{11.9}$$

$$\widehat{\eta}_i | \eta \sim N\left(\eta_i, \frac{1}{s_{1i}} + \frac{1}{s_{0i}} \right), \tag{11.10}$$

The normality assumption in both layers of models is approximately true under large samples, and such a model is referred to as the Normal-Normal model. Since sensitivity and specificity are proportions, another way is to assume binomial distributions in the first layer for modeling the with-in study variability, which would be more appropriate for smaller samples (Arends et al. 2008):

$$\widehat{\xi}_i \sim Binomial\left(\frac{1}{1 + e^{-\xi_i}}, n_{0i} \right), \tag{11.11}$$

$$\widehat{\eta}_i \sim Binomial\left(\frac{1}{1 + e^{-\eta_i}}, n_{1i} \right). \tag{11.12}$$

This type of model is referred to as Binomial-Normal model. Note that the 95% bivariate confidence region of sensitivity (TPR) and 1-specificity (FPR) using the bivariate model is plotted in Figure 11.5.

11.5 Joint Meta-Analysis of Sensitivity and Specificity Resulting in Summary ROC Curve

As we have discussed earlier, when sensitivity and specificity estimates from different DTA studies vary significantly, it is more meaningful to demonstrate and model the relation between the average sensitivity and average

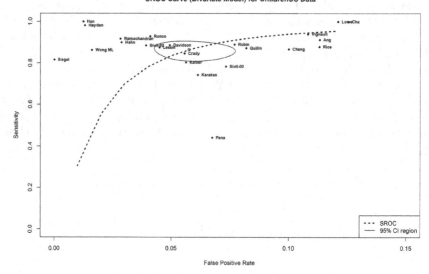

FIGURE 11.5
SROC curve for the ChildrenUS data.

specificity over potentially different choices of threshold values, heterogeneity
in populations, or variation in studies, etc. Given that the statistical analysis
based on the ROC curve considers the sensitivity and specificity together, we
can follow the regular ROC analysis to construct a summary of different values of sensitivity and specificity from different studies with different diagnostic
cut-off values. Such a "summary curve" adopting from the regular ROC curve
is designed particularly for MA of DTA studies and is referred to as a SROC
curve.

Figure 11.5 gives the reported sensitivity (or TPR) on the y-axis and the
reported FPR (or 1-specificity) on the x-axis as a point for each study. To
produce a smooth SROC curve (i.e., the dashed-line) from the observed data,
we can use variables $U = logit(FPR)$ and $V = logit(TPR)$ so that the
smooth SROC curve can be linearized through the logit transformation, and
thus linear regression model can be applied. Another popular method Moses
et al. (1993), referred as the Moses-Littenberg method in the MA literature,
projects (V, U) into the (S, B) space as $B = V - U$ and $S = U + V$, where S
and B are the linear functions of U and V and fit the linear regression as

$$B = \phi_0 + \phi_1 S \tag{11.13}$$

The interpretation of B, i.e., the outcome from the above regression model, is
the log of the DOR, as B is the difference between the logit functions of TPR
and FPR. If we simplify the equation, we can arrive at the conclusion. We can
transform back to the original SROC space expressing the TPR=SROC as a
function of FPR:

$$SROC\left(FPR\right) = \left[1 + e^{-\phi_0/(1-\phi_1)} \left(\frac{1 - FPR}{FPR}\right)^{(1+\phi_1)/(1-\phi_1)}\right]^{-1} \quad (11.14)$$

so that we can plot the smooth SROC curve (i.e., the dashed line) along with the observed scatter plot in Figure 11.5.

The above analysis of SROC assumes that the sensitivity and specificity pairs across all DTA studies are the same, such that the effect is fixed, and there is no heterogeneity between studies. If heterogeneity is detected between studies, the most straightforward idea is to consider adding a simple random intercept that is unique to each of the study, in the (S, B) linear regression model to account for the variability between studies other than pure random error. This approach is popular when heterogeneity exists, and we do not know or collect data for potential causes of such heterogeneity. Therefore, we could consider the random-effects model to account for the heterogeneity between studies as the following (Zhou et al. 2009):

$$B_i = \phi_{0i} + \phi_1 S_i + \varepsilon_i \quad (11.15)$$

$$\phi_{0i} \sim N\left(\phi, \sigma_{\phi_0}^2\right) \quad (11.16)$$

If more covariate data are collected across DTA studies, which can help explain the heterogeneity between studies, then we should include those covariates (z) in the regression model. We can transform the fitted regression line back to the original SROC space similarly to the fixed SROC method.

Furthermore, following the bivariate method in Section 11.4, we can transform the bivariate model of TPR and FPR into the logit space of (U, V). The logit space of (U, V) can be further transformed into the (B, S) space so that we can obtain a fitted linear regression line for the model of $B = \phi_0 + \phi_1 S$ and transform it back to the SROC space. The relation between the parameters in the bivariate model from Section 11.4 to the regression parameters is (Zhou et al. 2009):

$$\phi_1 = \frac{\sigma_\eta^2 - \sigma_\xi^2}{\sigma_\eta^2 + \sigma_\xi^2 + 2\sigma_{\eta\xi}} \text{ and } \phi_0 = \eta - \xi - \phi_1\left(\eta + \xi\right). \quad (11.17)$$

Additionally, another type of statistical model using the Bayesian approach for fitting the SROC curve with heterogeneity between studies is the HSROC model. HSROC model is hierarchical with random effects, which is similar to the bivariate model, and it fits for within-study variability in the first step of modeling and the between-study variability (heterogeneity) as the second. The HSROC model differs from the bivariate model in the parameterization at the second step: the bivariate model uses sensitivity and specificity as parameters directly, while the HSROC model uses a scale parameter α and location parameters β_i where β_i is unique for each DTA study. Both α and β_s are random and assumed to be distributed as uniform and normal distributions, respectively. The mean of the underlying normal distribution of β_i depends on some hyperparameters λ_0 and λ_1 as $E(\beta_i) = \lambda_0 + \lambda_1 Z_i$, which can account for heterogeneity due to different covariates values from each DTA study. In the third step of the HSROC model, the underlying distributions of the hyperparameters λ_0 and λ_1 and the hyperparameters for defining the variances are specified. The equation for the HSROC curve is as follows (Rutter and Gatsonis 2001):

$$SROC\left(FPR\right) = logit^{-1}\left[logit\left(FPR\right)e^{-E(\alpha)} + E\left(\lambda_0 + \lambda_1 Z_i\right)e^{-E(\alpha)/2}\right]$$

$$(11.18)$$

Note that when there are no covariates in the regression model, the HSROC model and bivariate model are mathematically equivalent.

11.6   R Demonstration

Many R packages were developed for DTA MA studies with a standard approach. For example, "mada" (Doebler and Holling 2015) and "mvmeta" (Gasparrini and Gasparrini 2019) for fitting the bivariate normal models, "lme4" (Bates et al. 2007) for bivariate binomial that fits the sensitivity and specificity (proportions) better than the normal models, and "HSROC" (Schiller and Dendukuri 2015) for fitting the HSROC models. In this chapter, we use "mada" and "lme4" packages for illustration of the R programming. It gives a summary of MA estimates of sensitivity and specificity, and it can also estimate the area under the summary ROC curve as a single accuracy measure and fit the meta-regression models. Other R packages use more advanced methods, such as "bamdit" (Verde 2018) using the Bayesian approach to fit the bivariate model and accounting for more challenging situations such as modeling multiple diagnostic thresholds (Steinhauser et al. 2016) and performing MA for DTA with an imperfect gold standard (Huang 2014).

We will demonstrate how to obtain the forest plot (Figure 11.4) and the SROC curve (Figure 11.5) in R with packages "mada" and "lme4." We will also fit the bivariate binomial model and HSROC models.

We set the working directory to the appropriate drive where the data file (normally a .csv file) is saved. And then, we read the data file to R.

```
setwd(".../Code")
```

```
##Read the dataset ChildrenUS.csv to R and name it as 'x.'
X <- read.csv(file = "ChildrenUS.csv", header = TRUE)
```

We need to install the packages "mada" and "lme4" for MA of DTA and load those packages.

```
#install.packages("mada")
#install.packages("lme4")

##Load the packages

library(mada)
library(lme4)
```

First, we will use function madad in the "mada" package to produce the forest plots for both sensitivity and specificity of the ChildrenUS data. We can save the plots in one file named "ChildrenUS Forestplots" with various formats, such as .png, .svg, .tiff, or .pdf.

```
png("ChildrenUS Forestplots.png", width=12, height=8, res=300,
 units="in") ##this line will output the plot
#svg(filename = "ChildrenUS Forestplot.svg", width=12, height=8)
#tiff("ChildrenUS Forestplot.tiff", width=12, height=8,
 compression = "lzw", res=300, units="in")
#pdf("ChildrenUS Forestplot.pdf", width=12, height=8)

par(mfrow=c(1,2))
forest(madad(X, correction.control = "single", method = "wald"),
 type = "sens", main = "Forest plot of sensitivities",
 snames=X$Study)
text(-0.2, 24.35, "Study", pos = 2)
text(1.05, 24.35, "Sensitivity [95% CI]", pos=4)

forest(madad(X, correction.control = "single", method = "wald"),
  type = "spec", main = "Forest plot of specificities",
  snames=X$Study)
text(0.3, 24.35, "Study", pos=2)
text(1.03, 24.35, "Specificity [95% CI]", pos=4)
dev.off()
```

Next, we use function "reitsma" to fit the bivariate binomial model with random effects. The SROC curve (Figure 11.5) for the ChildrenUS data can be plotted from the fitted model.

• Fitting bivariate binomial model

```
fit <- reitsma(X, correction.control="single")csummary(fit)
## Call:  reitsma.default(data = X, correction.control = "single")
##
## Bivariate diagnostic random-effects meta-analysis
## Estimation method: REML
##
## Fixed-effects coefficients
##                       Estimate Std. Error      z Pr(>|z|) 95%ci.lb 95%ci.ub
```

```
## tsens.(Intercept)     1.851     0.167  11.096   0.000     1.524    2.178 ***
## tfpr.(Intercept)     -2.797     0.130 -21.593   0.000    -3.051   -2.543 ***
## sensitivity           0.864        -       -       -      0.821    0.898
## false pos. rate       0.057        -       -       -      0.045    0.073
## ---
## Signif. codes:  0 '***' 0.001 '**' 0.01 '*' 0.05 '.' 0.1 ' ' 1
##
## Variance components: between-studies Std. Dev and correlation matrix
##        Std. Dev tsens  tfpr
## tsens    0.624  1.000     .
## tfpr     0.419 -0.223 1.000
##
##   logLik     AIC      BIC
##   72.176 -134.352 -125.209
##
## AUC:  0.965
## Partial AUC (restricted to observed FPRs and normalized):  0.818
##
## HSROC parameters
##      Theta     Lambda      beta sigma2theta sigma2alpha
##     -0.949      4.931    -0.399       0.101       0.638
```

- *SROC curve*

```
png(filename = "ChildrenUS SROC.png", width=12, height=8,res=300,
    units="in")
#svg(filename = "ChildrenUS SROC.svg", width=12, height=8)
#tiff("ChildrenUS SROC.tiff", width=12, height=8,
     compression = "lzw", res=300,  units="in")
#pdf("ChildrenUS SROC.pdf", width=12, height=8)
plot(fit, sroclwd=3,sroclty=3,xlim=c(0,0.15), ylim=c(0,1),
    main="SROC Curve (Bivariate Model with Random-effect)
        for ChildrenUS Data")
points(fpr(X), sens(X),pch=20)
text(fpr(X), sens(X), labels=X$Study,cex=0.7, font=2, pos=4)
legend("bottomright", c("SROC", "95% CI region"), lwd=c(3,1),
    lty=c(3,1))
dev.off()
```

Function "glmer" in package "lme4" is another function that can be used to fit bivariate models. It can also be used to fit HSROC models. The data should be in a long format. A new variable study_ID is created to assign a unique identifier for each study. Object Y is the reshaped data frame with the long format data. An indicator variable sens is defined to identify the sensitivity results. The data Y is then sorted by study_ID to cluster the two records per study together. Another indicator variable spec is defined to identify specificity results.

```
X$n1 <- X$TP+X$FN # number with the disease
X$n0 <- X$FP+X$TN # number without the disease
```

```
X$true1 <- X$TP   # number of true positive
X$true0 <- X$TN   # number of true negative
X$study_ID <-1:23 # unique identifier for each study
Y = reshape(X, direction = "long", varying = list( c("n1" ,
    "n0") ,   c( "true1","true0" ) ) ,
            timevar = "sens" , times = c(1,0) , v.names = c("n",
                "true") )
Y = Y[order(Y$id),]
Y$spec<- 1-Y$sens
```

Once the data set is reshaped, we fit a bivariate binomial model, HSROC model with unstructured variance-covariance matrix, and HSROC model with no correlation between sensitivity and specificity.

• Bivariate binomial model

```
model.bivariate= glmer( formula = cbind( true , n - true ) ~ 0
    + sens + spec + (0+sens + spec|study_ID),
                data = Y , family = binomial  )
##More detail can be obtained by using the summary command
(model.bivariate.summary = summary(model.bivariate))

## Generalized linear mixed model fit by maximum likelihood
    (Laplace
##    Approximation) [glmerMod]
##  Family: binomial  ( logit )
## Formula: cbind(true, n - true) ~ 0 + sens + spec + (0 + sens
            + spec |
##      study_ID)
##    Data: Y
##
##     AIC      BIC   logLik deviance df.resid
##    262.1    271.3   -126.1   252.1      41
##
## Scaled residuals:
##     Min      1Q   Median      3Q      Max
## -1.21238 -0.31455  0.00051  0.26401  1.87358
##
## Random effects:
##  Groups    Name Variance Std.Dev. Corr
##  study_ID sens 0.4649    0.6818
##           spec 0.2353    0.4851    0.20
## Number of obs: 46, groups:  study_ID, 23
##
## Fixed effects:
##       Estimate Std. Error z value Pr(>|z|)
```

```
## sens   1.9919     0.1785     11.16    <2e-16 ***
## spec   2.9541     0.1405     21.02    <2e-16 ***
## ---
## Signif. codes:  0 '***' 0.001 '**' 0.01 '*' 0.05 '.' 0.1 ' ' 1
##
## Correlation of Fixed Effects:
##        sens
## spec 0.123
```

• HSROC model with unstructured variance-covariance matrix

```
glmer( formula = cbind( true , n - true ) ~ 0 + sens + spec +
    (0+sens + spec|study_ID),
       data = Y, family = binomial  , nAGQ = 1 , verbose = 2  )
## Generalized linear mixed model fit by maximum likelihood
   (Laplace
##   Approximation) [glmerMod]
##  Family: binomial  ( logit )
## Formula: cbind(true, n - true) ~ 0 + sens + spec +
         (0 + sens + spec |
##      study_ID)
##    Data: Y
##       AIC        BIC     logLik  deviance  df.resid
##  262.1139   271.2571  -126.0569  252.1139        41
## Random effects:
##  Groups    Name Std.Dev. Corr
##  study_ID sens 0.6818
##           spec 0.4851    0.20
## Number of obs: 46, groups:  study_ID, 23
## Fixed Effects:
##  sens   spec
## 1.992  2.954
```

• HSROC model with no correlation

```
glmer( formula = cbind( true , n - true ) ~ 0 + sens + spec +
   (0+sens|study_ID) + (0+spec|study_ID),
       data = Y, family = binomial  , nAGQ = 1 , verbose = 2  )
## Generalized linear mixed model fit by maximum likelihood
     (Laplace
##   Approximation) [glmerMod]
##  Family: binomial  ( logit )
## Formula: cbind(true, n - true) ~ 0 + sens + spec +
         (0 + sens | study_ID) +
##      (0 + spec | study_ID)
##    Data: Y
##       AIC        BIC     logLik  deviance  df.resid
```

```
##   260.4165  267.7310 -126.2082  252.4165         42
## Random effects:
##  Groups      Name Std.Dev.
##  study_ID    sens 0.6846
##  study_ID.1  spec 0.4879
## Number of obs: 46, groups:   study_ID, 23
## Fixed Effects:
##  sens    spec
## 1.995   2.948
```

Function "metadiag" in the package "bamdit" uses JAGS to perform MCMC (Markov Chain Monte Carlo) sampling and can also fit the bivariate random-effects model. Bayesian SROC (BSROC) curves can be plotted from the fitted model using function "bsroc". However, in this example, the range of the observed FPR is less than 20%. Calculating the BSROC curve makes no sense.

11.7 Stata Demonstration

Stata is another data analysis tool that is generally more straightforward for practitioners to handle compared to other statistical software such as SAS and R. The Stata command "midas" (Dwamena 2009) gives an MA summary of diagnostic accuracy measures (sensitivity and specificity) from the bivariate model and provides the fitted SROC curve. Midas can consider heterogeneity between studies and fit meta-regression models. Stata command "metandi" (Harbord and Whiting 2009) uses the same bivariate method as midas, and it can also fit the HSROC model. We use "metandi" for illustrating the Stata programming in this chapter.

MA for ChildrenUS data is carried out with Stata (Version: Stata/SE 16.1 for Windows) as following. First, we need to set the working directory where the data file ChildrenUS.csv is saved.

```
. cd "C:\Code"
C:\Code
```

Second, we need to import the data set into Stata. The summary of the data set can be obtained by command "describe".

```
. insheet using "ChildrenUS.csv", comma clear
(5 vars, 23 obs)

. describe

Contains data
  obs:           23
  vars:           5
-----------------------------------------------------------------------
```

```
               storage    display    value
variable name  type       format     label      variable label
----------------------------------------------------------------------
study          str12      %12s                   Study
fp             byte       %8.0g                   FP
fn             byte       %8.0g                   FN
tp             int        %8.0g                   TP
tn             int        %8.0g                   TN
----------------------------------------------------------------------
Sorted by:
    Note: Dataset has changed since last saved.
```

Now, we do MA with the command "metandi" to fit the bivariate model and the HSROC model.

```
. *** Install gllamm and metandi if needed (to run each command
    statement remove the *) ***
. * ssc install gllamm, replace
. * ssc install metandi, replace
.
. *** Use metandi to meta-analyse studies
. metandi tp fp fn tn


Refining starting values:

Iteration 0: log likelihood = -131.48005
Iteration 1: log likelihood = -126.65195
Iteration 2: log likelihood = -126.4444
Iteration 3: log likelihood = -125.99882


Performing gradient-based optimization:

Iteration 0: log likelihood = -125.99882
Iteration 1: log likelihood = -125.99681
Iteration 2: log likelihood = -125.99681


Meta-analysis of diagnostic accuracy


Log likelihood   = -125.99681               Number of studies =   23
```

	Coef.	Std. Err.	z	P>|z|	[95% Conf. Interval]	
Bivariate						
E(logitSe)	1.992739	.1803329			1.639293	2.346185
E(logitSp)	2.954364	.1417309			2.676577	3.232152
Var(logitSe)	.4710237	.2042426			.201349	1.101884
Var(logitSp)	.2381015	.1396696			.0754137	.7517514
Corr(logits)	.2035082	.355215			-.4776218	.73184
HSROC						
Lambda	5.184033	.4150577			4.370535	5.997531
Theta	-.911742	.4655078			-1.82412	.0006365
beta	-.3411056	.3609704	-0.94	0.345	-1.048595	.3663834
s2alpha	.8060862	.3818046			.3185722	2.039647

s2theta	.1333687	.0768954		.0430807	.4128811
Summary pt.					
Se	.8800326	.0190387		.8374387	.9126305
Sp	.9504693	.0066723		.9356303	.9620264
DOR	140.7666	34.19156		87.44736	226.5962
LR+	17.76744	2.471126		13.52814	23.33519
LR-	.1262191	.0201608		.092292	.172618
1/LR-	7.922731	1.265485		5.793138	10.83518

Covariance between estimates of E(logitSe) & E(logitSp)   .0031953

Metandi gives the parameter estimates of the SROC model and produces a summary ROC plot as below:

```
. metandi tp fp fn tn, plot

. metandiplot tp fp fn tn [aw=1], conf(off) pred(off) ///
> summ(off) yscale(titlegap(3)) xscale(titlegap(3)) legend(off) ///
> title(SROC plot) scheme(s1mono)
```

The bivariate model can also be fitted with "xtmelogit". First, the data need to in a long format with two records per study—one for the diseased group and one for the nondiseased group. Here we use the unstructured variance-covariance matrix.

```
. *** Perform meta-analysis ***
. xtmelogit true sens spec , nocons|| study: sens spec, ///
> nocons cov(un) binomial(n) refineopts(iterate(3)) intpoints(5) variance

Refining starting values:

Iteration 0:   log likelihood = -131.48005
Iteration 1:   log likelihood = -126.65195
Iteration 2:   log likelihood = -126.55003
Iteration 3:   log likelihood = -125.99898

Performing gradient-based optimization:

Iteration 0:   log likelihood = -125.99898
Iteration 1:   log likelihood = -125.99681
Iteration 2:   log likelihood = -125.99681
```

```
Mixed-effects logistic regression        Number of obs    =    46
Binomial variable: n
Group variable: study                    Number of groups =    23

                                         Obs per group:
                                                     min =     2
                                                     avg =   2.0
                                                     max =     2

Integration points =   5                 Wald chi2(2)     = 506.95
Log likelihood = -125.99681              Prob > chi2      = 0.0000
```

```
----------------------------------------------------------------------
        true |   Coef.    Std. Err.     z    P>|z|    [95% Conf. Interval]
-------------+--------------------------------------------------------
        sens | 1.992739   .1803329   11.05   0.000    1.639293   2.346185
        spec | 2.954364   .1417309   20.84   0.000    2.676577   3.232152
----------------------------------------------------------------------


----------------------------------------------------------------------
  Random-effects Parameters  |   Estimate   Std. Err.    [95% Conf. Interval]
-----------------------------+----------------------------------------
study: Unstructured          |
                var(sens)    |   .4710237   .2042426    .2013491   1.101884
                var(spec)    |   .2381015   .1396696    .0754137   .7517515
          cov(sens,spec)     |   .0681529   .121746    -.1704648   .3067706
----------------------------------------------------------------------
LR test vs. logistic model: chi2(3) = 74.30          Prob > chi2 = 0.0000
```

Note: LR test is conservative and provided only for reference.

We can find the covariance between the logit sensitivity and logit specificity.

```
. matrix list e(V)

symmetric e(V)[5,5]
                      eq1:        eq1:   lns1_1_1:   lns1_1_2: atr1_1_1_2:
                     sens        spec      _cons       _cons       _cons
  eq1:sens      .03251994
  eq1:spec      .0031953    .02008764
lns1_1_1:_cons  .00842414   .00014766   .04700533
lns1_1_2:_cons  .00027696   .00307634   .00136484   .08602397
atr1_1_1_2:_cons -.00174594  .00410703   .00247981  -.00155442   .13731626


. *** Display the coefficient vector ***
. matrix list e(b)

e(b)[1,5]
           eq1:        eq1:   lns1_1_1:   lns1_1_2: atr1_1_1_2:
          sens        spec      _cons       _cons       _cons
y1     1.992739   2.9543642 -.37642343   -.7175291  .20638962
```

11.8   Other Statistical Packages for DTA

Many different packages are available for performing a MA of diagnostic accuracy studies (DTA). We will discuss popular alternative packages besides R and Stata in this section, and some of these are designed for specific DTA analysis, which requires less coding and more straightforward to apply.

Meta-DiSc (Zamora et al. 2006) is free software, which is easy to use even for beginners, for MA of diagnostic and screening tests. It is downloadable from https://meta-disc.software.informer.com/1.4/. Users can import data, such as TP, FP, TN, FN, and aggregate values of covariates from each DTA study from text files, or type in the software directly. This package can investigate the homogeneity of studies graphically and statistically, and compute the pooled indexes and fit the SROC curve.

Cochrane RevMan (Wang and Leeflang 2019) is another free software for MA of DTA studies. It is downloaded from https://community.cochrane. org/help/tools-and-software/revman-5. There are two versions of Cochrane RevMan: RevMan Web (online) and RevMan 5 (desktop). RevMan Web is the online platform designed to integrate with other systematic review software to prepare and manage systematic reviews for Cochrane users. RevMan 5 is the desktop version of the software used for other review formats (diagnostic, methodology, overviews), for non-Cochrane reviews, and offline working. RevMan 5 is compatible with RevMan Web, and you can use both if needed. RevMan only provides limited analyses, and sensitivities and specificities are studied individually. However, you can apply advanced statistical models in RevMan by importing the parameter estimates obtained from other statistical software such as SAS, Stata, or R.

Statistical Analysis System (SAS) is a popular statistical software for data management and analysis. The SAS University Edition for academic use is free. The SAS macro "MetaDAS" can be used for the fitting of bivariate and HSROC models and is downloadable from https://methods.cochrane.org/ sites/methods.cochrane.org.sdt/files/public/uploads/METADAS_v1.3_txt.txt.

12

Network Meta-Analysis

Lili Yu and Xinyan Zhang

In meta-analysis, we are interested in comparing the effectiveness of different interventions for some condition or population. However, individual randomized controlled clinical trials usually compare the effects of the subsets of the interventions, most often two interventions directly. Therefore, the direct comparisons between two or more interventions may not exist.

Network meta-analysis (also known as multiple treatment comparison or mixed treatment comparison) are proposed to compare all interventions. It is a generalization of pairwise meta-analysis to simultaneous analysis of several interventions by incorporating indirect comparisons. The indirect comparisons of the effects of different interventions were evaluated from separate randomized controlled trials. Each trial provides direct comparisons of different interventions with the same control group. In other words, the indirect comparison of the effects of different interventions can be obtained based on their direct comparisons with the same control condition.

However, heterogeneity and potential inconsistency (Salanti et al. 2014; Schwarzer, Carpenter, and Rücker 2015) may exist among these trials and potentially even more challenging than in pairwise meta-analysis. In Section 12.5, we therefore describe graphical tools for presenting and understanding heterogeneity.

There are a variety of different methods and software for network meta-analysis (Bafeta et al. 2013). In this chapter, we will discuss two major approaches, a frequentist as well as a Bayesian hierarchical model, and how they can be implemented in R and Stata.

12.1 Concepts and Challenges of Network Meta-Analysis

To describe the method, we first consider a simple pairwise comparison between two conditions. Assume in a randomized controlled trial i, we compare the effect of one treatment A to a control B. The comparison can be displayed in the following graph:

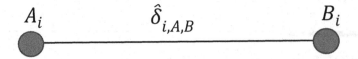

In this graph, there are two components. First, the two blue points (so-called nodes) represent the two conditions A and B in trial i. Second, the line is called an edge, which is connecting the two nodes. This edge shows how A and B relate to each other. On the edge, the effect size $\hat{\delta}_{i,A,B}$ represents the comparison between A and B. The effect size can be different metrics, such as the standardized mean difference, Odds Ratio, Incidence Rate Ratio, and so forth, depending on different situations.

Also assume we have another study j. In this trial, another treatment C is compared with the same control B in the first study i. We use $\hat{\delta}_{j,C,B}$ to represent the effect size by comparing C and B. We can add this information to our graph:

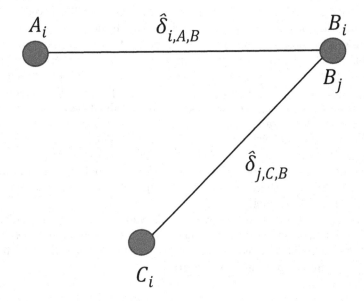

This creates our first small network. In this network, there are two effect size estimates in this network: $\hat{\delta}_{i,A,B}$, comparing A to B, and $\hat{\delta}_{j,C,B}$, comparing between C and B. These two effect size estimates are called direct effect because they are compared in real randomized trials directly. Therefore, we denote the two effect size estimates as $\hat{\delta}_{B,A}^{direct}$ and $\hat{\delta}_{B,C}^{direct}$, respectively. Note the reference condition is written as the first subscript in the notation. In our example, B is the reference condition, which is the first subscript in the effect size estimates.

In the above graph, we see condition B is directly connected to all other nodes, condition A and condition C. Although condition A and condition

C are not connected directly, they can be connected indirectly. Specifically, condition A is connected first to condition B, then condition B is connected to condition C. In this relationship, condition B serves as the link, or "bridge" between condition A and condition C. Therefore, the indirect connection can be derived from the information of the direct connection. Now we can make the network graph as

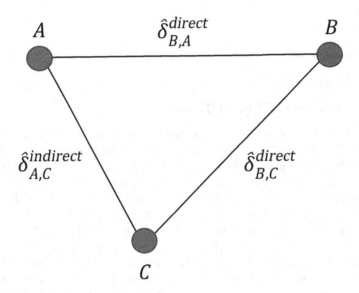

where $\hat{\delta}_{A,C}^{indirect}$ represents the indirect connection between A and C. It can be calculated using the following:

$$\hat{\delta}_{A,C}^{indirect} = \hat{\delta}_{B,A}^{direct} - \hat{\delta}_{B,C}^{direct}$$

with variance

$$\sigma^{2\,indirect}_{A,C} = \sigma^{2\,direct}_{B,A} + \sigma^{2\,direct}_{B,C}$$

Network meta-analysis can combine both direct and indirect evidence to estimate the effect sizes from several randomized trials. This means in addition to the direct evidence for a specific comparison, such as comparison between condition A and condition B, we can also derive indirect evidence to obtain more information about the comparison. Therefore, it is also called mixed-treatment comparison meta-analysis and it makes the effect size estimations more precise. In order to compare the direct and indirect evidence, we need the following assumptions:

1. the studies are independent, and

2. the underlying effects are consistent, which is also known as transitivity assumption (Salanti 2012; Veroniki et al. 2013).

In practice, consistency means the effect size estimate of a comparison is exchangeable between trials, no matter if a trial is direct or indirect. For the above example, we have three conditions, A, B, and C. In this example, consistency means $\hat{\delta}_{A,B}^{direct} = \hat{\delta}_{A,B}^{indirect}$ for the comparison A and B; $\hat{\delta}_{A,C}^{direct} = \hat{\delta}_{A,C}^{indirect}$ for the comparison A and C; and $\hat{\delta}_{B,C}^{direct} = \hat{\delta}_{B,C}^{indirect}$ for the comparison B and C.

12.2 Data Sets

12.2.1 Diabetes Clinical Trials

This study is to compare different treatments for the mean difference (MD) of HbA1c value of type 2 diabetes patients. The different treatments consist of adding different oral glucose-lowering agents to a baseline sulfonylurea therapy. To do network meta-analysis, we need to find randomized trials that compared the treatments for the type 2 diabetes patients. Then a systemic literature review was conducted to search for all relevant articles published from January 1993 to June 2009. The search is restricted to randomized controlled trials for humans. In addition, patients with type 2 diabetes should have been treated with sulfonylurea monotherapy for at least 4 weeks before inclusion and took at least half maximal recommended dose. Therefore, we excluded the trials that the patients treated with diet alone or with any other glucose-lowering agent. The trials must have a minimum of 50 randomized patients and measurements of HbA1c after a follow-up ranging from 3 to 12 months.

Finally, 26 studies were selected with 6646 patients in total. Among them, there are 53 arms including one with 3 arms and 10 treatment groups. The 10 treatment groups consist of acarbose, benfluorex, metformin, miglitol, pioglitazone, placebo, rosiglitazone, sitagliptin, sulfonylurea alone, and vildagliptin. The data are displayed in Table 12.1. Variable TE is the pairwise treatment effect comparing treatments treat 1 and treat 2; variable seTE is the corresponding standard error; variables treat1.long and treat2.long are the two treatments being compared. Variables treat1 and treat2 are a shortened name of the two treatments; the studlab column contains the unique study label, indicating in which study the comparison was made.

12.2.2 Parkinson's Clinical Trials

The second study is a meta-analysis review of seven clinical trials, which investigated four dopamine agonists compared with a placebo group as adjunct therapy for treating Parkinson's diseases. The four dopamine agonists are Ropinirole, Pramipexole, Bromocriptine, and Cabergoline. Each clinical trial in the meta-analysis compared any two dopamine agonists or any

TABLE 12.1
Diabetes Clinical Trial Data

	TE	seTE	treat1.long	treat2.long	treat1	treat2	studlab
1	-1.9	0.1414	Metformin	Placebo	metf	plac	DeFronzo1995
2	-0.82	0.0992	Metformin	Placebo	metf	plac	Lewin2007
3	-0.2	0.3579	Metformin	Acarbose	metf	acar	Willms1999
4	-1.34	0.1435	Rosiglitazone	Placebo	rosi	plac	Davidson2007
5	-1.1	0.1141	Rosiglitazone	Placebo	rosi	plac	Wolffenbuttel1999
6	-1.3	0.1268	Pioglitazone	Placebo	piog	plac	Kipnes2001
7	-0.77	0.1078	Rosiglitazone	Placebo	rosi	plac	Kerenyi2004
8	0.16	0.0849	Pioglitazone	Metformin	piog	metf	Hanefeld2004
9	0.1	0.1831	Pioglitazone	Rosiglitazone	piog	rosi	Derosa2004
10	-1.3	0.1014	Rosiglitazone	Placebo	rosi	plac	Baksi2004
11	-1.09	0.2263	Rosiglitazone	Placebo	rosi	plac	Rosenstock2008
12	-1.5	0.1624	Rosiglitazone	Placebo	rosi	plac	Zhu2003
13	-0.14	0.2239	Rosiglitazone	Metformin	rosi	metf	Yang2003
14	-1.2	0.1436	Rosiglitazone	Sulfonylurea	rosi	sulf	Vongthavaravat2002
15	-0.4	0.1549	Acarbose	Sulfonylurea	acar	sulf	Oyama2008
16	-0.8	0.1432	Acarbose	Placebo	acar	plac	Costa1997
17	-0.57	0.1291	Sitagliptin	Placebo	sita	plac	Hermansen2007
18	-0.7	0.1273	Vildagliptin	Placebo	vild	plac	Garber2008
19	-0.37	0.1184	Metformin	Sulfonylurea	metf	sulf	Alex1998
20	-0.74	0.1839	Miglitol	Placebo	migl	plac	Johnston1994
21	-1.41	0.2235	Miglitol	Placebo	migl	plac	Johnston1998a
22	0	0.2339	Rosiglitazone	Metformin	rosi	metf	Kim2007
23	-0.68	0.2828	Miglitol	Placebo	migl	plac	Johnston1998b
24	-0.4	0.4356	Metformin	Placebo	metf	plac	Gonzalez-Ortiz2004
25	-0.23	0.3467	Benfluorex	Placebo	benf	plac	Stucci1996
26	-1.01	0.1366	Benfluorex	Placebo	benf	plac	Moulin2006
27	-1.2	0.3758	Metformin	Placebo	metf	plac	Willms1999
28	-1	0.4669	Acarbose	Placebo	acar	plac	Willms1999

TABLE 12.2

Parkinson's Clinical Trial Data

Study	Treatment	Mean	std.dev	SampleSize
o	Placebo	−1.22	3.7	54
1	Ropinirole	−1.53	4.28	95
2	Placebo	−0.7	3.7	172
2	Pramipexole	−2.4	3.4	173
3	Placebo	−0.3	4.4	76
3	Pramipexole	−2.6	4.3	71
3	Bromocriptine	−1.2	4.3	81
4	Ropinirole	−0.24	3	128
4	Bromocriptine	−0.59	3	72
5	Ropinirole	−0.73	3	80
5	Bromocriptine	−0.18	3	46
6	Bromocriptine	−2.2	2.31	137
6	Cabergoline	−2.5	2.18	131
7	Bromocriptine	−1.8	2.48	154
7	Cabergoline	−2.1	2.99	143

one dopamine agonist and the placebo group. The outcome measured in all seven clinical trials is mean "off-time" reduction among Parkinson's disease patients. "Off-time" is the term used for the days when a medication for treating Parkinson's disease is not working well.

The data set is displayed in Table 12.2. The total sample size from all seven clinical trials is 1613. There are five variables in the data set, including study, treatment, mean, std.dev, and sampleSize. Study column listed the study id for each clinical trial; treatment column contains the treatment names in each clinical trial; mean is the mean "off-time" reduction; std.dev is the standard deviation of the mean; sampleSize is the column containing the sample sizes for each treatment being compared in each clinical trial.

12.3   Frequentist Network Meta-Analysis

Suppose we have data from K trials with N treatments. Let $\boldsymbol{\delta} = (\delta_1, \delta_2, \ldots, \delta_m)$ be a $m \times 1$ vector of effect sizes from the K trials with corresponding standard errors $\boldsymbol{\sigma} = (\sigma_1, \sigma_2, \ldots, \sigma_m)$. The m is the total number of pairwise comparisons. If all K trials are two-arm trials, $m = K$. Now we want to estimate N treatment effects $\boldsymbol{\delta}^{\text{treat}}$, a $N \times 1$ vector of the treatments. Then our model is

$$\hat{\boldsymbol{\delta}} = \boldsymbol{X}\boldsymbol{\delta}^{\text{treat}} + \boldsymbol{\epsilon}, \quad \boldsymbol{\epsilon} \sim N(0, \boldsymbol{\Sigma}) \tag{12.1}$$

where $\hat{\boldsymbol{\delta}}$ is a $m \times 1$ vector of observed effect sizes in a network meta-analysis consisting of all pairwise effect size; $\boldsymbol{X}$ is a $m \times N$ design matrix, in which the columns represent the different treatments and the rows represent the comparisons between treatments, which are 1 and -1; the $\boldsymbol{\Sigma}$ is a diagonal matrix with elements σ_i^2. In model (12.1), we can estimate the parameter $\boldsymbol{\delta}^{treat}$. Then the comparison of the effects of different treatments can be obtained.

Example:

Assume we have $K = 5$ studies and $N = 5$ treatment. The treatments are A, B, C, D, and E. Each study does a distinct two-arm comparison. They are A compared with B, A compared with C, A compared with D, B compared with C, B compared with D. We then have a vector of (observed) effect sizes $\hat{\boldsymbol{\delta}} = \left(\hat{\delta}_{1,A,B}, \hat{\delta}_{2,A,C}, \hat{\delta}_{3,A,D}, \hat{\delta}_{4,B,C}, \hat{\delta}_{5,B,D}\right)^T$. The parameters (treatment effects) we are estimating in our network are $\boldsymbol{\delta}^{treat} = (\delta_A, \delta_B, \delta_C, \delta_D)^T$. Using the model (12.1), we get the following equation:

$$\hat{\boldsymbol{\theta}} = \boldsymbol{X}\boldsymbol{\delta}^{treat} + \boldsymbol{\epsilon}$$

$$
\begin{pmatrix}
\hat{\delta}_{1,A,B} \\
\hat{\delta}_{2,A,C} \\
\hat{\delta}_{3,A,D} \\
\hat{\delta}_{4,B,C} \\
\hat{\delta}_{5,B,D}
\end{pmatrix}
=
\begin{pmatrix}
1 & -1 & 0 & 0 \\
1 & 0 & -1 & 0 \\
1 & 0 & 0 & -1 \\
0 & 1 & -1 & 0 \\
0 & 1 & 0 & -1
\end{pmatrix}
\begin{pmatrix}
\delta_A \\
\delta_B \\
\delta_C \\
\delta_D
\end{pmatrix}
+
\begin{pmatrix}
\epsilon_1 \\
\epsilon_2 \\
\epsilon_3 \\
\epsilon_4 \\
\epsilon_5
\end{pmatrix}
$$

Because we only have data on treatment differences, we have at most $(N-1)$ independent treatment comparisons. However, we have N parameters, which are the N treatment effect in δ^{treat}. Therefore, it is overparameterized in model (12.1) and we cannot estimate each of the elements in $\boldsymbol{\delta}^{treat}$. In the next subsection, we will explain how to estimate the fitted values from model (12.1), and then use these to estimate the treatment comparisons and assess the extent of heterogeneity.

12.3.1 Fixed-Effects Model

As model (1) has the overparameterized problem, the matrix $\boldsymbol{X}$ is not of full rank and hence its inverse does not exist. Then we cannot estimate δ^{treat} using the weighted least squares method. To deal with this problem, the Moore–Penrose pseudoinverse matrix (Albert 1972; Rucker and Schwarzer 2014) is applied. Let $\boldsymbol{L}$ be the $N \times N$ Laplacian matrix, which is calculated by

$$\boldsymbol{L} = \boldsymbol{X}^T \boldsymbol{W} \boldsymbol{X}$$

where $\boldsymbol{W}$ is a $m \times m$ diagonal matrix with elements $(1/\sigma_1^2, 1/\sigma_2^2, \ldots, 1/\sigma_m^2)$, the inverse variance of each comparison. Let $\boldsymbol{L}^+$ (Gutman and Xiao 2004; Rao and Mitra 1971) be the Moore-Penrose pseudoinverse of $\boldsymbol{L}$. It is calculated by

$$L^+ = \left(L - \frac{J}{N}\right)^{-1} + \frac{J}{N} \tag{12.2}$$

where $\mathbf{J}$ is the $N \times N$ matrix whose elements are all 1. Then the network estimate $\hat{\delta}^{nma}$ of the fitted values can be calculated as

$$\hat{\delta}^{nma} = \mathbf{X}\mathbf{L}^+\mathbf{X}^T\mathbf{W}\hat{\delta} = \mathbf{H}\hat{\delta}$$

and the variance–covariance matrix of $\hat{\delta}^{nma}$ is calculated by $\mathbf{X}\mathbf{L}^+\mathbf{X}^T$. Therefore, we can estimate treatment comparisons and the corresponding variance. These results are equivalent to those obtained by (weighted) maximum likelihood (Paterson 1983; Senn et al. 2013; Yates 1940).

To measure the heterogeneity in the network based on model (1), we can calculate Q_{total} as follows:

$$Q_{total} = \left(\hat{\delta} - \hat{\delta}^{nma}\right)^T \mathbf{W} \left(\hat{\delta} - \hat{\delta}^{nma}\right)$$

It is equivalent to Cochran's Q statistic (Higgins and Thompson 2002). When all studies are two-arm studies, it is approximately χ^2-distributed with $m - (N-1)$ degrees of freedom under the null hypothesis of no heterogeneity. Therefore, it can be used to test consistency in the network meta-analysis.

12.3.1.1 Multiarm Studies

Multiarm studies include more than two treatment groups. When there are multiarm studies in the network meta-analysis, we include them as a series of two-arm comparisons. Suppose we have a multiarm study with p treatments. Then we include this study as $p(p-1)/2$ possible pairwise comparisons in the network meta-analysis. For example, a three-arm study contributes 3 $(3(3-1)/2 = 3)$ pairwise comparisons in the network meta-analysis.

Because the pairwise comparisons from multiarm studies are correlated with each other, we need to adjust the variances of these pairwise comparisons. Gutman and Xiao (2004) proposed back-calculation to inflate the variance for comparisons within each multiarm study. Then the adjusted variances are used in the weighted least squares method for model (1). In this way, we obtain the results that can appropriately accommodate the correlations within multiarm studies.

To explain the back-calculation method, suppose we have S multiarm study. For each $s = 1, \ldots, S$, multiarm study, there are $p_s(p_s - 1)/2$ pairwise comparisons, where p_s is the number of treatments. Let σ^2_{sij} be the variance for the pairwise comparison of treatment i and treatment j $(i \neq j)$. Define $\mathbf{\Sigma}_s$ as a $p_s \times p_s$ symmetric matrix with zero as diagonal elements and σ^2_{sij} as off-diagonal element at ith row and jth column. Let $\mathbf{X}_s$ be design matrix for multiarm study s. Then we calculate

$$L^+_s = -\frac{1}{2p^2_s}\mathbf{X}^T_s\mathbf{X}_s\mathbf{\Sigma}_s\mathbf{X}^T_s\mathbf{X}_s$$

and $L_s = (L_s^+)^+$ using (2). Let l_{sij} be the elements of L_s at the *ith* row and *jth* column. Then the adjusted variance for the comparison of treatment i and treatment j ($i \neq j = 1, \ldots, p_s$) is $-1/l_{sij}^{-1}$. Rücker and Schwarzer (2014) showed that this method leads to the same results as those of the standard approach (Krahn, Binder, and Konig 2013; Senn et al. 2013).

12.3.1.2 I-Squared for Network Meta-Analysis

We can use the following I^2 value to measure the amount of inconsistency in our network:

$$I^2 = \max(\frac{Q_{total} - df}{Q_{total}}, 0)$$

in which the degrees of freedom (df) is calculated by:

$$df = \left(\sum_{k=1}^{K} p_k - 1\right) - (N - 1)$$

where K is the number of studies, p_k is the number of arms in each study k, and N is the total number of treatments in the entire network.

12.3.2 Random-Effects Model

A simple random-effects model can be used in network meta-analysis as well. It adds a common heterogeneity variance τ^2 to each pairwise comparison. Then the observed variance of each comparison is $\sigma_i^2 + \hat{\tau}^2$, $i = 1, \ldots, m$. We estimate τ^2 using a special case of the generalized DerSimonian–Laird estimate given (Jackson, White, and Riley 2013) as follows:

$$\hat{\tau}^2 = \max\left(\frac{Q_{total} - df}{tr\left((I - H)UW\right)}, 0\right),$$

where U is a block diagonal matrix and the diagonal blocks are obtained from the matrix $XX^T/2$ by selecting a $p \times p$ block for each p-arm study. Now the network meta-analysis is applied to the same observed effect sizes as in the standard pairwise meta-analysis but uses the new observed variances.

12.4 Network Meta-Analysis of Diabetes Clinical Trial Data

We illustrate the application of the R package *netmeta* for network meta-analysis. We install the package and load the library.

```
>install.packages("netmeta)
>library(netmeta)
```

We load the data in Table 12.1 into R as follows and then rename it as data

```
>data(Senn2013)
>data <- Senn2013
```

12.4.1   Network Meta-Analysis

First, we analyze the data using network meta-analysis based on fixed-effects model.

```
>nma_fixed <- netmeta(TE, seTE, treat1, treat2, studlab,
    data=data, sm='MD', comb.fixed=TRUE, comb.random=FALSE,
    reference.group = "plac")
```

In the R code above, sm='MD' means the MDs are compared between the treatments; comb.fixed=TRUE means fixed effect model is applied; comb.random=FALSE means random-effects model is not applied; reference.group = "plac" means the reference group is the placebo group and the results will show the comparisons of each treatment versus placebo. If we do not define reference.group here, the results will show all pairwise comparisons between the treatments.

Here is the output,

```
>nma_fixed
Original data (with adjusted standard errors for multi-arm
    studies):
```

\# First in addition to the data, it shows number of arms in each study with an asterisk indicating multiarm studies, which need the adjusted standard errors (seTE.adj). We can see the Willms1999 study has three arms. Its adjusted standard errors are different from the original standard errors (seTE).

	treat1	treat2	TE	seTE	seTE.adj	narms	multiarm
DeFronzo1995	metf	plac	-1.9000	0.1414	0.1414	2	
Lewin2007	metf	plac	-0.8200	0.0992	0.0992	2	
Willms1999	acar	metf	0.2000	0.3579	0.3884	3	*
Davidson2007	plac	rosi	1.3400	0.1435	0.1435	2	
Wolffenbuttel1999	plac	rosi	1.1000	0.1141	0.1141	2	
Kipnes2001	piog	plac	-1.3000	0.1268	0.1268	2	
Kerenyi2004	plac	rosi	0.7700	0.1078	0.1078	2	
Hanefeld2004	metf	piog	-0.1600	0.0849	0.0849	2	
Derosa2004	piog	rosi	0.1000	0.1831	0.1831	2	
Baksi2004	plac	rosi	1.3000	0.1014	0.1014	2	
Rosenstock2008	plac	rosi	1.0900	0.2263	0.2263	2	
Zhu2003	plac	rosi	1.5000	0.1624	0.1624	2	
Yang2003	metf	rosi	0.1400	0.2239	0.2239	2	
Vongthavaravat2002	rosi	sulf	-1.2000	0.1436	0.1436	2	
Oyama2008	acar	sulf	-0.4000	0.1549	0.1549	2	

Costa1997	acar	plac	-0.8000	0.1432	0.1432	2	
Hermansen2007	plac	sita	0.5700	0.1291	0.1291	2	
Garber2008	plac	vild	0.7000	0.1273	0.1273	2	
Alex1998	metf	sulf	-0.3700	0.1184	0.1184	2	
Johnston1994	migl	plac	-0.7400	0.1839	0.1839	2	
Johnston1998a	migl	plac	-1.4100	0.2235	0.2235	2	
Kim2007	metf	rosi	-0.0000	0.2339	0.2339	2	
Johnston1998b	migl	plac	-0.6800	0.2828	0.2828	2	
Gonzalez-Ortiz2004	metf	plac	-0.4000	0.4356	0.4356	2	
Stucci1996	benf	plac	-0.2300	0.3467	0.3467	2	
Moulin2006	benf	plac	-1.0100	0.1366	0.1366	2	
Willms1999	metf	plac	-1.2000	0.3758	0.4125	3	*
Willms1999	acar	plac	-1.0000	0.4669	0.8242	3	*

Next, it shows the number of arms (narms) for each study. Again, we can see only Willms1999 has three arms. All other studies have two arms.

Number of treatment arms (by study):

	narms
DeFronzo1995	2
Lewin2007	2
Willms1999	3
Davidson2007	2
Wolffenbuttel1999	2
Kipnes2001	2
Kerenyi2004	2
Hanefeld2004	2
Derosa2004	2
Baksi2004	2
Rosenstock2008	2
Zhu2003	2
Yang2003	2
Vongthavaravat2002	2
Oyama2008	2
Costa1997	2
Hermansen2007	2
Garber2008	2
Alex1998	2
Johnston1994	2
Johnston1998a	2
Kim2007	2
Johnston1998b	2
Gonzalez-Ortiz2004	2
Stucci1996	2
Moulin2006	2

The following table shows us the fitted values (MD) for each comparison in the network meta-analysis model. The Q column shows how much each comparison contributes to the overall inconsistency in our network. We can

see that the Q value of DeFronzo1995 study is high, with Q=30.89, which indicates it has the largest contribution among all studies to the overall inconsistency.

Results (fixed effect model):

	treat1	treat2	MD	95%-CI	Q	leverage
DeFronzo1995	metf	plac	-1.1141	[-1.2309; -0.9973]	30.89	0.18
Lewin2007	metf	plac	-1.1141	[-1.2309; -0.9973]	8.79	0.36
Willms1999	acar	metf	0.2867	[0.0622; 0.5113]	0.05	0.09
Davidson2007	plac	rosi	1.2018	[1.1084; 1.2953]	0.93	0.11
Wolffenbuttel1999	plac	rosi	1.2018	[1.1084; 1.2953]	0.80	0.17
Kipnes2001	piog	plac	-1.0664	[-1.2151; -0.9178]	3.39	0.36
Kerenyi2004	plac	rosi	1.2018	[1.1084; 1.2953]	16.05	0.20
Hanefeld2004	metf	piog	-0.0477	[-0.1845; 0.0891]	1.75	0.68
Derosa2004	piog	rosi	0.1354	[-0.0249; 0.2957]	0.04	0.20
Baksi2004	plac	rosi	1.2018	[1.1084; 1.2953]	0.94	0.22
Rosenstock2008	plac	rosi	1.2018	[1.1084; 1.2953]	0.24	0.04
Zhu2003	plac	rosi	1.2018	[1.1084; 1.2953]	3.37	0.09
Yang2003	metf	rosi	0.0877	[-0.0449; 0.2203]	0.05	0.09
Vongthavaravat2002	rosi	sulf	-0.7623	[-0.9427; -0.5820]	9.29	0.41
Oyama2008	acar	sulf	-0.3879	[-0.6095; -0.1662]	0.01	0.53
Costa1997	acar	plac	-0.8274	[-1.0401; -0.6147]	0.04	0.57
Hermansen2007	plac	sita	0.5700	[0.3170; 0.8230]	0.00	1.00
Garber2008	plac	vild	0.7000	[0.4505; 0.9495]	0.00	1.00
Alex1998	metf	sulf	-0.6746	[-0.8482; -0.5011]	6.62	0.56
Johnston1994	migl	plac	-0.9439	[-1.1927; -0.6952]	1.23	0.48
Johnston1998a	migl	plac	-0.9439	[-1.1927; -0.6952]	4.35	0.32
Kim2007	metf	rosi	0.0877	[-0.0449; 0.2203]	0.14	0.08
Johnston1998b	migl	plac	-0.9439	[-1.1927; -0.6952]	0.87	0.20
Gonzalez-Ortiz2004	metf	plac	-1.1141	[-1.2309; -0.9973]	2.69	0.02
Stucci1996	benf	plac	-0.9052	[-1.1543; -0.6561]	3.79	0.13
Moulin2006	benf	plac	-0.9052	[-1.1543; -0.6561]	0.59	0.87
Willms1999	metf	plac	-1.1141	[-1.2309; -0.9973]	0.04	0.02
Willms1999	acar	plac	-0.8274	[-1.0401; -0.6147]	0.04	0.02

```
Number of studies: k = 26
Number of treatments: n = 10
Number of pairwise comparisons: m = 28
Number of designs: d = 15
```

\# The next is the core results of the network model: the treatment estimates. It shows the treatment difference between all treatments and the placebo condition. This is because we specified reference.group. We can see in the row for plac, it shows "." because we do not compare plac with itself. If reference.group is not specified, then the output will show all comparisons between any two treatments (including placebo).

```
Fixed effects model

Treatment estimate (sm = 'MD', comparison: other treatments
    vs 'plac'):
```

```
            MD              95%-CI
acar -0.8274 [-1.0401; -0.6147]
benf -0.9052 [-1.1543; -0.6561]
metf -1.1141 [-1.2309; -0.9973]
migl -0.9439 [-1.1927; -0.6952]
piog -1.0664 [-1.2151; -0.9178]
plac        .                  .
rosi -1.2018 [-1.2953; -1.1084]
sita -0.5700 [-0.8230; -0.3170]
sulf -0.4395 [-0.6188; -0.2602]
vild -0.7000 [-0.9495; -0.4505]
```

\# The last part of the output shows heterogeneity/inconsistency of the network model. We also see that the heterogeneity/inconsistency in our network model is very high, with $I_2 = 81.4\%$. The tests of heterogeneity (Higgins et al. 2012) break down the total heterogeneity into within and between design variations. Designs refer to the subset of treatments compared in a study. That the studies have the same designs means these studies contain the same subset of treatments. For example, the study Costa 1997 and the study Willms 1999 are two different designs because they do not have the same subsets of the treatments. For the study Costa 1997, it contains the treatments acar and plac. However, the Willms 1999 study contains the treatments acar, plac, and metf. Although they have same treatments acar and plac, the Willms 1999 has one more treatment metf.

The output shows that the heterogeneity between designs is inconsistent in the network. It shows p-value = 0.0021, which indicates that the inconsistency is highly significant. The within design heterogeneity is the conventional heterogeneity between the designs with the same treatments. It shows p-value = 0.0001, which is highly significant as well. Based on this information, we conclude that the random-effects model may be more appropriate for this data set. Therefore, we should rerun the function setting comb.random to TRUE.

```
Quantifying heterogeneity / inconsistency:
tau^2 = 0.1087; tau = 0.3297; I^2 = 81.4% [72.0%; 87.7%]

Tests of heterogeneity (within designs) and inconsistency
   (between designs):
                    Q d.f.  p-value
Total           96.99   18 < 0.0001
Within designs  74.46   11 < 0.0001
Between designs 22.53    7   0.0021
```

To check if a random-effects model is appropriate for this data, we can calculate the total inconsistency from the full design-by-treatment interaction random-effects model (Higgins et al. 2012). It can be obtained by using the following R code:

```
>decomp.design(nma_fixed)
```

\# The first part of the output is again the Test of heterogeneity and inconsistency as the last output in nma_fixed.

```
Q statistics to assess homogeneity / consistency
```

	Q	df	p-value
Total	96.99	18	< 0.0001
Within designs	74.46	11	< 0.0001
Between designs	22.53	7	0.0021

\# Then it shows the decomposition of Q statistic within designs and between designs.

```
Design-specific decomposition of within-designs Q statistic
```

Design	Q	df	p-value
metf:rosi	0.19	1	0.6655
plac:benf	4.38	1	0.0363
plac:metf	42.16	2	< 0.0001
plac:migl	6.45	2	0.0398
plac:rosi	21.27	5	0.0007

\# The decomposition of Q statistic within designs indicates that there are five designs that have more than two studies. Except the design comparing metf versus rosi, all other designs have significant heterogeneity.

```
Between-designs Q statistic after detaching of single designs
```

Detached design	Q	df	p-value
acar:sulf	22.52	6	0.0010
metf:piog	17.13	6	0.0088
metf:rosi	22.52	6	0.0010
metf:sulf	7.51	6	0.2760
piog:rosi	22.48	6	0.0010
plac:acar	22.44	6	0.0010
plac:metf	22.07	6	0.0012
plac:piog	17.25	6	0.0084
plac:rosi	16.29	6	0.0123
rosi:sulf	6.77	6	0.3425
plac:acar:metf	22.38	5	0.0004

\# The last part is the most important part. It shows the test if a full design-by-treatment interaction random-effects model fits the data well. The $Q = 2.19$, p-value $= 0.9483$ suggesting that a random-effects model may be more appropriate for this data.

```
Q statistic to assess consistency under the assumption of
a full design-by-treatment interaction random effects model

                 Q df p-value tau.within tau2.within
Between designs 2.19  7  0.9483     0.3797      0.1442
```

12.4.2 The Treatment Ranking

To show which treatment is best, we can use netrank function to produce the ranking of the treatments from the most to the least beneficial. It calculates P-scores for each treatment with the largest one being the most beneficial one. The P-scores are equivalent to the SUCRA score (Rucker and Schwarzer 2015), which will be introduced in Bayesian network meta-analysis. We need to specify the small.values parameter in the netrank function to tell if smaller effect sizes in a comparison are good or bad. The R code and the output are as follows:

```
> netrank(nma_fixed,small.values = "good")

     P-score
rosi  0.9789
metf  0.8513
piog  0.7686
migl  0.6200
benf  0.5727
acar  0.4792
vild  0.3512
sita  0.2386
sulf  0.1395
plac  0.0000
```

It shows that rosi is the most beneficial treatment for diabetes based on the data we use.

12.4.3 Graphical Display of the Network Model

Now we illustrate a graphical representation of the network using R function netgraph.

```
> netgraph(nma_fixed, seq=c("plac", "benf", "migl", "acar",
  "sulf","metf", "rosi", "piog", "sita", "vild"))
```

This will provide a graph in Figure 12.1. The seq specifies the anti-clockwise order of the treatments that will show in Figure 12.1. A line connects the treatment which is compared with at least one other treatment directly. The thickness of the line is determined by the inverse standard error of the direct comparison of the treatment effect from all studies. Then a thicker line

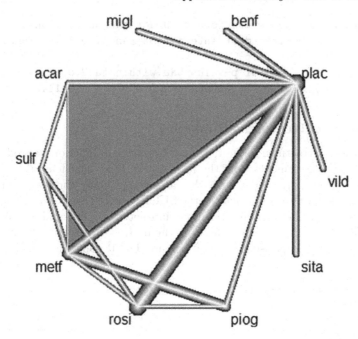

FIGURE 12.1
A graph representation of the network for the diabetes data. The treatments are equally spaced on the perimeter of the circle.

represents the treatment comparison has smaller standard error and therefore the comparison is more accurate. A shading area means that there is a multi-arm study. For example, the figure shows that the line between treatment rosi and plac is thickest. This means that there is a direct comparison between rosi and plac, and this comparison has smallest standard error among other direct comparison between other treatments. In addition, a shading area connecting the treatments acar, metf and plac means there is a three-arm study that includes these three treatments.

A good feature of the netgraph function is that it can produce a 3D graph, which may show you a better view of you network structure. It needs *rgl* package and uses the following R code (graphs not shown).

```
library(rgl)
netgraph(m.netmeta, dim = "3d")
```

12.4.4 Forest Plots

We see the results that compare each treatment with placebo in Section 12.4.1. Now we show how to make forest plots for fixed-effects and random-effects model. Here are the R codes.

```
> forest(nma_fixed, xlim=c(-1.5, 1), ref="plac",
    leftlabs="Contrast to Placebo",xlab="HbA1c difference")
> forest(nma_fixed, xlim=c(-1.5, 1), ref="plac",
    leftlabs="Contrast to Placebo",xlab="HbA1c difference",
    pooled="random")
```

Figures 12.2 and 12.3 are the outputs for fixed-effects model and random-effects model separately.

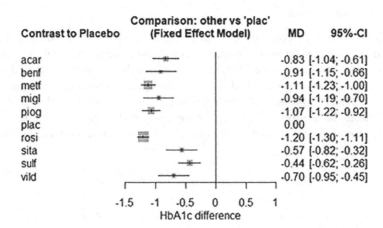

FIGURE 12.2
Forest plot for the Senn data example, fixed-effects model, with placebo as reference.

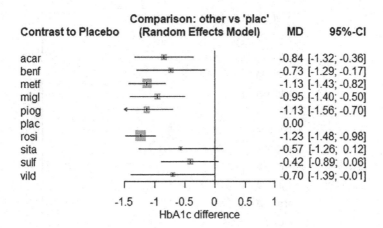

FIGURE 12.3
Forest plot for the Senn data example, random-effects model, with placebo as reference.

12.5   The Net Heat Plot

The net heat plot (Konig, Krahn, and Binder 2013; Krahn, Binder, and Konig 2013, 2014) can provide two types of information. First, it can tell the contribution of each design to the estimate for each network. Second, it can tell the extent of inconsistency due to each design for each network estimate. Figure 12.4 shows a net heat plot for the fixed effect analysis of the Senn data example. It is created by the following R code:

```
>netheat(nma_fixed)
```

The rows and the columns are treatment comparisons within designs which have more than two studies. In other words, the designs with only one study are omitted. The comparisons from the three-arm design use symbol "_" following the treatment comparison label. The gray squares represent how important the treatment comparisons in the column for the estimation of the treatment comparisons in the row. The larger of the area of the gray squares, the more importance of the treatment comparison in the column. For example, for the

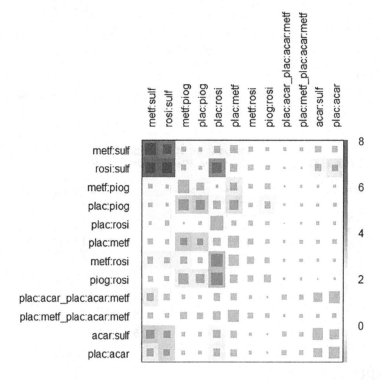

FIGURE 12.4
Net heat plot of the Senn data example based on a fixed-effects model.

plac:acar treatment comparison, the largest gray square is the one on the diagonal. It means that the direct comparison has the largest source of information. In addition, there are also moderate size squares in the same row and in the column of the metf:sulf, rosi:sulf, plac:rosi, metf:plac, and acar:sulf comparisons. It means there are other sources of indirect evidence from other studies.

Second, the color in Figure 12.4 shows the contribution of each design to the inconsistency between designs. The colors range from red to blue. Red means largest inconsistency and blue means consistency.

For the diagonal positions, it represents each design's contribution to the inconsistency between designs in the network. The (1,1) position (metf:sulf) and (2,2) position (rosi:sulf) are red, which mean these two designs contribute most of the inconsistency between designs. The (4,4) position (piog:plac) is orange, which means less contribution to the inconsistency. Then (3,3) and (5,5) positions are yellow, which means lesser contribution. All other diagonals are blue, which means few contributions.

For the off-diagonal positions, it represents the contribution of the design in the column to the inconsistency of the design in the row, when the "consistency" assumption is relaxed for the column. Red color indicates it will decrease the inconsistency of the design in the row. For example, for position (1,2), the associated column is rosi:sulf and the associated row is metf:sulf. The color in this position means when we relax the "consistency" assumption for the design rosi:sulf, what the change of the between-design inconsistency of the design meft:sulf. Because the color is red, it means it will decrease a lot. This indicates the treatment comparison metf:sulf from the design rosi:sulf is inconsistent with the others. On the other hand, blue color indicates the consistency between the design in the column and in the row. For example, the position (2,8), the associated column is arar:sulf and the associated row is rosi:sulf. The color in this position is blue which means these two designs are consistent.

The contributions of each design to the inconsistency can also be obtained using the following R code:

```
>round(decomp.design(nma_fixed)$Q.inc.design, 2)
```

acar:sulf	metf:piog	metf:rosi	metf:sulf
0.01	1.75	0.01	6.62
piog:rosi	plac:acar	plac:benf	plac:metf
0.04	0.04	0.00	0.20
plac:migl	plac:piog	plac:rosi	plac:sita
0.00	3.39	1.05	0.00
plac:vild	rosi:sulf	plac:acar:metf	plac:acar:metf
0.00	9.29	0.14	-0.01

The output shows that the largest two contributors of the inconsistency are rosi:sulf (9.29) and metf:sulf (6.62). This agrees with the results from

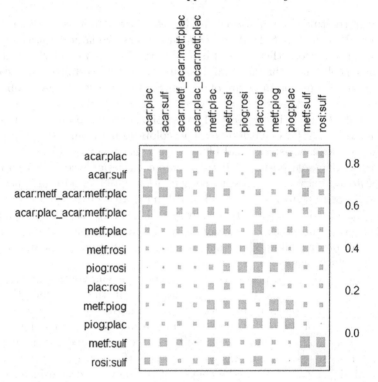

FIGURE 12.5
Net heat plot of the Senn data example from a random-effects model

Figure 12.4. The inconsistency in the network can be largest reduced by removing the design rosi:sulf.

Because inconsistency is large for fixed-effects model, we can try a random-effects model. The net heat plot for the random-effect model can be obtained by the following R code. The corresponding net heat plot is shown in Figure 12.5. It shows a considerable reduction in inconsistency.

```
> netheat(mn, random=TRUE)
```

12.6 Bayesian Network Meta-Analysis

In this section, we will discuss how to perform a network meta-analysis under the Bayesian framework. First, we will briefly introduce the concepts of Bayesian inference in general.

12.6.1 Introduction to Bayesian Inference

Bayesian inference involves a process of fitting a probability model to a set of observed data and summarizes the results for the unobserved parameters or unobserved data given the observed data (Gelman 2014). The essential characteristic of Bayesian methods is that the use of probability for quantifying uncertainty in inferences based on statistical data analysis and the process of Bayesian data analysis can be divided into three steps as following: (1) setting up a joint probability model for all observable data and unobservable parameters in a problem; (2) calculating and interpreting the appropriate posterior distribution, which is known as the conditional probability distribution of the unobserved parameters of interest, given the observed data; (3) evaluating the model fitting and the implications of the resulting posterior distribution (Gelman 2014).

12.6.1.1 Baye's Theorem

The fundamental concepts of Bayesian statistics evolve from Bayes' theorem. It differs from frequentist's statistics as it incorporates "subjective" prior information into statistical inference. In Bayesian statistics, conclusions are made in terms of probability statements for a parameter θ or unobserved data $\tilde{y}$. The probability statements are conditional on the observed data, noted as y, which are written as $p(\theta|y)$ or $p(\tilde{y}|y)$. Through Bayes' theorem, the condition probability $p(\theta|y)$ can be expressed as:

$$p(\theta|y) = \frac{p(y|\theta)\,p(\theta)}{p(y)}$$

As the data is fixed, $p(y)$ is a fixed constant and the above formula could be simplified as:

$$p(\theta|y) \propto (y|\theta)\,p(\theta)$$

Specifically, $p(y|\theta)$ is known as the likelihood of the data, while $p(\theta)$ is the prior probability for parameter θ; $p(\theta|y)$ is called the posterior probability. The prior probability $p(\theta)$ could be determined based on previous knowledge. By taking the likelihood of the data and the prior knowledge about the parameters into account, we estimate the posterior distribution $p(\theta|y)$. Moreover, the posterior is a distribution, meaning the results of Bayesian inference are still measures of uncertainty for our subjective belief in the true parameter values.

12.6.1.2 Prediction

Bayesian inference can also be used in terms of unobserved data $\tilde{y}$, known as predictive inferences. The distribution of $\tilde{y}$ is called the posterior predictive distribution since it is also conditional on the observed data y. And it is expressed as an average of conditional predictions over the posterior distribution of θ:

$$p(\tilde{y}|y) = \int p(\tilde{y}, \theta|y)\, d\theta = \int p(\tilde{y}|\theta, y)\, p(\theta|y)\, d\theta = \int p(\tilde{y}|\theta)\, p(\theta|y)\, d\theta$$

12.6.1.3   Bayesian Computation with Simulation

Bayesian computation focuses on computation for the posterior distribution, $p(\theta|y)$, or the predictive posterior distribution, $p(\tilde{y}|y)$. Many methods have been used in the sampling for those posterior distributions in Bayesian computation. Among them, Markov Chain Monte Carlo (MCMC) is the most widely used. Gibbs sampler is the simplest MCMC algorithm that has been found to be useful in many multidimensional problems. It could be considered as a special case of Metropolis Hastings Algorithm, which is another type of MCMC algorithm. Except those, there are also modal and distributional approximation algorithms (for details, see (Gelman 2014)).

12.6.2   Bayesian Meta-Analysis Models

The objective in Bayesian meta-analysis is the same as previous stated in Chapter 3 under a frequentist's framework, which to demonstrate that the new drug is effective in treating the disease. In Bayesian meta-analysis, we will formulate the meta-analysis model through Bayesian hierarchical modeling structure (Efthimiou et al. 2016). The word "hierarchical" means a "multilevel" structure in the model. And Bayesian meta-analysis can be directly applicable to network meta-analysis without any other extension (Dias, Sutton, Ades, et al. 2013). In this section, we will discuss the formulation of meta-analysis under Bayesian framework with objective to identify the efficacy of a drug in a pairwise comparative study. We will define the Bayesian meta-analysis by first identifying a common measure of treatment effect size δ in clinical studies, such as the difference in means if response is continuous. Alternatively, if the response is dichotomous or binary, the effect size can be difference in proportions, log-odds ratio, or relative risk.

12.6.2.1   Fixed-Effects Models

Suppose that we want to conduct a pairwise meta-analysis among K studies. We collect a treatment effect size $\hat{\delta}_i$ from each of studies $i = 1, \ldots, K$. In the fixed-effects model, we model the treatment effect size following a normal distribution as:

$$\hat{\delta}_i \sim N(\delta, \sigma_i^2)$$

where δ is the true value of the treatment effect size and σ_i^2 is the variance for each study. The fixed-effects model only considers within-study variations and assumes only one true value of the treatment effect size across all the studies, meaning δ remains the same for K studies. Besides, if the true effect size δ is unknown, under Bayesian framework, it can be modeled with a prior for true value of the treatment effect size δ as:

$$\delta \sim N(0, \tau^2)$$

where we need to pre-specify the variance τ^2 for true effect δ. If the variance τ^2 is set to be very large, we have an "uninformative prior," which means that our prior information will not have a big impact on the posterior results. In another words, it is equivalent to the fixed-effects model under frequentist's framework.

12.6.2.2 Random-Effects Models

In fixed-effects model, it is assumed that the true effect size is the same for all the studies. However, it is not practical to use a fixed-effects model when we want to meta-analyze with different studies, such as separate clinical trials. Thus, a random-effects meta-analysis model should be used instead. The random-effects model assumes the true treatment effect size to be different for each study. The model can be written as:

$$\hat{\delta}_i \sim N(\delta_i, \sigma_i^2)$$

where δ_i is the true effect size for study i. Moreover, to address the between-study variation, in the random-effects model, δ_i is assumed to follow a normal distribution as:

$$\delta_i \sim N(\delta, \tau^2)$$

where δ denotes the overall mean treatment effect of the population and τ^2 denotes the between-study variance. For both overall mean treatment effect δ and between-study variance τ^2, we can incorporate pre-specified values as prior information. Alternatively, we can further model both parameters δ and τ^2 to follow hyperprior distributions through a hierarchical model as:

$$\delta \sim N(\delta_0, \eta_0^2)$$
$$\tau^2 \sim Unif(u, v)$$

where δ_0, η_0^2, u, v are called hyperparameters in the hierarchical model.

12.6.3 Bayesian Network Meta-Analysis Model

Under Bayesian framework, we can easily extend and adapt the Bayesian meta-analysis model to the network meta-analysis. We can extend the above-mentioned random-effects model for a pairwise comparative study to network meta-analysis, which compare multiple different treatments. Suppose K studies provided mixed comparisons among N studies. We denote an effect size from study i as $\hat{\delta}_{i,bn}$, which compares treatment b to treatment n in that study, $b = 1, \ldots, N; n = 2, \ldots, N; b < n$. The study-specific effect size $\hat{\delta}_{i,bn}$ can be modeled as:

$$\hat{\delta}_{i,bn} \sim N(\delta_{i,bn}, \sigma_i^2)$$

where $\delta_{i,bn}$ is the true treatment effects of treatment n compared to treatment b for study i. It is assumed to be a random effect following a normal distribution:

$$\delta_{i,bn} \sim N(\delta_{bn}, \tau_{bn}^2)$$

δ_{bn} denotes the overall true mean effect size between treatment n and treatment b; τ_{bn}^2 denotes the between-trial variance between treatment n and treatment b, and we can assume $\tau_{bn}^2 = \tau^2$ as equal between-trial variance.

$$\delta_{i,bn} \sim N(\delta_{bn}, \tau^2)$$

Moreover, $\delta_{i,bn}$ follows the transition relationship as: $\delta_{i,bn} = \delta_{i,b1} - \delta_{i,n1}$. Treatment 1 could be viewed as reference treatment. This relationship also holds for $\delta_{bn} = \delta_{b1} - \delta_{n1}$. Under Bayesian hierarchical model structure, we can also specify prior information for unknown parameters δ_{bn} and τ^2:

$$\delta_{bn} \sim N(\delta_0, \eta_0^2)$$
$$\tau^2 \sim Unif(u, v)$$

According to Dias, Sutton, Ades, et al. (2013), we can use weakly informative priors for both parameters as: $\delta_{bn} \sim N(0, 100^2)$ and $\tau \sim Unif(0, 5)$.

12.6.4 Multiarm Trials

Within Bayesian framework, it is easy to extend a network meta-analysis to multiarm trials. Suppose we are interested in a number of multiarm trials with a total of N treatments. To compare N treatments, we will have a vector δ_i of *N-1* random treatments effects, $\delta_i = (\delta_{i,12}, \ldots, \delta_{i,bN})^T$. For multiarm trials, the between-trial variance needs to include the random effect covariance which can vary from constant and equal structure to totally unrestricted positive-definite matrix (Greco et al. 2016; Dias, Sutton, Ades, et al. 2013). Assuming homogeneous between-trial variance, the vector of *N-1* random treatments effects, δ_i, is assumed to follow a multivariate normal distribution:

$$\delta_i = \begin{pmatrix} \delta_{i,12} \\ \vdots \\ \delta_{i,bN} \end{pmatrix} \sim N_{N-1} \left(\begin{pmatrix} \delta_{12} \\ \vdots \\ \delta_{bN} \end{pmatrix}, \begin{pmatrix} \tau^2 & \cdots & \tau^2/2 \\ \vdots & \ddots & \vdots \\ \tau^2/2 & \cdots & \tau^2 \end{pmatrix} \right).$$

12.7 Bayesian Network Meta-Analysis of Parkinson's Clinical Trial Data in R

Currently, there are two R packages *bnma* and *gemtc* available for Bayesian network meta-analysis. The capabilities of these two R packages are similar. Both packages *bnma* and *gemtc* work with the software called JAGS ("Just Another Gibbs Sampler") (Plummer 2003), which uses MCMC algorithm to simulate a sequence of dependent samples from the posterior distribution of the parameters. JAGS needs to be installed on our computer before we can fit a Bayesian network meta-analysis using the above two R packages. The software is freely available for both Windows and Mac/Unix from https://sourceforge.net/projects/mcmc-jags/files/. Next, we will demonstrate how to run a Bayesian network meta-analysis for continuous outcome using the R package *gemtc*. First, we need to install and load the package.

```
install.packages("gemtc")
library(gemtc)
```

In order to connect *gemtc* with JAGS, an R package *rjags* is required, which provides an interface from R to JAGS. Thus, we need to install and load R package *rjags*.

```
install.packages("rjags")
library(rjags)
```

12.7.1 Data Preparation and Visualization

We will use the Parkinson's disease data set as displayed in Table 12.2 for this demonstration. The data set is named as **parkinson** and ready in the format to be analyzed in the R package *gemtc*. The data set contains fifteen rows of arm-based data including mean off-time reductions, standard deviations for the reductions, and sample size for each comparison. Instead of calling the data object parkinson from *gemtc*, we will first show how to prepare the input data in a format as required by the package. The input data are the arm-level data with following input variable names: study, treatment, mean, std.dev, and sampleSize.

```
# Create a new network by specifying all information.
data <- read.table(textConnection('study treatment  mean std.dev
   sampleSize

       1        Placebo -1.22   3.70        54
       1        Ropinirole -1.53    4.28        95
       2        Placebo -0.70   3.70       172
       2        Pramipexole -2.40    3.40        173
       3        Placebo -0.30   4.40        76
```

```
3          Pramipexole -2.60    4.30        71
3          Bromocriptine -1.20   4.30          81
4          Ropinirole -0.24    3.00       128
4          Bromocriptine -0.59    3.00         72
5          Ropinirole -0.73    3.00       80
5          Bromocriptine -0.18    3.00         46
6          Bromocriptine -2.20    2.31        137
6          Cabergoline -2.50    2.18       131
7          Bromocriptine -1.80    2.48       154
7          Cabergoline -2.10    2.99       143'), header=TRUE)
```

Now we need to prepare the data with the function mtc.network() for downstream modeling analysis. As we are using arm-level data, we have to use data.ab argument. We save the result as an object network and first take a look at it by printing it out.

```
network <- mtc.network(data.ab = data)
```

```
# Print the network
print(network)
#> MTC dataset: Network
#> Arm-level data:
#>      study      treatment   mean std.dev sampleSize
#> 1       1         Placebo -1.22    3.70         54
#> 2       1       Ropinirole -1.53    4.28         95
#> 3       2         Placebo -0.70    3.70        172
#> 4       2     Pramipexole -2.40    3.40        173
#> 5       3 Bromocriptine -1.20    4.30         81
#> 6       3         Placebo -0.30    4.40         76
#> 7       3     Pramipexole -2.60    4.30         71
#> 8       4 Bromocriptine -0.59    3.00         72
#> 9       4       Ropinirole -0.24    3.00        128
#> 10      5 Bromocriptine -0.18    3.00         46
#> 11      5       Ropinirole -0.73    3.00         80
#> 12      6 Bromocriptine -2.20    2.31        137
#> 13      6     Cabergoline -2.50    2.18        131
#> 14      7 Bromocriptine -1.80    2.48        154
#> 15      7     Cabergoline -2.10    2.99        143
```

We can also use the function summary() to provide some more insights about the structure of the network. It is clear to see the number of studies for each treatment and the numbers of different n-arm studies from the output. Also, the number of studies for each treatment comparison is available.

```
summary(network)
#> $Description
#> [1] "MTC dataset: Network"
```

```
#>
#> $`Studies per treatment`
#> Bromocriptine   Cabergoline      Placebo   Pramipexole    Ropinirole
#>             5             2            3             2             3
#>
#> $`Number of n-arm studies`
#> 2-arm 3-arm
#>     6     1
#>
#> $`Studies per treatment comparison`
#>              t1            t2 nr
#> 1 Bromocriptine Cabergoline  2
#> 2 Bromocriptine     Placebo  1
#> 3 Bromocriptine Pramipexole  1
#> 4 Bromocriptine  Ropinirole  2
#> 5       Placebo Pramipexole  2
#> 6       Placebo  Ropinirole  1
```

To visualize the structure of the network, we can use the function `plot()` to generate a network plot as shown in Figure 12.6, which displays various pairs of treatment comparison. Similar as the other R package *netmeta*, the edge thickness of the network plot reflects the number of comparisons between the compared two treatments.

```
plot(network)
```

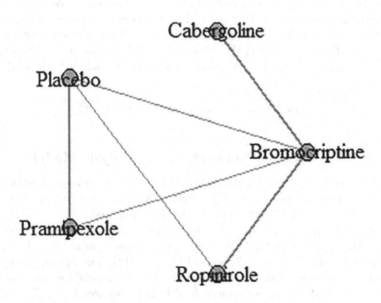

FIGURE 12.6
Network Plot for Parkinson data.

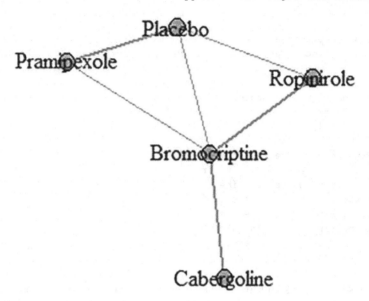

FIGURE 12.7
Network plot for Parkinson's data, generated with Fruchterman-Reingold algorithm.

We can also improve the visualization of the network plot as displayed in Figure 12.7 using the Fruchterman-Reingold algorithm. We can do that by specifying the option `layout` as `layout.fruchterman.reingold`. The Fruchterman-Reingold algorithm is inherently random in generating the network plots. Thus, we can run the same code multiple times to get the results. Also, it requires a dependent R package *igraph* to be installed and loaded.

```
library(igraph)
plot(network, layout=layout.fruchterman.reingold)
```

12.7.2   Generate the Network Meta-Analysis Model

To run the Bayesian network model, we will use the function `mtc.network()` with the generated and saved object `network`. There are five types of network models that available through the function, including "consistency," "nodesplit," "regression," "ume," or "use." The option "consistency" refers to the ordinary consistency model without any additional parameters (Dias, Sutton, Ades, et al., 2013; van Valkenhoef et al., 2012). The option "nodesplit" refers to a node-splitting model, which is used to access the inconsistency of the model and will be introduced in details in Section 12.7.6. The option "regression" refers to a network meta-regression model, similar as a traditional meta-regression. For details, please refer to (Dias, Sutton, Welton, et al., 2013) or https://github.com/gertvv/gemtc. The options "ume" refers to unrelated study effects models, which assume the studies are independent and model the effects within each study (Valkenhoef). The options "use" refer unrelated mean effects model, which assume the comparisons are independent and model the effects within each comparison (Dias, Sutton, Welton, et al., 2013; Valkenhoef). By default, if left unspecified, the model will be a consistency model. We also need to specify the number of Markov chains we need for running Bayesian network meta-analysis model. By default, 4 chains will be run. Besides, we can specify a model to be either "fixed" or "random" through the option `linearModel` in this function. Also, the package *getmc* can analyze continuous data, dichotomous data, and rate/survival data. For various types of outcome, we can specify a corresponding likelihood/link for the outcome through options `likelihood` and `link`. For our example data, we can specify them to be `normal` and `identify` for MD which is continuous data. Below is an example to run a Bayesian network model for continuous data using random model.

```
model <- mtc.model(network, likelihood = 'normal',
                   link = 'identity', linearModel = "random",
                   n.chain = 4)
```

12.7.3   Specify the Priors

In the function `mtc.model`, we can specify hyperpriors for the heterogeneity parameters in the Bayesian network meta-analysis model through the option `hy.prior`. If left unspecified, default values are used. By default, a uniform distribution will be specified. To specify a hyperprior for heterogeneity parameters of the random-effects model, we need to provide a vector of length 4 for the function `mtc.hy.prior`, where the first element should be type of hyperparameter, such as variance, standard deviation, or precision. The second element is where we can specify the prior distribution, including "dunif" (uniform), "dgamma" (Gamma), or "dlnorm" (log-normal). And the next two are the parameters associated with the distribution. Below is an example of using a hyperprior of uniform(0, 5).

```
model <- mtc.model(network, likelihood = 'normal',
                   link = 'identity', hy.prior=mtc.hy.prior
                   ("std.dev", "dunif", 0, 5), linearModel = "random",
                   n.chain = 4)
```

12.7.4   Markov Chain Monte Carlo Simulation

Once we set up the Bayesian network meta-analysis model for a data, we can use Gibbs Sampling Method, the MCMC simulation from software JAGS, to estimate the posterior distributions for all the parameters. Then we can summarize the results of the Bayesian network meta-analysis model for the parameters of interest. In running any MCMC simulation, we have three options that we need to specify in the function `mtc.run` to improve the accuracy of the MCMC simulation.

1. In any MCMC simulation chain, the first few runs will normally likely produce inaccurate posterior samples. Thus, a procedure called burn-in is commonly used to eliminate that inaccuracy by getting rid of certain number of first simulation draws for the posterior samples. It can be achieved by using `n.adapt` option in the function `mtc.run`.

2. It is also important to determine how many iterations we need to run for a MCMC simulation chain. We want the MCMC simulation chain to run long enough so we have accurate estimates of the parameters of interest, which is known as that the chain reaches convergence. It can be achieved by using `n.adapt` option in the function `mtc.run`. It can be achieved by using `n.iter` option in the function `mtc.run`.

3. A third option `thin` is also available in the function `mtc.run`. We can specify a thinning factor through this option to only use the values of every ith iteration to summarize the posterior samples for the parameters. By doing this, it could reduce the risk of having autocorrelation in the simulated posterior samples.

In the following example, we are showing a simulation in the function `mtc.run`. The simulation chain, saved as object `chain`, will extract every 5th iteration for the posterior samples. The burn-in is 500 and the number of iterations is set to be 10,000. We need to provide the name for the `model` object as we have set up in the above section and specify the other previous described parameters. In the output below, the compiled model graph contains 15 observed stochastic nodes and 20 unobserved stochastic nodes, with a total graph size of 446.

```
chain <- mtc.run(model, n.adapt = 500, n.iter = 10000, thin = 5)
#> Compiling model graph
#>     Resolving undeclared variables
#>     Allocating nodes
#> Graph information:
#>     Observed stochastic nodes: 15
#>     Unobserved stochastic nodes: 20
#>     Total graph size: 446
#>
#> Initializing model
```

12.7.5 Assessing the Convergence

After we generated a sequence of posterior samples for a parameter, it is necessary to check the convergence of the simulated samples. To do so, we can generate a trace plot in the fashion of a "time series" plot to check the mix of our simulated samples over all iterations. We can use the function plot to examine the outputs of object chain. The trace plots for the simulated samples stored in the object chain are displayed in Figure 12.8.

```
plot(chain)
```

In Figure 12.8, five trace plots are shown to examine if the mix of the simulated samples reached to a convergence or not for four mean treatments difference parameters and a standard deviation parameter. Based on all the four chains, the convergence of this Bayesian network meta-analysis model does not show any problematic signs. We can also evaluate the density plots of posterior samples for all those five parameters as shown on the right panel in Figure 12.8. The density plots are displaying distributions close to the assumptions which suggest convergence is met in this model.

We can also use Gelman-Rubin-Brooks Plot to examine the convergence of the posterior samples. The plot shows Potential Scale Reduction Factor (PSRF), PSRF is a measure comparing the within-chain variation to the

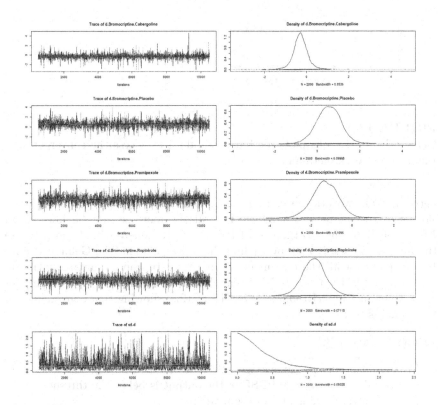

FIGURE 12.8
Trace and density plots for Parkinson data with Bayesian network meta-analysis model.

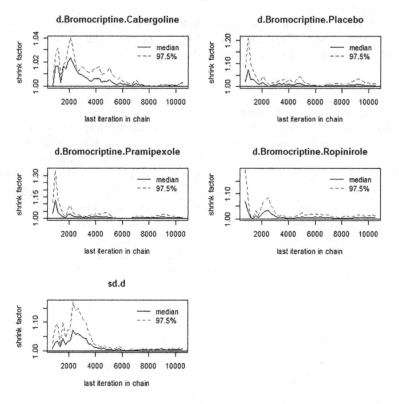

FIGURE 12.9
Gelman-Rubin-Brooks plots for Parkinson data to access the convergence of
Bayesian network meta-analysis model.

between-chain variation over time. To satisfy convergence, the PRSF should
slowly go to one as the number of iterations increase and be lower than
1.05 when it reaches to the end of the chain. To generate that plot, we use
the function `gelman.plot` by feeding the object `chain`. The Gelman-Rubin-
Brooks plots for all the treatment comparison MDs and standard deviation
are displayed in Figure 12.9. It is clear that the PRSF goes to 1 at the end of
every Gelman-Rubin-Brooks plot in Figure 12.9, showing that convergence in
the model is met.

```
gelman.plot(chain)
```

We can also output the average PSRF of `chain` using the following code
and we see that the average PRSF in the output is below the threshold 1.05,
indicating convergence is met in the model.

```
gelman.plot(chain)
#> [1] 1.005185
```

12.7.6 Assessing Inconsistency: The Nodesplit Method

Similar as in running a network meta-analysis model under frequentist's framework, we need to evaluate the consistency of the Bayesian network meta-analysis model as well. We can use nodesplit method to achieve that (Dias et al., 2010). The nodesplit method removes both arms in estimating the direct evidence from indirect evidence in the network and examines all relevant network models using MCMC simulations (van Valkenhoef et al., 2016; Dias et al., 2010). Using this method, a three-arm trial will not contribute any evidence to the network of indirect evidence. We can use the function `mtc.nodesplit` in the package *gemtc* to implement the method. Except that plugging in the object network which was generated by the function `mtc.network`, we also need to specify the parameters as we have specified in the function `mtc.run`. Below is the example how we can use the same MCMC simulation options that we have used for generating the object `chain` to examine the model inconsistency. We first generate an object named `nodesplit` with the function `mtc.nodesplit`:

```
nodesplit <- mtc.nodesplit(network,
                   linearModel = "random",
                   n.adapt = 500,
                   n.iter = 10000,
                   thin = 5)
```

Then we can use the function `summary` to summarize by feeding the object `nodesplit` and interpret the results of the nodesplit model. The output below summarized the results of direct only, indirect only, and network (direct and indirect combined) evidence for the treatment effects comparisons. If there are different estimates using direct and indirect evidence, it suggests the possibility of inconsistency in the network model. Also, one or more comparisons with $p < 0.05$ would suggest a problematic amount of inconsistency in the network. All p-values in the following output are greater than 0.05, suggesting our network model is not problematic with inconsistency.

```
summary(nodesplit)
#> Node-splitting analysis of inconsistency
#> =========================================
#>
#>     comparison                 p.value CrI
#> 1   d.Bromocriptine.Placebo    0.65900
#> 2   -> direct                          0.88 (-1.3, 3.1)
#> 3   -> indirect                        0.27 (-2.3, 2.7)
#> 4   -> network                         0.53 (-0.65, 1.7)
#> 5   d.Bromocriptine.Pramipexole 0.98750
#> 6   -> direct                          -1.4 (-3.6, 0.67)
#> 7   -> indirect                        -1.4 (-4.7, 1.5)
#> 8   -> network                         -1.3 (-2.6, -0.071)
```

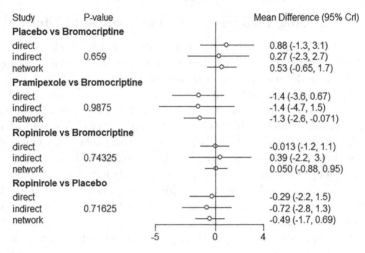

FIGURE 12.10
Forest plot of Parkinson data to access inconsistency of the Bayesian network meta-analysis model.

```
#> 9   d.Bromocriptine.Ropinirole  0.74325
#> 10 -> direct                              -0.013 (-1.2, 1.1)
#> 11 -> indirect                             0.39 (-2.2,  3.)
#> 12 -> network                              0.050 (-0.88, 0.95)
#> 13 d.Placebo.Ropinirole       0.71625
#> 14 -> direct                              -0.29 (-2.2, 1.5)
#> 15 -> indirect                            -0.72 (-2.8, 1.3)
#> 16 -> network                             -0.49 (-1.7, 0.69)
```

We can also use the function plot to generate a forest plot as shown in Figure 12.10 for the above summarized nodesplit model for better visualization of the results. It is clear that no *p*-value is less than 0.05, indicating that our model does not have the inconsistency problem.

```
plot(summary(nodesplit))
```

12.7.7   Summarize the Network Meta-Analysis Results

After we build and validate a Bayesian network meta-analysis model, we can now summarize and report the Bayesian network meta-analysis model results. A forest plot is a commonly used approach to summarize and present the meta-analysis results, which could also be used in reporting Bayesian network meta-analysis models. The example code below is to generate a forest plot as displayed in Figure 12.11 for the objects chain. We chose placebo as the reference treatment for comparison specified in the function relative.effect

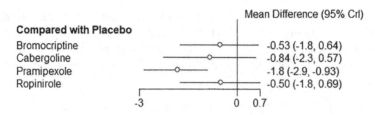

FIGURE 12.11
Forest plot of Parkinson data with Bayesian network meta-analysis model.

so the forest plot shows four treatments as compared with placebo. It is clear that only the treatment Pramipexole is significant different in treatment effect as compared with placebo (MD = -1.8 with 95% Confidence interval $(-2.9, -0.93)$).

```
forest(relative.effect(chain, t1 = "Placebo"))
```

Besides visualizing the meta-analysis results with forest plots to show various pairwise comparisons, we also need to determine the ranking of all treatments in the network meta-analysis. It can be achieved by calculating rank-probabilities using *gemtc*. The treatments are ranked based on their effect to a chosen baseline for each MCMC iteration. Rank-probabilities are calculated from the rankings and the number of iterations. We can use the function `rank.probability` to calculate the rank probabilities for all the treatments and placebo. The option `preferredDirection` needs to be set as 1 if higher MD is preferred; otherwise it needs to be set as -1 if lower MD is preferred. The following example is the code to generate an object rank for calculating and plotting rank-probabilities. The output below includes a table and a corresponding plot as in Figure 12.12 of the rank probabilities for all four treatments and placebo. It can be seen that the probability for Pramipexole

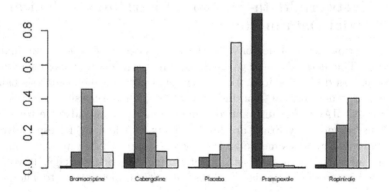

FIGURE 12.12
Rank probabilities for Parkinson data.

to be the best treatment is 0.8996; the probability for Cabergoline to be the second best treatment is 0.5835; the probability for Bromocriptine to be the third best treatment is 0.4574; the probability for Ropinirole to be the fourth best treatment is 0.4040; the probability for Placebo to be the worst treatment is 0.7300.

```
rank <- rank.probability(chain, preferredDirection=-1)
rank
#> Rank probability; preferred direction = -1
#>                    [,1]      [,2]      [,3]      [,4]      [,5]
#> Bromocriptine 0.005125 0.089750 0.457375 0.357375 0.090375
#> Cabergoline   0.079250 0.583500 0.198375 0.092375 0.046500
#> Placebo       0.000625 0.057500 0.077000 0.134875 0.730000
#> Pramipexole   0.899625 0.066875 0.021625 0.011375 0.000500
#> Ropinirole    0.015375 0.202375 0.245625 0.404000 0.132625
plot(rank, beside=TRUE, cex.names=0.5)
```

Alternatively, a metric, named Surface Under the Cumulative Ranking (SUCRA) score, can be calculated to evaluate the most efficacious treatment in a network (Rucker and Schwarzer 2015; Salanti, Ades, and Ioannidis, 2011). The function sucra is available to calculate the SUCRA scores as shown below. And we can see that Pramipexole is most likely to be the best treatment, then followed in sequence by Cabergoline, Ropinirole, Bromocriptine, and Placebo.

```
sucra(rank)
#> Bromocriptine  Cabergoline     Placebo  Pramipexole    Ropinirole
#>     0.3904688    0.6391562   0.1159688    0.9634375     0.3909687
```

12.8   Network Meta-Analysis of Parkinson's Clinical Trial Data in Stata

In this section, we will demonstrate how to perform network meta-analysis in Stata. The network package in Stata can perform frequentist's network meta-analysis directly. Alternatively, Bayesian network meta-analysis can be summarized in Stata, by working externally with a Bayesian software like WinBugs or JAGs. Because network meta-analysis is an advance topic, the functions provided by Stata are not as many as those by R, especially for Bayesian meta-analysis methods. Here, we only present how to carry out frequentist network meta-analysis in Stata using network package. If you are interested in running Bayesian analysis with Stata, please refer to Thompson (2014).

To perform network meta-analysis in Stata, we need to install the *network* package first (White 2015). Besides, we need to install two other packages, *network graphs* and *mvmeta* packages. Below is the code to install those three packages, which only needs to be run once.

```
. net install network,
       from(http://www.homepages.ucl.ac.uk/~rmjwiww/stata/meta)
. net from http://www.clinicalepidemio.fr/Stata
. net install mvmeta,
       from(http://www.homepages.ucl.ac.uk/~rmjwiww/stata/meta)
```

Next, we need to prepare and load the data set into Stata. We will use the same data set as shown in Section 12.2.2 and demonstrated the analysis of it in Section 12.7. The input data set is formatted the same as what we input in Section 12.7, which can be saved as a data object in Stata, named as "*Parkinson.dta.*" The following command is to load the Parkinson data into Stata:

```
. use " Parkinson.dta"
```

Then, the data need to be set up using command:

```
. network setup mean stddev samplesize,
  studyvar(study) trtvar(treatment) ref(Placebo)
```

In the command, *network setup* means that we are using network package to set up a data set. Mean is the variable name in the data set for means of treatment effects. `stddev` is the variable name in the data set for the standard deviations of means of treatment effects. `samplesize` is the variable name in the data set for sample size for each treatment compared. After a comma, we specify `studyvar(study) trtvar(treatment) ref(Placebo)`. `studyvar()` is the function to include the variable name for study title. `trtvar()` is the function to include the variable name for treatment. `Ref()` is the function to specify the name of treatment that is chosen as the reference treatment in the analysis. Below is the output to show the structure of the input data:

```
Treatments used
A:                               Bromocriptine
B:                               Cabergoline
C (reference):                   Placebo
D:                               Pramipexole
E:                               Ropinirole

Measure                          Mean difference
Standard deviation pooling:      off

Studies
ID variable:                     study
Number used:                     7
IDs with augmented reference arm: 4 5 6 7
```

```
observations added:                0.00001
mean in augmented observations:    study-specific mean
SD in augmented observations:      study-specific within-arms SD


Network information
Components:                        1 (connected)
D.f. for inconsistency:            2
D.f. for heterogeneity:            2


Current data
Data format:                       augmented
Design variable:                   _design
Estimate variables:                _y*
Variance variables:                _S*
Command to list the data:          list study _y* _S*,
                                   noo sepby(_design)
```

As we can see from the above output, for studies with no information on the reference treatment, 4, 5, 6, 7, an extremely small amount of data is generated by Stata using augmented method. The advantage of the augmented method is that the overall effect size is not affected and all studies will be analyzed.

Next, we can use the following command to create a network plot as shown in Figure 12.13. There are five nodes, one for each treatment. The size of the

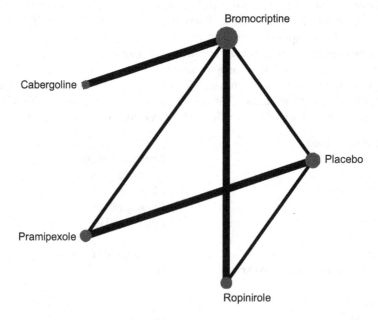

FIGURE 12.13
Network plot of Parkinson data generated from Stata.

nodes indicates the number of studies and the lines connecting nodes indicate the amount of relevant treatments.

. network map

After we visualize the network with the above network plot, we need to test the consistency among three network meta-analysis assumptions. The following command is the command for the inconsistency test in Stata. And the output of the following command for this example is presented in Figure 12.14.

```
Command is: mvmeta _y _S  , bscovariance(exch 0.5) longparm suppress(uv mm) eq(_
> y_D: des_CD, _y_E: des_CE) vars(_y_A _y_B _y_D _y_E)
Note: using method reml
Note: regressing _y_A on (nothing)
Note: regressing _y_B on (nothing)
Note: regressing _y_D on des_CD
Note: regressing _y_E on des_CE
Note: 7 observations on 4 variables
Note: variance-covariance matrix is proportional to .5*I(4)+.5*J(4,4,1)

initial:      log likelihood = -33.558486
rescale:      log likelihood = -33.558486
rescale eq:   log likelihood = -32.173319
Iteration 0:  log likelihood = -32.173319
Iteration 1:  log likelihood = -32.146166
Iteration 2:  log likelihood = -32.146166

Multivariate meta-analysis
Variance-covariance matrix = proportional .5*I(4)+.5*J(4,4,1)
Method = reml                              Number of dimensions    =    4
Restricted log likelihood = -32.146166     Number of observations  =    7
```

		Coef.	Std. Err.	z	P>|z|	[95% Conf. Interval]	
_y_A							
	_cons	-.8999974	.6949872	-1.29	0.195	-2.262147	.4621525
_y_B							
	_cons	-1.199997	.7255239	-1.65	0.098	-2.621998	.2220033
_y_D							
	des_CD	.5999984	.8133713	0.74	0.461	-.9941801	2.194177
	_cons	-2.299998	.7177458	-3.20	0.001	-3.706754	-.8932425
_y_E							
	des_CE	.5891405	1.024155	0.58	0.565	-1.418167	2.596448
	_cons	-.8991404	.7762413	-1.16	0.247	-2.420545	.6222646

```
Estimated between-studies SDs and correlation matrix:
          SD         _y_A       _y_B       _y_D       _y_E
_y_A  4.076e-07       1          .          .          .
_y_B  4.076e-07      .5          1          .          .
_y_D  4.076e-07      .5         .5          1          .
_y_E  4.076e-07      .5         .5         .5          1

Testing for inconsistency:
 ( 1)  [_y_D]des_CD = 0
 ( 2)  [_y_E]des_CE = 0

          chi2( 2) =     0.68
        Prob > chi2 =    0.7121
```

FIGURE 12.14

Output of inconsistency test for network meta-analysis of Parkinson data from Stata.

The *p*-value for the consistency test at the overall level is presented at the bottom of Figure 12.14. We fail to reject the null hypothesis and the consistency assumption could be accepted at the overall level of each treatment.

```
. network meta inconsistency
```

Meanwhile, we can test locally on loop inconsistency using the following command. It will output the estimates of direct, indirect, and difference between direct and indirect evidence for each treatments comparison and test results as below. None of the treatments in this example showed statistical significance in inconsistency, which infers the consistency assumption is accepted in both global and local tests.

```
. network sidesplit all
Side      Direct                 Indirect               Difference
          Coef.      Std. Err.   Coef.      Std. Err.   Coef.      Std. Err.  P>|z|
C D *    -1.832787   .3376548   -1.116554   1.92139    -.7162326   1.950188   0.713
C E       -.3099999   .6680897   -.6681133   .7102573   .3581134    .9750945   0.713
A C       .8939593    .6947998   .1816914    .6680047   .7122679    .9696232   0.463
A B *     -.3         .2082732   1.033686    1164.672  -1.333686    1164.672   0.999
A D      -1.382778    .6987335  -1.164448    .7956367  -.2183295    1.06462    0.838
A E       .0008568    .3457508   .3589709    .9117379  -.3581141    .9750947   0.713
```

Since the assumptions are satisfied, we can use the following command to fit the consistency network meta-analysis model to our example data. The Figure 12.15 displays the output of fitting a network meta-analysis model for Parkinson data with estimated coefficient, standard error, *z* value, *p*-value, and 95% confidence intervals for each treatment.

```
. network meta consistency
```

We can also display the effect sizes from Figure 12.15 in two other plots: network forest plot and interval plot. To generate a network forest plot for example data as shown in Figure 12.16, the command as below is used:

```
. network forest, msize (*0.15) diamond eform xlabel
  (0.1 1 10 100) colors (black blue red) list
```

The main command is `network forest` to generate forest plots, which will be followed by a comma and then options to customize the forest plot. `msize` (*0.15) is the option to decrease the value of individual studies' effect size by 0.15 times. `Diamond` is the option to use a diamond shape for summary effect sizes. `eform` is to generate transformed indices for easy interpretation. `xlabel` (0.1 1 10 100) is to set up the labels on the *x*-axis and `colors` (black blue red) is to specify the colors for the treatment effects. As shown in Figure 12.16, black lines are for the effects of each study within a treatment in the comparison set. Blue diamond is labeled as pooled within design, which is the pooled effect of a treatment in the comparison set and shows the results of the test for the inconsistency model. And red diamond is for the pooled

```
Command is: mvmeta _y _S  , bscovariance(exch 0.5) longparm suppress(uv mm) vars(_y_A _y_B _y_D _y_E)
Note: using method reml
Note: using variables _y_A _y_B _y_D _y_E
Note: 7 observations on 4 variables
Note: variance-covariance matrix is proportional to .5*I(4)+.5*J(4,4,1)

initial:      log likelihood = -36.593785
rescale:      log likelihood = -36.593785
rescale eq:   log likelihood = -34.142529
Iteration 0:  log likelihood = -34.142529
Iteration 1:  log likelihood = -34.091776
Iteration 2:  log likelihood = -34.091772
Iteration 3:  log likelihood = -34.091772

Multivariate meta-analysis
Variance-covariance matrix = proportional .5*I(4)+.5*J(4,4,1)
Method = reml                            Number of dimensions    =    4
Restricted log likelihood = -34.091772   Number of observations  =    7
```

		Coef.	Std. Err.	z	P>|z|	[95% Conf. Interval]	
_y_A							
	_cons	-.523993	.4786352	-1.09	0.274	-1.462101	.4141148
_y_B							
	_cons	-.8239929	.521986	-1.58	0.114	-1.847067	.1990808
_y_D							
	_cons	-1.811553	.3326681	-5.45	0.000	-2.463571	-1.159536
_y_E							
	_cons	-.4781112	.4866355	-0.98	0.326	-1.431899	.4756768

```
Estimated between-studies SDs and correlation matrix:
           SD      _y_A    _y_B    _y_D    _y_E
_y_A  1.710e-09     1       .       .       .
_y_B  1.710e-09    .5       1       .       .
_y_D  1.710e-09    .5      .5       1       .
_y_E  1.710e-09    .5      .5      .5       1
```

FIGURE 12.15
Output of a consistency model for Parkinson data from Stata.

overall effect, which is labeled as pooled overall and shows the result of the test for the consistency model. Besides, the p-value at the left bottom of Figure 12.16 is the p-value of the global test for inconsistency, the same as presented in Figure 12.14. The x-axis is based on exponential of the MD so we make inferences based on the confidence intervals containing 1 or not. We can also investigate if the consistency model is supported or not based on the similarity between blue diamond (pooled within design) and red diamond (pooled overall effect).

When the number of studies is large, the network forest plot will be difficult to read. As an alternative, we can generate interval plots as in Figure 12.17 for our example data using the following command:

```
. intervalplot, eform null (1) labels (Placebo IV_single
    IV_double Topical Combination) margin (10 8 15 10) textsize
    (2) xlabel(0.03 0.1 1 18)
```

The main command to generate interval plots is **intervalplot**, which will be followed by a comma and then other options. **eform** is the option to

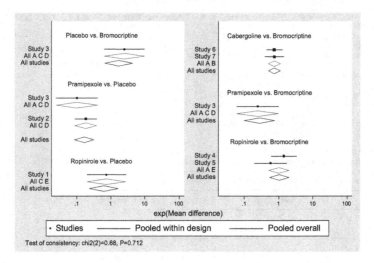

FIGURE 12.16
Network forest plot of consistency network meta-analysis model for Parkinson
data from Stata.

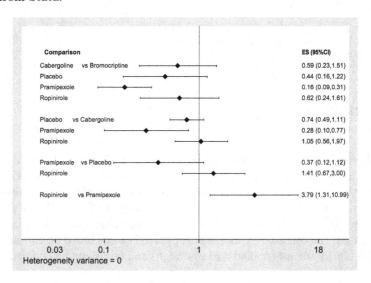

FIGURE 12.17
Interval plot of consistency network meta-analysis model for Parkinson data
from Stata.

transform the original logarithmic data into indices so that interpretation is
easier; null() is the function to input the value to show statistically significant
difference in a ratio such as 1 for odds ratio; labels() is the function to add
the labels for all the treatments. margin() sets the appropriate ranges to

display plots. `textsize()` is the option to set the size of the text that will be used in generating the plots. `xlabel()` is to set the values shown on the *x*-axis. As shown in Figure 12.17, it is easy to compare the effect sizes of each treatment comparison and interpret the results using this interval plot.

After we compared the effectiveness of the treatments, we have to rank the treatments to identify which treatment intervention shows the most superior treatment effect (Tonin et al., 2017). We can use the following command to generate a table as shown in Figure 12.18 and a figure as shown in Figure 12.19 to evaluate the treatment superiority.

```
Estimated probabilities (%) of each treatment being the best (and other ranks)
- assuming the minimum parameter is the best
- using 10000 draws
- allowing for parameter uncertainty
```

study and			Treatment		
Rank	Placebo	Bromocriptine	Cabergoline	Pramipexole	Ropinirole
1					
Best	0.0	0.1	3.6	96.1	0.3
2nd	4.0	4.0	72.3	3.2	16.5
3rd	6.8	49.5	17.8	0.6	25.4
4th	11.3	37.9	5.4	0.2	45.2
Worst	77.9	8.5	0.9	0.0	12.6
MEAN RANK	4.6	3.5	2.3	1.0	3.5
SUCRA	0.1	0.4	0.7	1.0	0.4

FIGURE 12.18
Results of network rank test for Parkinson data generated from Stata.

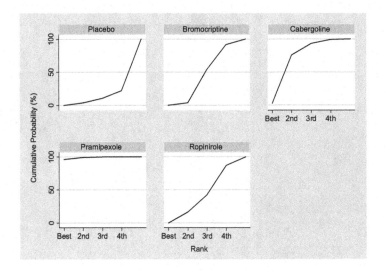

FIGURE 12.19
Network rank test plot for Parkinson data generated from Stata.

```
. network rank min, line cumulative xlabel (1/4) seed (10000)
  reps (10000) meanrank
```

The main command is `network rank min`, which specifies superiority will be determined by using ascending order of effect size; if `network rank max` is used, superiority will be determined by using descending order of effect size. The options after the comma will be used to customize the plots as shown in Figure 12.19. As shown in Figures 12.18 and 12.19, the probability of treatment Pramipexole being the best is 96.1% and the probability of Place being the worst is 77.9%. In SCURA, the surface area for Pramipexole is 1, confirming it to be the best treatment in the multiple treatment comparisons.

13

Meta-Analysis for Rare Events

All the methods presented thus far for meta-analysis in this book are based on large sample theory as well as the theory of large sample approximations. For rare events, these methods usually break down. For example, when events are zeros, the methods for risk-ratio and odds-ratio (OR) discussed in Section 4.2 cannot be used and when the events are rare, but not all zeros, the variance estimates for these methods are not robust which may lead to unreliable statistical inferences. The typical remedies are to remove the studies with zero events from the meta analysis, or add a small value, say 0.5, to the rare events which could lead to biased statistical inferences as pointed out by Tian et al. (2009) and Cai et al. (2010).

In this chapter, we use the well-known Rosiglitazone meta-analysis data to illustrate the bias when classical meta-analysis methods are used for rare events. We then introduce a R package `gmeta` which implements a novel `confidence distributions` (CDs) approach proposed in Singh et al. (2005), Xie et al. (2011) and Xie and Singh (2013) to unify the framework for meta-analysis where two methods are implemented for meta-analysis of rare events. The general introduction to this package can be found from http://stat.rutgers.edu/home/gmeta/. As seen from this link, methods implemented in `gmeta` include:

1. Combination of p-values: Fisher's method, Stouffer (normal) method, Tippett (min) method, Max method, Sum method;

2. Model based meta-analysis methods: Fixed-effect model, Random-effect model, Robust method1 (a small number of large studies), Robust method2 (a large number of small studies);

3. Combine evidence from 2 by 2 tables: Mantel-Haenszel Odd Ratio, Peto's Log Odd Ratio, Exact method1 (Odd Ratio), Exact method2 (Risk Difference)

Among these methods, the "Exact method1" (i.e., `exact1`) for OR and the "Exact method2" (i.e., `exact2`) in Tian et al. (2009) for risk-difference can be used for rare event meta-analysis.

13.1   The Rosiglitazone Meta-Analysis

In a meta-analysis for the effect of rosiglitazone on the risk of myocardial infarction (MI) and death from cardiovascular causes, Nissen and Wolski (2007) searched the available published literature and found 116 potentially relevant studies where 42 of these met the inclusion criteria. Data were then extracted from the 42 publications and combined using a fixed-effects meta-analysis model. This yielded an OR for the rosiglitazone group to the control group of 1.43 with 95% confidence interval (CI) of (1.03, 1.98) and p-value = 0.03 for MI; and 1.64 with 95% CI of (0.98, 2.74) and p-value = 0.06 for death from cardiovascular causes. Based on these results, the authors concluded that rosiglitazone use was statistically significantly associated with the risk of MI and was borderline statistically significant with death from cardiovascular causes. Therefore, using rosiglitazone for the treatment of Type 2 diabetes could lead to serious adverse cardiovascular effects.

Since its publication, numerous authors questioned the validity of the analysis and interpretation of the results. For example, Shuster and Schatz (2008) (which is online available at http://care.diabetesjournals.org/ content/31/3/e10.full.pdf) pointed out that the fixed-effects meta-analysis was inappropriate. They reanalyzed 48 (not 42) eligible studies via a new random-effects method (Shuster et al., 2007) that yielded different conclusions; i.e., a strong association with cardiac death was found, but there was no significant association with MI. Other meta-analyses of data from the studies can be found from Dahabreh (2008), Tian et al. (2009), Cai et al. (2010), and Lane (2012) (online publication available at http://www.ncbi.nlm.nih.gov/ pubmed/22218366).

In this chapter, we further illustrate meta-analysis for rare events using this data with R implementations in `gmeta`.

13.2   Step-by-Step Data Analysis in R

13.2.1   Load the Data

The data from Tian et al. (2009), which is available as the supplementary material at http://www.ncbi.nlm.nih.gov/pmc/articles/PMC2648899/bin/ kxn034_index.html, are re-entered into our Excel databook (i.e., `dat4Meta`). This data can be loaded into R with the following R code chunk:

```
> # Load the Rosiglitazone data from excel file
> require(gdata)
> # Get the data path
> datfile = "Your Data Path/dat4Meta.xls"
```

```
> # Call "read.xls" to read the Excel data
> dat  = read.xls(datfile, sheet="Data.Rosiglitazone",
                perl="c:/perl64/bin/perl.exe")
> # Print the first 6 studies
> head(dat)

ID  Study    n.TRT MI.TRT Death.TRT n.CTRL MI.CTRL Death.CTRL
1 49653/011  357    2        1       176     0       0
2 49653/020  391    2        0       207     1       0
3 49653/024  774    1        0       185     1       0
4 49653/093  213    0        0       109     1       0
5 49653/094  232    1        1       116     0       0
6  100684     43    0        0        47     1       0
```

With this dataframe, we perform meta-analyses of both the risk difference (RD) and OR for MI and cardiovascular death (Death). We contrast the results from the classical fixed-effects and random-effects models using the R package `meta` to the results from the *CD* implemented in the R package `gmeta`.

13.2.2 Data Analysis for MI

To analyze the data for MI, we first create a dataframe (only for MI) as follows:

```
> datMI  = dat[,c("MI.TRT","MI.CTRL","n.TRT","n.CTRL")]
```

For classical fixed-effects and random-effects meta-analysis, we make use of the R library `meta`, introduced in previous chapters, and use the inverse weighting method to combine studies. This is implemented in the following R code chunk:

```
> # Load the library
> library(meta)
> # Call metabin with RD=risk difference
> MI.RD.wo = metabin(MI.TRT,n.TRT,MI.CTRL,n.CTRL,data=datMI,
        incr=0, method="Inverse", sm="RD")
> # Print the summary
> summary(MI.RD.wo)

Number of studies combined: k=48

                      RD         95%-CI    z  p.value
Fixed effect model   0.002  [0.001; 0.003] 3.24  0.0012
Random effects model 0.002  [0.001; 0.003] 3.24  0.0012

Quantifying heterogeneity:
tau^2 < 0.0001; H = 1 [1; 1]; I^2 = 0% [0%; 0%]
```

```
Test of heterogeneity:
  Q d.f.  p.value
27.9   47   0.9879
```

Details on meta-analytical method:
- Inverse variance method
- DerSimonian-Laird estimator for tau^2

As seen from the summary, the combined RD = 0.0018 with 95% CI of (7e-04, 0.0028) and a p-value = 0.0012 for both fixed-effects and random-effects models – since the `Test of heterogeneity` – is not statistically significant (p-value = 0.9879 and $\hat{\tau}^2 \approx 0$). Even though the RD is small and the left endpoint of the CI is just to the right of 0, these results are consistent with the conclusion that MIs in rosiglitazone group are statistically significantly higher than in the control group.

Note that in the above R code chunk, the option `incr` is set to zero which means no value is added to the zero MIs. In this dataframe, there are 10 studies with zero MIs for both rosiglitazone and control. The standard errors for the RD corresponding to these studies cannot be computed which is set to zero as default in this R function call.

A typical way to adjust the zero MIs is to add a small increment of 0.5 to them as a correction for lack of continuity, which is the default setting in the R function call to `metabin` as follows:

```
> # Call metabin with default setting to add 0.5
> MI.RD = metabin(MI.TRT,n.TRT,MI.CTRL,n.CTRL,data=datMI,
        method="Inverse", sm="RD")
> # Print the summary
> summary(MI.RD)
```

```
Number of studies combined: k=48

                        RD      95%-CI     z   p.value
Fixed effect model    0.001  [0; 0.003] 1.73   0.0834
Random effects model  0.001  [0; 0.003] 1.73   0.0834
```

Quantifying heterogeneity:
tau^2 < 0.0001; H = 1 [1; 1]; I^2 = 0% [0%; 0%]

```
Test of heterogeneity:
    Q d.f.  p.value
17.98   47      1
```

Details on meta-analytical method:
- Inverse variance method
- DerSimonian-Laird estimator for tau^2

With 0.5 added to the zero cells, we see from the output that the combined RD is now 0.0014 with 95% CI of $(-2e-04, 0.0029)$ and p-value $= 0.0834$ for both fixed-effects and random-effects models. The conclusion changed from statistically significant to statistically non-significant. Readers may want to try to add different increments to the zero cells and examine the effects of this artificial correction (although well founded in history of the analysis of contingency table data) for lack of continuity. In fact, Sweeting et al. (2004) provided compelling evidence that imputing arbitrary numbers to zero cells in continuity correction can result in very different conclusions.

Tian et al. (2009) developed an exact and efficient inference procedure to use all the data without this artificial continuity correction. This is a special case of the *CD* framework as proved in the **Supplementary Notes** at http://stat.rutgers.edu/home/gyang/researches/gmetaRpackage/. This method is implemented into gmeta as method="exact2". The R code to implement this method is as follows:

```
> # Call "gmeta" with method="exact2"
> MI.exactTianRD =  gmeta(datMI,gmi.type="2x2",method="exact2",
        ci.level=0.95,n=2000)
```

The summary of this modeling can be printed as follows:

```
> summary(MI.exactTianRD)
```

```
        Exact Meta-Analysis Approach through CD-Framework
Call:
gmeta.default(gmi = datMI, gmi.type = "2x2", method = "exact2",
    n = 2000, ci.level = 0.95)
```

Combined CD Summary:

	mean	median	stddev	CI.1	CI.2
exp1	-4.53e-03	-5.81e-03	0.00619	-0.01777	0.020567
exp2	6.12e-04	-1.16e-03	0.00878	-0.01396	0.018077
exp3	5.97e-03	3.73e-03	0.00727	-0.00565	0.025406
exp4	1.12e-02	1.05e-02	0.01256	-0.01489	0.044330
exp5	-2.44e-03	-4.30e-03	0.00819	-0.01949	0.031133
exp6	1.75e-02	1.95e-02	0.03239	NA	NA
exp7	-7.89e-03	-7.47e-03	0.01245	-0.03842	0.029153
exp8	-2.24e-02	-3.27e-02	0.02650	NA	0.027238
exp9	-2.50e-03	-2.56e-03	0.00389	-0.01194	0.009509
exp10	-1.84e-03	-4.05e-03	0.00694	-0.01605	0.026811
exp11	3.49e-03	3.79e-03	0.00504	-0.01164	0.016145
exp12	-1.53e-03	-3.44e-03	0.00622	-0.01209	0.017555
exp13	-3.08e-03	-5.39e-03	0.01073	-0.02021	0.012985
exp14	-3.91e-03	-4.61e-03	0.00536	-0.01519	0.017104
exp15	1.00e-03	-1.08e-03	0.00861	-0.01378	0.019149

```
exp16          5.87e-03  5.62e-03 0.01363 -0.01808 0.039631
exp17          9.03e-03  6.97e-03 0.02226 -0.03358 0.055565
exp18         -7.81e-03 -9.18e-03 0.01055 -0.02966 0.033602
exp19         -1.35e-02 -1.61e-02 0.01769 -0.05159 0.025194
exp20          2.48e-03 -3.53e-04 0.00951 -0.01477 0.030524
exp21          8.63e-03  7.78e-03 0.01272 -0.02793 0.040218
exp22          6.09e-03  5.53e-03 0.00878 -0.01952 0.028042
exp23         -1.46e-02 -1.71e-02 0.02632       NA       NA
exp24         -1.49e-02 -2.85e-02 0.03846       NA 0.049259
exp25          8.28e-03  7.01e-03 0.00615 -0.00254 0.023689
exp26          7.00e-03  5.72e-03 0.02451 -0.04541       NA
exp27         -6.34e-03 -7.63e-03 0.01003 -0.03105 0.025329
exp28         -4.22e-03 -4.17e-03 0.00649 -0.01995 0.015046
exp29         -1.03e-02 -1.18e-02 0.01668 -0.05235 0.040833
exp30         -5.72e-03 -5.40e-03 0.00893 -0.02750 0.021104
exp31          2.79e-03 -1.43e-06 0.01502 -0.02461 0.047615
exp32         -9.28e-05 -8.58e-04 0.00241 -0.00421 0.009685
exp33          8.12e-04 -8.25e-05 0.00287 -0.00417 0.009115
exp34          5.67e-03  3.73e-03 0.01191 -0.01673 0.030232
exp35         -3.27e-03 -3.84e-03 0.00512 -0.01577 0.013017
exp36         -3.90e-03 -4.15e-03 0.00592 -0.01818 0.013397
exp37         -1.72e-03 -3.43e-03 0.00589 -0.01445 0.023542
exp38          1.56e-04 -1.94e-04 0.00651 -0.01712 0.018428
exp39          6.13e-04 -2.07e-03 0.00806 -0.01238 0.024941
exp40         -2.41e-04 -2.33e-03 0.00715 -0.01234 0.021490
exp41         -2.39e-03 -2.52e-03 0.00200 -0.00651 0.001540
exp42         -4.70e-03 -4.70e-03 0.00445 -0.01419 0.003493
exp43          2.94e-03 -6.03e-07 0.01802 -0.02813 0.056682
exp44          2.10e-03 -1.27e-04 0.00812 -0.01255 0.025546
exp45         -3.43e-04 -5.37e-04 0.01453 -0.03956 0.038902
exp46         -8.29e-05 -4.24e-03 0.04255       NA       NA
exp47          1.16e-04 -5.10e-07 0.00532 -0.01408 0.015145
exp48          1.43e-03 -1.07e-05 0.00424 -0.00507 0.013882
combined.cd -1.77e-03 -2.21e-03 0.00188 -0.00386 0.000878
```

```
Confidence level= 0.95
```

The last row contains the combined estimates and can be produced as follows:

```
> summary(MI.exactTianRD)$mms[49,]

                mean    median  stddev    CI.1     CI.2
combined.cd -0.00177 -0.00221 0.00188 -0.00386 0.000878
```

We see that the mean difference is −0.00177 with 95% CI of (−0.00386, 0.00088), indicating no statistically significant difference between rosiglitazone group and the control group on MI.

We now analyze the MI dataframe using the OR. Similarly, the classical fixed-effects and random-effects models can be implemented as follows:

```
> # Call metabin without 0.5 correction
> MI.OR.wo = metabin(MI.TRT,n.TRT,MI.CTRL,n.CTRL,data=datMI,
        incr=0,method="Inverse", sm="OR")
> # Summary
> summary(MI.OR.wo)

Number of studies combined: k=38

                        OR        95%-CI     z  p.value
Fixed effect model    1.29   [0.895; 1.85] 1.36   0.1736
Random effects model  1.29   [0.895; 1.85] 1.36   0.1736

Quantifying heterogeneity:
tau^2 < 0.0001; H = 1 [1; 1]; I^2 = 0% [0%; 0%]

Test of heterogeneity:
  Q d.f. p.value
 5.7   37       1

Details on meta-analytical method:
- Inverse variance method
- DerSimonian-Laird estimator for tau^2

> # Call metabin with default 0.5 correction
> MI.OR = metabin(MI.TRT,n.TRT,MI.CTRL,n.CTRL,data=datMI,
            method="Inverse", sm="OR")
> # Print the Summary
> summary(MI.OR)

Number of studies combined: k=38

                        OR        95%-CI     z  p.value
Fixed effect model    1.29    [0.94; 1.76] 1.57   0.1161
Random effects model  1.29    [0.94; 1.76] 1.57   0.1161

Quantifying heterogeneity:
tau^2 < 0.0001; H = 1 [1; 1]; I^2 = 0% [0%; 0%]
```

```
Test of heterogeneity:
     Q d.f.  p.value
  16.22   37  0.9988
```

```
Details on meta-analytical method:
- Inverse variance method
- DerSimonian-Laird estimator for tau^2
```

We see that with or without the default 0.5 continuity correction, the 95% CIs and *p*-values are slightly different, but yield the same conclusion that there is no statistically significant difference between the rosiglitazone group and the control group on MI.

We now can call `gmeta` for the exact method using the OR, which is implemented as follows:

```
> # Call "gmeta" for "exact1" on OR
> MI.exactLiuOR = gmeta(datMI,gmi.type="2x2",
        method="exact1", ci.level=0.95,n=2000)
> # Print the summary
> summary(MI.exactLiuOR)
```

```
        Exact Meta-Analysis Approach through CD-Framework
Call:
gmeta.default(gmi = datMI, gmi.type = "2x2", method = "exact1",
    n = 2000, ci.level = 0.95)
```

```
Combined CD Summary:
             mean  median stddev   CI.1   CI.2
exp1          Inf      NA    Inf -1.951    Inf
exp2       0.1141 -0.0044  1.360 -2.525  3.446
exp3      -1.4316 -1.4333  1.631 -5.110  2.233
exp4         -Inf      NA    Inf   -Inf  2.274
exp5          Inf      NA    Inf -3.636    Inf
exp6         -Inf      NA    Inf   -Inf  3.033
exp7          Inf      NA    Inf -2.920    Inf
exp8       0.9942  0.9346  0.888 -0.669  3.002
exp9          Inf      NA    Inf -2.939    Inf
exp10         Inf      NA    Inf -3.687    Inf
exp11        -Inf      NA    Inf   -Inf  2.971
exp12         Inf      NA    Inf -2.625    Inf
exp13      0.7556  0.6374  1.360 -1.882  4.088
exp14         Inf      NA    Inf -1.922    Inf
exp15      0.0593 -0.0592  1.360 -2.581  3.392
exp16     -0.6514 -0.6520  1.634 -4.320  3.018
exp17     -0.8065 -0.6886  1.366 -4.143  1.840
exp18         Inf      NA    Inf -1.928    Inf
```

```
exp19          1.1847  1.0326  1.266 -1.135 4.398
exp20          NaN       NA    Inf   -Inf   Inf
exp21          -Inf      NA    Inf   -Inf 2.928
exp22          -Inf      NA    Inf   -Inf 2.933
exp23          Inf       NA    Inf -2.909   Inf
exp24          Inf       NA    Inf -2.970   Inf
exp25          -Inf      NA    Inf   -Inf 0.534
exp26        -0.4690 -0.4347  0.978 -2.603 1.466
exp27          Inf       NA    Inf -2.979   Inf
exp28          Inf       NA    Inf -2.898   Inf
exp29          Inf       NA    Inf -2.956   Inf
exp30          Inf       NA    Inf -2.921   Inf
exp31          NaN       NA    Inf   -Inf   Inf
exp32          Inf       NA    Inf -4.084   Inf
exp33          NaN       NA    Inf   -Inf   Inf
exp34        -0.8514 -0.7333  1.362 -4.183 1.788
exp35          Inf       NA    Inf -2.973   Inf
exp36          Inf       NA    Inf -2.876   Inf
exp37          Inf       NA    Inf -3.656   Inf
exp38          NaN       NA    Inf   -Inf   Inf
exp39          Inf       NA    Inf -4.306   Inf
exp40          Inf       NA    Inf -4.107   Inf
exp41          0.5133  0.5055  0.428 -0.314 1.385
exp42          0.2739  0.2760  0.251 -0.226 0.762
exp43          NaN       NA    Inf   -Inf   Inf
exp44          NaN       NA    Inf   -Inf   Inf
exp45          NaN       NA    Inf   -Inf   Inf
exp46          NaN       NA    Inf   -Inf   Inf
exp47          NaN       NA    Inf   -Inf   Inf
exp48          NaN       NA    Inf   -Inf   Inf
combined.cd    0.3300  0.3301  0.184 -0.028 0.694
```

```
Confidence level= 0.95
```

The combined results from this summary are on the log scale, and we transform back to the OR as follows:

```
> # Use `exp' function to transform back
> exp(summary(MI.exactLiuOR)$mms[49,])
```

```
              mean median stddev CI.1 CI.2
combined.cd   1.39   1.39    1.2 0.972    2
```

This gives the OR of 1.39 with 95% CI of (0.972, 2) which again indicates that there is no statistically significant difference between the rosiglitazone group and the control group on MI.

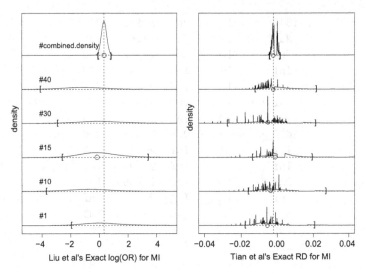

FIGURE 13.1
CDs from both exact methods.

We summarize the analyses using the novel *CDs* approach implemented in gmeta in Figure 13.1 with the following R code chunk where we only include the CDs for studies 1, 10, 15, 30, 40 as well as the combined CD:

```
> # Plot the gmeta confidence distributions
> par(mfrow=c(1,2))
> plot(MI.exactLiuOR,  trials=c(1,10,15,30,40), option=T,
    xlim=c(-5,5),xlab="Liu et al's Exact log(OR) for MI")
> plot(MI.exactTianRD, trials=c(1,10,15,30,40), option=T,
    xlim=c(-0.04,0.04), xlab="Tian et al's Exact RD for MI")
```

13.2.3   Data Analysis for Cardiovascular Death (Death)

Similarly, we use the same steps to analyze the data for cardiovascular death (Death). We first create a dataframe only for Death as follows:

```
> datDeath    = dat[,c("Death.TRT","Death.CTRL","n.TRT","n.CTRL")]
```

For RD, the classical fixed-effects and random-effects meta-analysis can be performed using the following R code chunk:

```
> # Call metabin with RD=risk difference
> Death.RD.wo = metabin(Death.TRT,n.TRT,Death.CTRL,n.CTRL,
    data=datDeath,incr=0, method="Inverse", sm="RD")
> # Print the summary
> summary(Death.RD.wo)
```

Number of studies combined: k=48

```
                          RD       95%-CI    z  p.value
Fixed effect model     0.001  [0; 0.002]  2.6   0.0094
Random effects model   0.001  [0; 0.002]  2.6   0.0094
```

Quantifying heterogeneity:
tau^2 < 0.0001; H = 1 [1; 1]; I^2 = 0% [0%; 0%]

Test of heterogeneity:
```
    Q  d.f.  p.value
13.69   47        1
```

Details on meta-analytical method:
- Inverse variance method
- DerSimonian-Laird estimator for tau^2

```
> # Call metabin with default setting to add 0.5
> Death.RD = metabin(Death.TRT,n.TRT,Death.CTRL,n.CTRL,
      data=datDeath, method="Inverse", sm="RD")
> # Print the summary
> summary(Death.RD)
```

Number of studies combined: k=48

```
                          RD         95%-CI       z  p.value
Fixed effect model     0.001  [-0.001;0.002]  0.943   0.3455
Random effects model   0.001  [-0.001;0.002]  0.943   0.3455
```

Quantifying heterogeneity:
tau^2 < 0.0001; H = 1 [1; 1]; I^2 = 0% [0%; 0%]

Test of heterogeneity:
```
   Q  d.f.  p.value
7.92   47        1
```

Details on meta-analytical method:
- Inverse variance method
- DerSimonian-Laird estimator for tau^2

Again, we see from the summaries that the combined RD = 0.001 with 95% CI of $(0, 0.002)$ and a p-value = 0.0094 for both fixed-effects and random-effects models without continuity correction. This statistical significance vanishes when 0.5 is added to the zero cells in 25 studies. The combined RD is now 0.001 with 95% CI of $(-0.001, 0.002)$ and a p-value = 0.943 for both fixed-effects and random-effects models.

With `gmeta` the RD is implemented as follows:

```
> # Call "gmeta" with method="exact2"
> Death.exactTianRD = gmeta(datDeath,gmi.type="2x2",
      method="exact2", ci.level=0.95,n=2000)
```

The summary for this modeling is printed as follows:

```
> summary(Death.exactTianRD)
```

        Exact Meta-Analysis Approach through CD-Framework

```
Call:
gmeta.default(gmi = datDeath, gmi.type = "2x2", method = "exact2",
    n = 2000, ci.level = 0.95)
```

Combined CD Summary:

	mean	median	stddev	CI.1	CI.2
exp1	-1.55e-03	-2.97e-03	0.005132	-0.01274	0.02063
exp2	1.08e-03	-1.15e-06	0.004528	-0.00749	0.01427
exp3	2.08e-03	-9.16e-07	0.005188	-0.00554	0.01723
exp4	1.81e-03	-4.80e-07	0.008317	-0.01362	0.02693
exp5	-2.94e-03	-4.31e-03	0.008163	-0.01947	0.03113
exp6	1.31e-04	-1.19e-03	0.023533	NA	NA
exp7	6.87e-05	-5.92e-07	0.008521	-0.02292	0.02371
exp8	-6.73e-03	-1.45e-02	0.026914	NA	NA
exp9	4.45e-05	3.23e-05	0.002701	-0.00718	0.00772
exp10	1.78e-03	-4.23e-04	0.006930	-0.01028	0.02180
exp11	-3.02e-03	-5.11e-03	0.010069	-0.01917	0.01200
exp12	2.52e-03	-3.20e-07	0.006694	-0.00725	0.02227
exp13	3.81e-03	4.10e-03	0.005403	-0.01231	0.01747
exp14	1.11e-03	-4.11e-07	0.004256	-0.00700	0.01394
exp15	-4.12e-03	-5.03e-03	0.005708	-0.01607	0.01830
exp16	4.84e-03	5.62e-03	0.013645	-0.01808	NA
exp17	2.48e-04	-1.00e-03	0.010064	-0.02675	0.02961
exp18	-3.44e-03	-4.51e-03	0.009007	-0.02128	0.03371
exp19	-6.44e-03	-7.02e-03	0.010694	-0.03353	0.02605
exp20	-3.97e-03	-5.54e-03	0.009487	-0.02297	0.03750
exp21	1.54e-04	-3.44e-04	0.008721	-0.02279	0.02449
exp22	1.47e-04	-1.65e-04	0.006004	-0.01583	0.01705
exp23	8.78e-05	-7.53e-07	0.018110	NA	NA
exp24	-3.63e-05	-1.75e-03	0.026734	NA	NA
exp25	-9.62e-04	-1.89e-03	0.003275	-0.00815	0.01320
exp26	-4.80e-03	-1.32e-02	0.025969	NA	0.03232
exp27	-1.21e-02	-1.46e-02	0.012116	NA	0.02518
exp28	-4.21e-03	-4.17e-03	0.006489	-0.01995	0.01505
exp29	1.58e-04	-3.29e-04	0.011882	-0.03109	0.03325

```
exp30           -5.62e-03 -5.39e-03 0.008944 -0.02750 0.02110
exp31            1.27e-03 -9.28e-07 0.015018 -0.02465      NA
exp32           -9.40e-05 -8.58e-04 0.002395 -0.00421 0.00968
exp33           -6.91e-04 -1.52e-03 0.002826 -0.00651 0.01123
exp34            5.64e-03  4.19e-03 0.008280 -0.01679 0.02624
exp35           -3.28e-03 -3.86e-03 0.005116 -0.01577 0.01302
exp36           -7.01e-05 -1.60e-04 0.003964 -0.01086 0.01088
exp37            1.57e-03 -1.90e-04 0.006005 -0.00930 0.01914
exp38            1.51e-04 -1.95e-04 0.006493 -0.01709 0.01843
exp39            3.30e-04 -2.08e-03 0.008065 -0.01239 0.02494
exp40           -6.02e-04 -2.33e-03 0.007125 -0.01233 0.02149
exp41           -8.61e-04 -9.91e-04 0.001884 -0.00499 0.00301
exp42            1.71e-04  1.26e-04 0.001499 -0.00377 0.00351
exp43            8.82e-04 -3.89e-07 0.018000 -0.02815      NA
exp44            1.87e-03 -1.20e-04 0.008131 -0.01253 0.02555
exp45           -3.66e-04 -5.37e-04 0.014531      NA      NA
exp46           -3.34e-04 -4.23e-03 0.042551      NA      NA
exp47            1.23e-04 -5.15e-07 0.005314 -0.01412 0.01515
exp48            1.43e-03 -6.97e-06 0.004238 -0.00507 0.01388
combined.cd -7.59e-04 -8.93e-04 0.000622 -0.00233 0.00135
```

```
Confidence level= 0.95
```

The last row contained the combined estimates and is produced as follows:

```
> summary(Death.exactTianRD)$mms[49,]
```

```
                 mean    median   stddev    CI.1    CI.2
combined.cd -0.000759 -0.000893 0.000622 -0.00233 0.00135
```

We see that the mean difference is -0.000759 with 95% CI of $(-0.00233, 0.00135)$, indicating no statistically significant difference between rosiglitazone group and the control group on cardiovascular death.

Similarly for the OR, the classical fixed-effects and random-effects models are implemented as follows:

```
> # Call metabin without 0.5 correction
> Death.OR.wo = metabin(Death.TRT,n.TRT,Death.CTRL,n.CTRL,
      data=datDeath,incr=0,method="Inverse", sm="OR")
> # Summary
> summary(Death.OR.wo)
```

```
Number of studies combined: k=23
```

```
                       OR        95%-CI     z  p.value
Fixed effect model    1.2  [0.642; 2.24] 0.568   0.5699
Random effects model  1.2  [0.642; 2.24] 0.568   0.5699
```

```
Quantifying heterogeneity:
tau^2 < 0.0001; H = 1 [1; 1]; I^2 = 0% [0%; 0%]

Test of heterogeneity:
    Q d.f. p.value
 1.02    22       1

Details on meta-analytical method:
- Inverse variance method
- DerSimonian-Laird estimator for tau^2

> # Call metabin with default 0.5 correction
> Death.OR = metabin(Death.TRT,n.TRT,Death.CTRL,n.CTRL,
      data=datDeath, method="Inverse", sm="OR")
> # Print the Summary
> summary(Death.OR)

Number of studies combined: k=23

                        OR        95%-CI      z   p.value
Fixed effect model    1.31   [0.805; 2.13] 1.08    0.2783
Random effects model  1.31   [0.805; 2.13] 1.08    0.2783

Quantifying heterogeneity:
tau^2 < 0.0001; H = 1 [1; 1]; I^2 = 0% [0%; 0%]

Test of heterogeneity:
    Q d.f. p.value
 4.79    22       1

Details on meta-analytical method:
- Inverse variance method
- DerSimonian-Laird estimator for tau^2
```

We see that with or without the default 0.5 continuity correction, the 95% CIs and *p*-values are slightly different, but yield the same conclusion that there is no statistically significant difference between the rosiglitazone group and the control group on cardiovascular death.

Now we call gmeta for the exact method for the OR which is implemented as follows:

```
> # Call "gmeta" for "exact1" on OR
> Death.exactLiuOR  =  gmeta(datDeath,gmi.type="2x2",
        method="exact1",  ci.level=0.95,n=2000)
> # Print the summary
> summary(Death.exactLiuOR)
```

Exact Meta-Analysis Approach through CD-Framework

Call:
gmeta.default(gmi = datDeath, gmi.type = "2x2", method = "exact1",
    n = 2000, ci.level = 0.95)

Combined CD Summary:

	mean	median	stddev	CI.1	CI.2
exp1	Inf	NA	Inf	-3.651	Inf
exp2	NaN	NA	Inf	-Inf	Inf
exp3	NaN	NA	Inf	-Inf	Inf
exp4	NaN	NA	Inf	-Inf	Inf
exp5	Inf	NA	Inf	-3.636	Inf
exp6	NaN	NA	Inf	-Inf	Inf
exp7	NaN	NA	Inf	-Inf	Inf
exp8	0.461	0.426	0.979	-1.473	2.59
exp9	NaN	NA	Inf	-Inf	Inf
exp10	NaN	NA	Inf	-Inf	Inf
exp11	0.779	0.661	1.360	-1.859	4.11
exp12	NaN	NA	Inf	-Inf	Inf
exp13	-Inf	NA	Inf	-Inf	2.95
exp14	NaN	NA	Inf	-Inf	Inf
exp15	Inf	NA	Inf	-1.934	Inf
exp16	-0.651	-0.652	1.634	-4.320	3.02
exp17	NaN	NA	Inf	-Inf	Inf
exp18	Inf	NA	Inf	-3.627	Inf
exp19	Inf	NA	Inf	-2.937	Inf
exp20	Inf	NA	Inf	-3.657	Inf
exp21	NaN	NA	Inf	-Inf	Inf
exp22	NaN	NA	Inf	-Inf	Inf
exp23	NaN	NA	Inf	-Inf	Inf
exp24	NaN	NA	Inf	-Inf	Inf
exp25	Inf	NA	Inf	-3.653	Inf
exp26	0.712	0.594	1.365	-1.934	4.05
exp27	Inf	NA	Inf	-1.278	Inf
exp28	Inf	NA	Inf	-2.898	Inf
exp29	NaN	NA	Inf	-Inf	Inf
exp30	Inf	NA	Inf	-2.921	Inf
exp31	NaN	NA	Inf	-Inf	Inf
exp32	Inf	NA	Inf	-4.084	Inf
exp33	Inf	NA	Inf	-3.719	Inf
exp34	-Inf	NA	Inf	-Inf	2.85
exp35	Inf	NA	Inf	-2.973	Inf
exp36	NaN	NA	Inf	-Inf	Inf
exp37	NaN	NA	Inf	-Inf	Inf

```
exp38           NaN     NA    Inf   -Inf  Inf
exp39           Inf     NA    Inf -4.306  Inf
exp40           Inf     NA    Inf -4.107  Inf
exp41         0.183  0.180  0.435 -0.672 1.05
exp42        -0.246 -0.186  0.877 -2.235 1.40
exp43           NaN     NA    Inf   -Inf  Inf
exp44           NaN     NA    Inf   -Inf  Inf
exp45           NaN     NA    Inf   -Inf  Inf
exp46           NaN     NA    Inf   -Inf  Inf
exp47           NaN     NA    Inf   -Inf  Inf
exp48           NaN     NA    Inf   -Inf  Inf
combined.cd   0.385  0.385  0.343 -0.268 1.09
```

```
Confidence level= 0.95
```

The combined results from this summary are on the log scale. We transform back to the OR as follows:

```
> exp(summary(Death.exactLiuOR)$mms[49,])
```

```
              mean median stddev  CI.1 CI.2
combined.cd   1.47   1.47   1.41 0.765 2.97
```

This gives an OR of 1.47 with 95% CI of (0.765, 2.97), which again indicates that there is no statistically significant difference between the rosiglitazone group and the control group on cardiovascular death. A figure similar to Figure 13.1 can be produced and we leave this as an exercise for interested readers.

13.3   Discussion

In this chapter, we discussed meta-analysis of rare events based upon the well-known rosiglitazone data set using the novel *CD* approach developed to unify the framework of meta-analysis. We pointed out that the classical fixed-effects and random-effects models are not appropriate for rare events. We recommend the new *CD* procedure which can combine test results based on exact distributions. The application of this new procedure is made easy with the R package gmeta.

For further reading, we recommend Sutton et al. (2002) which provides a review of meta-analyses for rare and adverse event data from the aspects of model choice, continuity corrections, exact statistics, Bayesian methods, and sensitivity analysis. There are other newly developed methods for meta-analysis of rare-events. Cai et al. (2010) proposed some approaches based on

Poisson random-effects models for statistical inference about the relative risk between two treatment groups. To develop fixed-effects and random-effects moment-based meta-analytic methods to analyze binary adverse-event data, Bhaumik et al. (2012) derived three new methods which include a simple (unweighted) average treatment effect estimator, a new heterogeneity estimator, and a parametric bootstrapping test for heterogeneity. Readers may explore these methods for other applications.

14

Meta-Analyses with Individual Patient-Level Data versus Summary Statistics

There are extensive discussions about the relative merits of performing meta-analysis with individual patient-level data (IPD) versus meta-analysis with summary statistics (SS) in those cases where IPD are accessible. Some favor IPD and others favor SS.

Traditionally, meta-analysis is aimed to analyze the SS from publications which is to combine the estimates of the effect size from several studies as discussed in the previous chapters. Since data sharing has been increasingly encouraged, original data at the individual level may be accessible for some research studies. When original individual data are available, it is known from the theory of statistics that the meta-analysis with IPD may reduce bias and gain efficiency in statistical inference.

One of the most important questions in meta-analysis is then to investigate their relative efficiency between the meta-analysis with IPD and the meta-analysis with SS to have a better understanding of how much efficiency could be potentially lost from meta-analysis with SS to meta-analysis with IPD. This chapter is designed to give an overview of this topic to interested readers.

A series of research has rigorously examined their relative efficiency as seen in (Chen et al., 2020; Lin and Zeng, 2010; Liu et al., 2015; Mathew and Nordstrom, 1999; Olkin and Sampson, 1998; Simmonds et al., 2005), to list a few. Specifically, in fixed-effects meta-analysis models, Olkin and Sampson (1998) and Mathew and Nordstrom (1999) focused on analysis of variance models. Lin and Zeng (2010) extended all of these settings to a general likelihood inference setting. Their result was further extended by Liu et al. (2015) to a more complex setting of analyzing heterogeneous studies and achieving complex evidence synthesis. All of these studies are restricted to fixed-effects meta-analysis models with the assumption of no between-study heterogeneity.

To accommodate between-study variations, random-effects meta-analysis models should be used as discussed in the previous chapters. For random-effects meta-analysis models on the relative efficiency between IPD versus SS, Zeng and Lin (2015) showed a surprising result that the meta-analysis with SS is always at least as efficient as the meta-analysis with IPD analysis. This conclusion relies on a critical assumption that the between-study variability is of order n^{-1}, where n is the median sample size of studies. In the recent study, Chen et al. (2020) systematically investigated the relative efficiency of IPD versus SS under a general likelihood inference setting. They showed theoretically and numerically that meta-analysis with SS (referenced as SS below) is at most as efficient as the meta-analysis with IPD (referenced as IPD below).

In this chapter, we use a real data set from placebo-controlled clinical studies of lamotrigine in the treatment of bipolar depression to illustrate the pros and cons of IPD and SS. Two clinical outcome measures, the Hamilton Rating Scale for Depression (HAMD) and the Montgomery-Asberg Depression Rating Scale (MADRS), are used. This chapter is organized as follows. In Section 14.1, we introduce this data as well as the descriptive statistics for the data. We then present data analysis from both IPD and SS on treatment comparisons for changes in HAMD in Section 14.2 and changes in MADRS in Section 14.3 – both of which led to the same conclusions as summarized in Section 14.4. Based on these conclusions, we then formulate a simulation to compare the efficiency of IPD to SS in Section 14.5 followed by some discussions in Section 14.6.

14.1   IPD with Five Studies of Lamotrigine

In Chapter 4, we referred to a meta-analysis using five studies of lamotrigine in the treatment of bipolar depression which was analyzed by Geddes et al. (2009). The studies were conducted by GlaxoSmithKline(GSK). We requested the individual patient-level data (IPD) from the company so that we can use the data in this chapter to illustrate the meta-analyses with IPD and SS. (Note to the interested readers, we cannot share the data to you directly since this is owned by GSK and you need to sign confidentiality with GSK so to get the IPD data.)

Five studies were reported in Geddes et al. (2009) as Study 1 (GW602/SCAB2001), Study 2 (GW603/SCAA2010), Study 3 (SCA40910), Study 4 (SCA10022), and Study 5 (SCA30924). In communication with GSK, we realized that Study 4 (SCA100222) should be SCA100223 which was an acute bipolar depression study. We excluded Study 2 (GW603/SCAA2010) due to a different dosing scheme and different lengths of the treatment phase.

We therefore requested the IPD from 4 studies from GSK which included data on:

- Subject as patient subject de-identified ID,
- Age as patient's age,
- Sex as patient's sex,
- MADRS0 as baseline MADRS,

- MADRS1 as the final MADRS,
- HAMD0 as the baseline HAMD,
- HAMD1 as the final HAMD,
- Study as the indicator of 4 studies and
- TRT as the treatment of lamotrigine vs placebo.

Readers interested in analyzing these data or reproducing the results in this chapter should request the IPD directly from the company (not from us).

We obtained the data and named it as datGSK with summary structure as follows:

```
> # Summary of GSK data
> summary(datGSK)

 Safety  Efficacy       Age           Sex         MADRS0
 N: 24   N: 38    Min.    :18.0   F:499   Min.    :10.0
 Y:842   Y:828    1st Qu.:29.0    M:367   1st Qu.:26.0
                  Median :38.0            Median :30.0
                  Mean   :38.6            Mean   :29.8
                  3rd Qu.:47.0            3rd Qu.:34.0
                  Max.   :79.0            Max.   :45.0

     MADRS1          HAMD0           HAMD1
 Min.   : 0     Min.   :18.0    Min.    : 0.0
 1st Qu.: 8     1st Qu.:21.0    1st Qu.: 8.0
 Median :17     Median :24.0    Median :15.0
 Mean   :18     Mean   :24.4    Mean   :14.9
 3rd Qu.:27     3rd Qu.:27.0    3rd Qu.:22.0
 Max.   :47     Max.   :37.0    Max.    :38.0
 NA's   :29                     NA's    :29
        Study        TRT          Duration        Subject
 SCA100223:221   LTG:438   >12 - 24 :163   Min.    :  1
 SCA30924 :259   PBO:428   8 - 12   :160   1st Qu.: 55
 SCA40910 :257             >24 - 52 :158   Median :109
 SCAB2001 :129             >8 - 24  :119   Mean   :115
                           >8 - <=24: 54   3rd Qu.:174
                           >52      : 51   Max.   :259
                           (Other)  :161

> # Print the first 6 observarons
> #head(datGSK)
```

Data for MADRS and HAMD are continuous. And we analyze these data using continuous measures – which is different from Geddes et al. (2009) where numbers of events were aggregated and reported.

The data are loaded into R and we analyze the difference between the final and baseline values for both HAMD and MADRS as defined as:

```
> # Make the difference between final to baseline
> datGSK$dMADRS = datGSK$MADRS1-datGSK$MADRS0
> datGSK$dHAMD  = datGSK$HAMD1-datGSK$HAMD0
```

There are some missing values in the final MADRS1 and HAMD1 and we remove them to consider the complete data as follows:

```
> # Remove missing values
> datGSK = datGSK[complete.cases(datGSK),]
```

We check our data with the data reported in Table 1 from Geddes et al. (2009). For the Age, the means and standard deviations can be calculated as:

```
> # Calculate the mean
> tapply(datGSK$Age,datGSK[,c("TRT","Study")],mean)
```

	Study			
TRT	SCA100223	SCA30924	SCA40910	SCAB2001
LTG	38.1	40.4	37.6	42.2
PBO	36.8	38.1	37.2	42.4

```
> # Calculate the SD
> tapply(datGSK$Age,datGSK[,c("TRT","Study")],sd)
```

	Study			
TRT	SCA100223	SCA30924	SCA40910	SCAB2001
LTG	11.5	12.4	12.7	11.5
PBO	11.9	12.0	11.5	12.8

We see that the values of these means and SDs by treatment from these 4 studies are quite similar, but not exactly the same. To further verify the data, we can check the number of participants in the studies reported in Geddes et al. (2009). The number of patients for each sex by treatment and study can be calculated as follows:

```
> # The number of females
> nF= xtabs(~TRT+Study, datGSK[datGSK$Sex=="F",])
> nF
```

	Study			
TRT	SCA100223	SCA30924	SCA40910	SCAB2001
LTG	70	70	73	35
PBO	68	65	62	39

```
> # The number of males
> nM= xtabs(~TRT+Study, datGSK[datGSK$Sex=="M",])
> # The percentage of females
> pctF = nF/(nF+nM)
> pctF
```

```
        Study
TRT    SCA100223  SCA30924  SCA40910  SCAB2001
  LTG      0.642     0.556     0.575     0.556
  PBO      0.642     0.533     0.521     0.600
```

Comparing these numbers from this calculation with the values from Table 1 in Geddes et al. (2009), we see that there are a few minor differences: (1) there are 68 (not 69) female participants in Study (SCA10023) for placebo, (2) there are 70 and 65 (not 69 and 66) females for Study SCA30924 from lamotrigine and placebo, and (3) there are 73 (not 74) females for Study SCA40910 from lamotrigine. These differences may be the result of the two analyses using different methods for handling missing data. We will proceed with the data for the comparison between IPD and SS.

14.2 Treatment Comparison for Changes in HAMD

14.2.1 Meta-Analysis with IPD

14.2.1.1 IPD Analysis by Each Study

Before we analyze the data, we make distribution plots to investigate the treatment differences graphically. The following R code chunk can be used for this purpose and produces Figure 14.1:

```
> # Load the ``lattice" library
> library(lattice)
> # call boxplot
> print(bwplot(dHAMD~TRT|Study, datGSK, xlab="Treatment",
  ylab="Changes in HAMD", strip=strip.custom(bg="white")))
```

Figure 14.1 illustrates the boxplot for the changes in HAMD by treatment for the four studies. It can be seen that the distributions heavily overlap indicating possible statistically nonsignificant difference.

This non-significance can be statistically tested using the linear model for each study. The analysis for the first data can be implemented using the following R code chunk:

```
> # Test for "SCA100223"
> mStudy1 = lm(dHAMD~TRT,
```

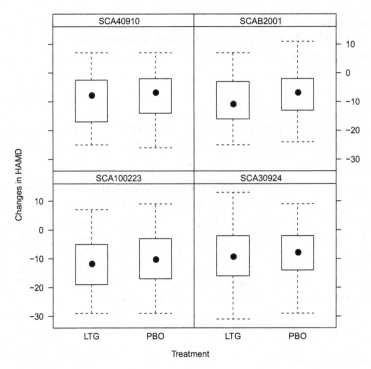

FIGURE 14.1
Boxplot by treatment for four studies.

```
        datGSK[datGSK$Study==levels(datGSK$Study)[1],])
> summary(mStudy1)

Call:
lm(formula = dHAMD ~ TRT, data = datGSK[datGSK$Study
                              == levels(datGSK$Study)[1], ])

Residuals:
    Min      1Q  Median      3Q     Max
-19.255  -7.255  -0.459   6.745  18.745

Coefficients:
            Estimate Std. Error t value Pr(>|t|)
(Intercept)  -11.541      0.831  -13.89   <2e-16 ***
TRTPBO         1.796      1.183    1.52     0.13
---
Signif. codes: 0 *** 0.001 ** 0.01 * 0.05 . 0.1
```

Residual standard error: 8.67 on 213 degrees of freedom
Multiple R-squared: 0.0107,   Adjusted R-squared: 0.00606
F-statistic: 2.3 on 1 and 213 DF, p-value: 0.131

It can be seen that the associated p-value is 0.131 which indicates a statistically insignificant difference between lamotrigine and placebo in study SCA100223.

Similarly, the analyses for other three studies are performed as follows:

```
> # Test for Study "SCA30924"
> mStudy2 = lm(dHAMD~TRT,
       datGSK[datGSK$Study==levels(datGSK$Study)[2],])
> summary(mStudy2)

Call:
lm(formula = dHAMD ~ TRT, data = datGSK[datGSK$Study
                   == levels(datGSK$Study)[2], ])

Residuals:
    Min      1Q  Median      3Q     Max
-21.746  -6.512   0.566   7.254  22.254

Coefficients:
            Estimate Std. Error t value Pr(>|t|)
(Intercept)   -9.254      0.749  -12.36   <2e-16 ***
TRTPBO         0.688      1.068    0.64     0.52
---
Signif. codes: 0 *** 0.001 ** 0.01 * 0.05 . 0.1

Residual standard error: 8.41 on 246 degrees of freedom
Multiple R-squared: 0.00169,       Adjusted R-squared: -0.00237
F-statistic: 0.416 on 1 and 246 DF, p-value: 0.52

> # Test for Study "SCA40910"
> mStudy3 = lm(dHAMD~TRT,
       datGSK[datGSK$Study==levels(datGSK$Study)[3],])
> summary(mStudy3)

Call:
lm(formula = dHAMD ~ TRT, data = datGSK[datGSK$Study
                   == levels(datGSK$Study)[3], ])

Residuals:
   Min     1Q Median     3Q    Max
-17.35  -6.35   1.41   6.65  16.17
```

```
Coefficients:
            Estimate Std. Error t value Pr(>|t|)
(Intercept)   -9.173      0.726   -12.6   <2e-16 ***
TRTPBO         0.526      1.044     0.5     0.61
```

```
Residual standard error: 8.19 on 244 degrees of freedom
Multiple R-squared: 0.00104, Adjusted R-squared: -0.00305
F-statistic: 0.254 on 1 and 244 DF,  p-value: 0.615
```

```
> # Test for Study "SCAB2001"
> mStudy4 = lm(dHAMD~TRT,
       datGSK[datGSK$Study==levels(datGSK$Study)[4],])
> summary(mStudy4)
```

```
Call:
lm(formula = dHAMD ~ TRT, data = datGSK[datGSK$Study
                  == levels(datGSK$Study)[4], ])
```

```
Residuals:
    Min      1Q  Median      3Q     Max
-16.185  -5.261   0.162   6.585  18.815
```

```
Coefficients:
            Estimate Std. Error t value Pr(>|t|)
(Intercept)   -10.51       1.01   -10.4   <2e-16 ***
TRTPBO          2.69       1.41     1.9    0.059 .
```

```
Residual standard error: 8 on 126 degrees of freedom
Multiple R-squared:  0.028,       Adjusted R-squared:  0.0203
F-statistic: 3.63 on 1 and 126 DF,  p-value: 0.0592
```

The associated *p*-values are 0.52 for study SCA30924, 0.615 for study SCA40910 and 0.059 for study SCAB2001, respectively. None are statistically significant at the 0.05 level, indicating that lamotrigine is not statistically more effective than the placebo in treating bipolar depression if the data are analyzed by study.

14.2.1.2   IPD Analysis with Pooled Data

For the IPD analysis, we pool the four studies together to test treatment and study interaction effects as follows:

```
> # Model the interaction
> m1 = lm(dHAMD~TRT*Study, datGSK)
> # Print the ANOVA result
> anova(m1)
```

```
Analysis of Variance Table

Response: dHAMD
           Df Sum Sq Mean Sq F value Pr(>F)
TRT         1    316   315.5    4.52  0.034 *
Study       3    465   154.9    2.22  0.084 .
TRT:Study   3    134    44.8    0.64  0.588
Residuals 829  57820    69.7
---
Signif. codes: 0 *** 0.001 ** 0.01 * 0.05 . 0.1
```

We see that the treatment is now statistically significant (p-value $=0.0337$) and the interaction is not (p-value $= 0.5883$). We then reduce the model by excluding the interaction term – which is to regard study as a block. In this situation, the test for treatment effect is carried out using the following R code chunk:

```
> # Model the main effect
> m2 = lm(dHAMD~TRT+Study, datGSK)
> # Print the ANOVA result
> anova(m2)

Analysis of Variance Table

Response: dHAMD
           Df Sum Sq Mean Sq F value Pr(>F)
TRT         1    316   315.5    4.53  0.034 *
Study       3    465   154.9    2.22  0.084 .
Residuals 832  57954    69.7
---
Signif. codes: 0 *** 0.001 ** 0.01 * 0.05 . 0.1
```

Again the treatment effect is statistically significant (p-value $= 0.0336$) and there is no statistically significant difference among the four studies (p-value $= 0.0839$). A Tukey multiple comparison procedure can be further performed to confirm this conclusion which can be done as follows:

```
> TukeyHSD(aov(dHAMD~TRT+Study, datGSK))

  Tukey multiple comparisons of means
    95% family-wise confidence level

Fit: aov(formula = dHAMD ~ TRT + Study, data = datGSK)

$TRT
         diff    lwr  upr p adj
PBO-LTG 1.23 0.0955 2.36 0.034
```

```
$Study
                             diff    lwr   upr p adj
SCA30924-SCA100223    1.74183 -0.260 3.74 0.114
SCA40910-SCA100223    1.74852 -0.257 3.75 0.112
SCAB2001-SCA100223    1.49703 -0.902 3.90 0.375
SCA40910-SCA30924     0.00669 -1.927 1.94 1.000
SCAB2001-SCA30924    -0.24480 -2.583 2.09 0.993
SCAB2001-SCA40910    -0.25149 -2.593 2.09 0.993
```

In summary, when data are pooled from the four studies, the treatment effect is now statistically significant in contrast to nonsignificance in the IPD analysis for each study in Section 14.2.1.1. This is expected since when data are pooled, statistical power is usually increased.

14.2.1.3   IPD Analysis Incorporating Covariates

It is well-known that the major advantage in IPD analysis is the capacity to incorporate covariates. For this data, we have IPD from Age and Sex. We incorporate these covariates into the linear model. We model the interactions between TRT and Study as follows:

```
> # Full model
> mAllStudy1 = lm(dHAMD~(Age+Sex)*TRT*Study, datGSK)
> # Print the ANOVA
> anova(mAllStudy1)

Analysis of Variance Table

Response: dHAMD
              Df Sum Sq Mean Sq F value Pr(>F)
Age            1    160     160    2.30  0.130
Sex            1     10      10    0.14  0.706
TRT            1    334     334    4.81  0.029 *
Study          3    435     145    2.08  0.101
Age:TRT        1      8       8    0.11  0.737
Sex:TRT        1     22      22    0.31  0.578
Age:Study      3    299     100    1.43  0.231
Sex:Study      3    310     103    1.48  0.217
TRT:Study      3    116      39    0.56  0.643
Age:TRT:Study  3    240      80    1.15  0.327
Sex:TRT:Study  3    227      76    1.09  0.353
Residuals    813  56572      70
---
Signif. codes: 0 *** 0.001 ** 0.01 * 0.05 . 0.1
```

From the results, we see that all 2-way and 3-way interactions are statistically nonsignificant. We reduce the model to the main effects as follows:

```
> # Fit the main effect model
> mAllStudy2 = lm(dHAMD~TRT+Study+Age+Sex, datGSK)
> # Print the ANOVA
> anova(mAllStudy2)
```

```
Analysis of Variance Table
```

```
Response: dHAMD
          Df Sum Sq Mean Sq F value Pr(>F)
TRT        1    316   315.5    4.53  0.034 *
Study      3    465   154.9    2.23  0.084 .
Age        1    158   157.7    2.27  0.133
Sex        1      1     1.3    0.02  0.891
Residuals 830 57795    69.6
---
Signif. codes: 0 *** 0.001 ** 0.01 * 0.05 . 0.1
```

The Sex and Age are not statistically significant which indicates that we can further reduce the model to the main effects of TRT and Study which is the model m2 above.

14.2.1.4 IPD Analysis with Linear Mixed-Effects Model

A more advanced statistical analysis for all the data together is to use mixed-effects modeling. In this mixed-effects modeling, we can pool all studies together to estimate the between-study heterogeneity along with the within-study variability.

To implement this, we make use of the R package lmerTest as follows:

```
> # Load the lmerTest package
> library(lmerTest)
```

Then we use the function lmer to fit linear mixed-effects model as follows:

```
> # Fit the random-intercept and random-slope model
> HAMD.Slope.lme = lmer(dHAMD~TRT+(TRT|Subject), datGSK)
> # Print the model summary
> summary(HAMD.Slope.lme)
```

```
Linear mixed model fit by REML. t-tests use
  Satterthwaite's method [lmerModLmerTest]
Formula: dHAMD ~ TRT + (TRT | Subject)
   Data: datGSK
```

```
REML criterion at convergence: 5928
```

Scaled residuals:
```
    Min      1Q   Median      3Q      Max
-2.5056  -0.7928  0.0083   0.8248  2.7475
```

Random effects:
```
 Groups    Name           Variance Std.Dev. Corr
 Subject  (Intercept)     0.527    0.726
           TRTPBO         0.317    0.563    1.00
 Residual                 68.883   8.300
Number of obs: 837, groups:  Subject, 259
```

Fixed effects:
```
             Estimate Std. Error      df t value Pr(>|t|)
(Intercept)   -10.007      0.406 358.383  -24.65   <2e-16 ***
TRTPBO          1.232      0.579 716.093    2.13    0.034 *
---
Signif. codes: 0 *** 0.001 ** 0.01 * 0.05 . 0.1
```

Correlation of Fixed Effects:
```
       (Intr)
TRTPBO -0.689
convergence code: 0
boundary (singular) fit: see ?isSingular
```

For model selection and model parsimony, we fit a simplified random-intercept only model as follows:

```
> # Fit the random-intercept and random-slope model
> HAMD.Int.lme = lmer(dHAMD~TRT+(1|Subject), datGSK)
> # Print the summary
> summary(HAMD.Int.lme)
```

Linear mixed model fit by REML. t-tests use
   Satterthwaite's method [lmerModLmerTest]
Formula: dHAMD ~ TRT + (1 | Subject)
   Data: datGSK

REML criterion at convergence: 5929

Scaled residuals:
```
    Min      1Q   Median      3Q      Max
-2.4882  -0.7744  0.0109   0.8189  2.7262
```

Random effects:
```
 Groups    Name           Variance Std.Dev.
 Subject  (Intercept)     0.935    0.967
```

```
Residual                 69.032   8.309
Number of obs: 837, groups:  Subject, 259

Fixed effects:
            Estimate Std. Error      df t value Pr(>|t|)
(Intercept)  -10.007      0.409 486.519  -24.47   <2e-16 ***
TRTPBO         1.235      0.578 834.605    2.14    0.033 *
---
Signif. codes: 0 *** 0.001 ** 0.01 * 0.05 . 0.1

Correlation of Fixed Effects:
       (Intr)
TRTPBO -0.696
```

The model selection based on likelihood-ratio test can be done as follows:

```
> anova(HAMD.Int.lme, HAMD.Slope.lme)
```

```
Data: datGSK
Models:
HAMD.Int.lme: dHAMD ~ TRT + (1 | Subject)
HAMD.Slope.lme: dHAMD ~ TRT + (TRT | Subject)
               Df  AIC  BIC logLik deviance Chisq Df Pr(>Chisq)
HAMD.Int.lme    4 5937 5956  -2964     5929
HAMD.Slope.lme 6 5941 5969  -2964     5929  0.08  2    0.96
```

From this likelihood-ratio test, we see that the associated $\chi^2 = 0.08$ with 2 degrees of freedom, which yielded p-value of 0.96. Therefore, the simplified random-intercept model is sufficient to fit the data.

With this model, the estimated between-study variance is 0.935 and within-study variance is 69.032, which is much larger than the between-study variance. We calculate the intraclass correlation (i.e., ICC) as:

```
> # Calculate ICC
> ICC.HAMD = 0.935/(0.935+69.032)
> # Print the ICC
> ICC.HAMD
```

```
[1] 0.0134
```

We see that the ICC is 1.34% which is very minimal. This indicates that the between-study variation is rather small and statistically not insignificant, which justifies the pooled analysis.

14.2.1.5 Summary of IPD Analysis

In summary, when the data from each study are analyzed separately, lamotrigine is not statistically more effective than the placebo. When the

data from all four studies are combined as a pooled IPD analysis with
regression model and linear mixed-effects model, lamotrigine is statistically
more effective than the placebo. In addition, Age and Sex are not significant
covariates.

Furthermore, there is no statistically significant difference among the
studies indicating no statistically significant heterogeneity among the four
studies, which justifies the fixed-effects meta-analysis we will perform in next
Section 14.2.2.

14.2.2   Meta-Analysis with SS

14.2.2.1   Generate the SS

For meta-analysis with SS, we need to generate SS from the IPD data for each
study and treatment. For this purpose, we **aggregate** the IPD into study-level
summaries as follows:

```
> # Get the number of observations
> nHAMD = aggregate(datGSK$dHAMD,
        list(Study=datGSK$Study,TRT = datGSK$TRT), length)
> nHAMD

        Study TRT   x
1 SCA100223 LTG 109
2   SCA30924 LTG 126
3   SCA40910 LTG 127
4   SCAB2001 LTG  63
5 SCA100223 PBO 106
6   SCA30924 PBO 122
7   SCA40910 PBO 119
8   SCAB2001 PBO  65

> # Calculate the means
> mHAMD = aggregate(datGSK$dHAMD,
        list(Study=datGSK$Study,TRT = datGSK$TRT), mean)
> mHAMD

        Study TRT       x
1 SCA100223 LTG -11.54
2   SCA30924 LTG  -9.25
3   SCA40910 LTG  -9.17
4   SCAB2001 LTG -10.51
5 SCA100223 PBO  -9.75
6   SCA30924 PBO  -8.57
7   SCA40910 PBO  -8.65
8   SCAB2001 PBO  -7.82

> # Calculate the SD
```

```
> sdHAMD = aggregate(datGSK$dHAMD,
         list(Study=datGSK$Study,TRT = datGSK$TRT), sd)
> sdHAMD

      Study TRT    x
1 SCA100223 LTG 8.75
2  SCA30924 LTG 8.11
3  SCA40910 LTG 8.42
4  SCAB2001 LTG 8.11
5 SCA100223 PBO 8.60
6  SCA30924 PBO 8.70
7  SCA40910 PBO 7.93
8  SCAB2001 PBO 7.89
```

14.2.2.2 Calculate the Effect Size: Mean Difference

To carry out the meta-analysis, we make use of R library `metafor`. With these study-level summaries, we first calculate the effect-size(ES). Since HAMD is reported with the same unit from all studies, we use the simple mean difference(MD) which can be specified in `measure="MD"`. The R code chunk is as follows:

```
> # Load the library
> library(metafor)
> # Calculate the effect size
> esHAMD = escalc(measure="MD",
         n1i= nHAMD$x[nHAMD$TRT=="LTG"],
         n2i= nHAMD$x[nHAMD$TRT=="PBO"],
         m1i= mHAMD$x[mHAMD$TRT=="LTG"],
         m2i= mHAMD$x[mHAMD$TRT=="PBO"],
         sd1i= sdHAMD$x[sdHAMD$TRT=="LTG"],
         sd2i= sdHAMD$x[sdHAMD$TRT=="PBO"], append=T)
> # Use the study name as row name
> rownames(esHAMD) = nHAMD$Study[nHAMD$TRT=="LTG"]
> # Print the calculated ESs and SDs
> esHAMD

               yi      vi
SCA100223 -1.7960  1.3993
SCA30924  -0.6884  1.1425
SCA40910  -0.5262  1.0866
SCAB2001  -2.6926  2.0015
```

Based on these ESs, we calculate the p-values associated with each study as follows:

```
> # Calculate the z-values
> z = esHAMD$yi/sqrt(esHAMD$vi)
```

```
> # Calculate the p-values
> pval = 2*(1-pnorm(abs(z)))
> # Print the p-values
> pval

[1] 0.129 0.520 0.614 0.057
attr(,"ni")
[1] 215 248 246 128
attr(,"measure")
[1] "MD"
```

We see from these studywise p-values that none of the four studies demonstrated statistical significance for lamotrigine as compared to placebo – which is similar to the IPD analysis of each study.

14.2.2.3 Meta-Analysis with Fixed-Effects Model

Now we perform the meta-analysis. We fit the fixed-effects meta-model and the series of random-effects meta-models to compare the results.

The fixed-effects meta-analysis can be carried out by following R code chunk:

```
> # The fixed-effects meta-analysis
> metaHAMD.MD.FE = rma(yi,vi,measure="MD",
                 method="FE", data=esHAMD)
> metaHAMD.MD.FE

Fixed-Effects Model (k = 4)

I^2 (total heterogeneity / total variability):   0.00%
H^2 (total variability / sampling variability):  0.67

Test for Heterogeneity:
Q(df = 3) = 2.0102, p-val = 0.5703

Model Results:
estimate      se     zval     pval    ci.lb    ci.ub
 -1.2345  0.5764  -2.1416   0.0322  -2.3642  -0.1047  *
---
Signif. codes:  0 *** 0.001 ** 0.01 * 0.05 . 0.1
```

We see that the associated p-value is 0.032 for the MD of -1.234 indicating statistically significant treatment effect.

14.2.2.4 Meta-Analysis with Random-Effects Model

We fit a series of random-effects models using different estimation methods to estimate between-study heterogeneity. These model-fittings are easily implemented as follows:

```
> # The random-effects meta-analysis with "DL"
> metaHAMD.MD.DL = rma(yi,vi,measure="MD",
                 method="DL", data=esHAMD)
> metaHAMD.MD.DL


Random-Effects Model (k = 4; tau^2 estimator: DL)

tau^2 (estimated amount of total heterogeneity): 0 (SE = 1.1027)
tau (square root of estimated tau^2 value):      0
I^2 (total heterogeneity / total variability):   0.00%
H^2 (total variability / sampling variability):  1.00

Test for Heterogeneity:
Q(df = 3) = 2.0102, p-val = 0.5703

Model Results:

estimate     se     zval    pval    ci.lb    ci.ub
 -1.2345  0.5764  -2.1416  0.0322  -2.3642  -0.1047  *


---
Signif. codes:  0 *** 0.001 ** 0.01 * 0.05 . 0.1

> # The random-effects meta-analysis with "HS"
> metaHAMD.MD.HS = rma(yi,vi,measure="MD",
                 method="HS", data=esHAMD)
> metaHAMD.MD.HS


Random-Effects Model (k = 4; tau^2 estimator: HS)

tau^2 (estimated amount of total heterogeneity): 0 (SE = 0.8138)
tau (square root of estimated tau^2 value):      0
I^2 (total heterogeneity / total variability):   0.00%
H^2 (total variability / sampling variability):  1.00

Test for Heterogeneity:
Q(df = 3) = 2.0102, p-val = 0.5703

Model Results:

estimate     se     zval    pval    ci.lb    ci.ub
 -1.2345  0.5764  -2.1416  0.0322  -2.3642  -0.1047  *


---
Signif. codes:  0 *** 0.001 ** 0.01 * 0.05 . 0.1
```

```
> # The random-effects meta-analysis with "HE"
> metaHAMD.MD.HE = rma(yi,vi,measure="MD",
                method="HE", data=esHAMD)
> metaHAMD.MD.HE

Random-Effects Model (k = 4; tau^2 estimator: HE)

tau^2 (estimated amount of total heterogeneity): 0 (SE = 1.1744)
tau (square root of estimated tau^2 value):      0
I^2 (total heterogeneity / total variability):  0.00%
H^2 (total variability / sampling variability): 1.00

Test for Heterogeneity:
Q(df = 3) = 2.0102, p-val = 0.5703

Model Results:

estimate      se     zval    pval    ci.lb    ci.ub
 -1.2345  0.5764  -2.1416  0.0322  -2.3642  -0.1047  *

---

Signif. codes:  0 *** 0.001 ** 0.01 * 0.05 . 0.1

> # The random-effects meta-analysis with "SJ"
> metaHAMD.MD.SJ = rma(yi,vi,measure="MD",
                method="SJ", data=esHAMD)
> metaHAMD.MD.SJ

Random-Effects Model (k = 4; tau^2 estimator: SJ)

tau^2 (estimated amount of total heterogeneity): 0.3428
                                         (SE = 0.5050)
tau (square root of estimated tau^2 value):      0.5855
I^2 (total heterogeneity / total variability):  20.24%
H^2 (total variability / sampling variability): 1.25

Test for Heterogeneity:
Q(df = 3) = 2.0102, p-val = 0.5703

Model Results:

estimate      se     zval    pval    ci.lb    ci.ub
 -1.2686  0.6491  -1.9545  0.0506  -2.5408   0.0036  .

---

Signif. codes: 0 *** 0.001 ** 0.01 * 0.05 . 0.1
```

```
> # The random-effects meta-analysis with "ML"
> metaHAMD.MD.ML = rma(yi,vi,measure="MD",
                  method="ML", data=esHAMD)
> metaHAMD.MD.ML


Random-Effects Model (k = 4; tau^2 estimator: ML)

tau^2 (estimated amount of total heterogeneity): 0 (SE = 0.9180)
tau (square root of estimated tau^2 value):      0
I^2 (total heterogeneity / total variability):   0.00%
H^2 (total variability / sampling variability):  1.00

Test for Heterogeneity:
Q(df = 3) = 2.0102, p-val = 0.5703

Model Results:

estimate     se     zval    pval    ci.lb    ci.ub
 -1.2345  0.5764  -2.1416  0.0322  -2.3642  -0.1047  *


---
Signif. codes:  0 *** 0.001 ** 0.01 * 0.05 . 0.1

> # The random-effects meta-analysis with "REML"
> metaHAMD.MD.REML = rma(yi,vi,measure="MD",
                  method="REML", data=esHAMD)
> metaHAMD.MD.REML


Random-Effects Model (k = 4; tau^2 estimator: REML)

tau^2 (estimated amount of total heterogeneity): 0 (SE = 1.0827)
tau (square root of estimated tau^2 value):      0
I^2 (total heterogeneity / total variability):   0.00%
H^2 (total variability / sampling variability):  1.00

Test for Heterogeneity:
Q(df = 3) = 2.0102, p-val = 0.5703

Model Results:

estimate     se     zval    pval    ci.lb    ci.ub
 -1.2345  0.5764  -2.1416  0.0322  -2.3642  -0.1047  *


---
Signif. codes:  0 *** 0.001 ** 0.01 * 0.05 . 0.1
```

```
> # The random-effects meta-analysis with "EB"
> metaHAMD.MD.EB = rma(yi,vi,measure="MD",
                    method="EB", data=esHAMD)
> metaHAMD.MD.EB

Random-Effects Model (k = 4; tau^2 estimator: EB)

tau^2 (estimated amount of total heterogeneity): 0 (SE = 1.0851)
tau (square root of estimated tau^2 value):      0
I^2 (total heterogeneity / total variability):   0.00%
H^2 (total variability / sampling variability):  1.00

Test for Heterogeneity:
Q(df = 3) = 2.0102, p-val = 0.5703

Model Results:

estimate     se     zval     pval    ci.lb    ci.ub
 -1.2345  0.5764  -2.1416  0.0322  -2.3642  -0.1047  *

---
Signif. codes: 0 *** 0.001 ** 0.01 * 0.05 . 0.1
```

From the above model-fittings, no **Test of Heterogeneity** is statistically significant and the treatment effect is significant with p-value of 0.0322 from all models which yields the same conclusion as the IPD pooled data analysis.

The conclusion can be illustrated using the forest plot from DL with a simple R code *forest(metaHAMD.MD.DL, slab=rownames(esHAMD))* which is shown in Figure 14.2.

14.3   Treatment Comparison for Changes in MADRS

We follow the same procedure as in the last section to analyze the MADRS without further explanation.

14.3.1   Meta-Analysis with IPD

14.3.1.1   IPD Analysis for Each Study

We first test the significance using data from each study as follows:

```
> # Test for Study "SCA100223"
> mStudy1 = lm(dMADRS~TRT,
```

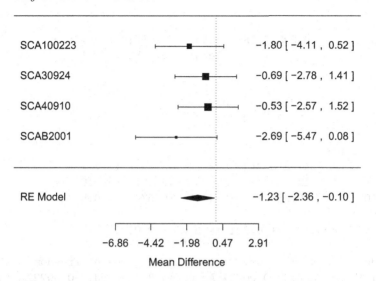

FIGURE 14.2
Forest plot for HAMD.

```
        datGSK[datGSK$Study==levels(datGSK$Study)[1],])
> summary(mStudy1)

Call:
lm(formula = dMADRS ~ TRT, data = datGSK[datGSK$Study
                      == levels(datGSK$Study)[1], ])

Residuals:
   Min     1Q Median     3Q    Max
-20.35  -9.24  -1.35  10.21  26.65

Coefficients:
            Estimate Std. Error t value Pr(>|t|)
(Intercept)  -13.651      1.052  -12.98   <2e-16 ***
TRTPBO         0.887      1.498    0.59     0.55
---
Signif. codes: 0 *** 0.001 ** 0.01 * 0.05 . 0.1

Residual standard error: 11 on 213 degrees of freedom
Multiple R-squared: 0.00164,Adjusted R-squared:-0.00304
F-statistic: 0.351 on 1 and 213 DF,  p-value: 0.554

> # Test for Study "SCA30924"
> mStudy2 = lm(dMADRS~TRT,
      datGSK[datGSK$Study==levels(datGSK$Study)[2],])
> summary(mStudy2)
```

```
Call:
lm(formula = dMADRS ~ TRT, data = datGSK[datGSK$Study
                    == levels(datGSK$Study)[2], ])


Residuals:
   Min    1Q Median    3Q    Max
-24.98  -8.22   1.07  9.07  26.02


Coefficients:
            Estimate Std. Error t value Pr(>|t|)
(Intercept)  -12.016      0.989  -12.15   <2e-16 ***
TRTPBO         0.950      1.410    0.67      0.5
---
Signif. codes: 0 *** 0.001 ** 0.01 * 0.05 . 0.1


Residual standard error: 11.1 on 246 degrees of freedom
Multiple R-squared: 0.00184,Adjusted R-squared: -0.00222
F-statistic: 0.454 on 1 and 246 DF,  p-value: 0.501

> # Test for Study "SCA40910"
> mStudy3 = lm(dMADRS~TRT,
      datGSK[datGSK$Study==levels(datGSK$Study)[3],])
> summary(mStudy3)

Call:
lm(formula = dMADRS ~ TRT, data = datGSK[datGSK$Study
                    == levels(datGSK$Study)[3], ])


Residuals:
    Min     1Q  Median     3Q     Max
-27.975 -8.940   0.595  9.130  31.165


Coefficients:
            Estimate Std. Error t value Pr(>|t|)
(Intercept)   -12.17       1.04  -11.71   <2e-16 ***
TRTPBO          1.14       1.49    0.76     0.45
---
Signif. codes: 0 *** 0.001 ** 0.01 * 0.05 . 0.1


Residual standard error: 11.7 on 244 degrees of freedom
Multiple R-squared: 0.00238,Adjusted R-squared:-0.00171
F-statistic: 0.583 on 1 and 244 DF,  p-value: 0.446

> # Test for Study "SCAB2001"
> mStudy4 = lm(dMADRS~TRT,
      datGSK[datGSK$Study==levels(datGSK$Study)[4],])
> summary(mStudy4)
```

```
Call:
lm(formula = dMADRS ~ TRT, data = datGSK[datGSK$Study
                     == levels(datGSK$Study)[4], ])

Residuals:
     Min      1Q  Median      3Q     Max
 -23.215  -8.851  -0.473   8.270  23.270

Coefficients:
            Estimate Std. Error t value Pr(>|t|)
(Intercept)   -13.27       1.38   -9.63   <2e-16 ***
TRTPBO          5.49       1.93    2.84   0.0053 **
---
Signif. codes: 0 *** 0.001 ** 0.01 * 0.05 . 0.1

Residual standard error: 10.9 on 126 degrees of freedom
Multiple R-squared: 0.06,Adjusted R-squared: 0.0526
F-statistic: 8.05 on 1 and 126 DF,  p-value: 0.00531
```

We can see that when data are analyzed for each study, there is no statistically significant treatment effect for the first three studies (i.e., SCA100223, SCA30924, and SCA40910); however, treatment effect is statistically significant in the fourth study (i.e., SCAB2001).

14.3.1.2 IPD Analysis for All Four Studies

We pool the four studies together to test treatment and study interaction as follows:

```
> # Model the interaction
> m1 = lm(dMADRS~TRT*Study, datGSK)
> # Print the ANOVA result
> anova(m1)

Analysis of Variance Table

Response: dMADRS
           Df Sum Sq Mean Sq F value Pr(>F)
TRT         1    599     599    4.75   0.03 *
Study       3    668     223    1.77   0.15
TRT:Study   3    548     183    1.45   0.23
Residuals 829 104515     126
```

We see that the treatment effect is now statistically significant (p-value $=$ 0.02952) and the interaction is not (p-value $=$ 0.22727). We then exclude the interaction and test the main effect as follows:

```
> # Model the main effect
> m2 = lm(dMADRS~TRT+Study, datGSK)
> # Print the ANOVA result
> anova(m2)

Analysis of Variance Table

Response: dMADRS
          Df Sum Sq Mean Sq F value Pr(>F)
TRT        1    599     599    4.75   0.03 *
Study      3    668     223    1.76   0.15
Residuals 832 105063    126
```

Again the treatment effect is statistically significant (p-value $= 0.02965$) and there is no statistically significant difference among the four studies (p-value $= 0.1525$). A Tukey multiple comparison procedure can be further performed to confirm this conclusion which can be done as follows:

```
> TukeyHSD(aov(dMADRS~TRT+Study, datGSK))

  Tukey multiple comparisons of means
    95% family-wise confidence level

Fit: aov(formula = dMADRS ~ TRT + Study, data = datGSK)

$TRT
        diff   lwr  upr p adj
PBO-LTG 1.69 0.168 3.22  0.03

$Study
                       diff     lwr  upr p adj
SCA30924-SCA100223    1.6674 -1.028 4.36 0.384
SCA40910-SCA100223    1.6158 -1.085 4.32 0.414
SCAB2001-SCA100223    2.7045 -0.525 5.93 0.137
SCA40910-SCA30924    -0.0516 -2.655 2.55 1.000
SCAB2001-SCA30924     1.0371 -2.111 4.19 0.831
SCAB2001-SCA40910     1.0887 -2.064 4.24 0.811
```

14.3.1.3   IPD Analysis with Covariates

Similarly, we incorporate the covariates Age and Sex to test their TRT and Study significance as follows:

```
> # Full model
> mAllStudy1 = lm(dMADRS~(Age+Sex)*TRT*Study, datGSK)
> # Print the ANOVA
> anova(mAllStudy1)
```

```
Analysis of Variance Table
```

```
Response: dMADRS
                Df Sum Sq Mean Sq F value Pr(>F)
Age              1    173     173    1.37  0.242
Sex              1     55      55    0.44  0.510
TRT              1    623     623    4.93  0.027 *
Study            3    584     195    1.54  0.202
Age:TRT          1     26      26    0.21  0.650
Sex:TRT          1      0       0    0.00  0.993
Age:Study        3    578     193    1.53  0.206
Sex:Study        3    285      95    0.75  0.521
TRT:Study        3    499     166    1.32  0.267
Age:TRT:Study    3    159      53    0.42  0.739
Sex:TRT:Study    3    759     253    2.01  0.112
Residuals      813 102589     126
```

Since there is no statistical significance for all the 2-way and 3-way interactions, we fit the main effect model as follows:

```
> # Fit the main effect model
> mAllStudy2 = lm(dMADRS~TRT+Study+Age+Sex, datGSK)
> # Print the ANOVA
> anova(mAllStudy2)
```

```
Analysis of Variance Table
```

```
Response: dMADRS
            Df Sum Sq Mean Sq F value Pr(>F)
TRT          1    599     599    4.74   0.03 *
Study        3    668     223    1.76   0.15
Age          1    137     137    1.08   0.30
Sex          1     31      31    0.24   0.62
Residuals  830 104896     126
```

Again, `Sex` and `Age` are not statistically significant which indicates that we can further reduce the model to the main effects `TRT` and `Study` which is the model m2 above.

14.3.2 Meta-Analysis with SS

14.3.2.1 Generate SS

Similarly, we first aggregate the IPD into study-level summaries as follows:

```
> # Get the number of observations
> nMADRS = aggregate(datGSK$dMADRS,
```

```
        list(Study=datGSK$Study,TRT = datGSK$TRT), length)
> nMADRS

        Study TRT   x
1 SCA100223 LTG 109
2  SCA30924 LTG 126
3  SCA40910 LTG 127
4  SCAB2001 LTG  63
5 SCA100223 PBO 106
6  SCA30924 PBO 122
7  SCA40910 PBO 119
8  SCAB2001 PBO  65

> # Calculate the means
> mMADRS = aggregate(datGSK$dMADRS,
      list(Study=datGSK$Study,TRT = datGSK$TRT), mean)
> mMADRS

        Study TRT      x
1 SCA100223 LTG -13.65
2  SCA30924 LTG -12.02
3  SCA40910 LTG -12.17
4  SCAB2001 LTG -13.27
5 SCA100223 PBO -12.76
6  SCA30924 PBO -11.07
7  SCA40910 PBO -11.03
8  SCAB2001 PBO  -7.78

> # Calculate the SD
> sdMADRS = aggregate(datGSK$dMADRS,
      list(Study=datGSK$Study,TRT = datGSK$TRT), sd)
> sdMADRS

        Study TRT    x
1 SCA100223 LTG 11.1
2  SCA30924 LTG 10.8
3  SCA40910 LTG 11.8
4  SCAB2001 LTG 11.5
5 SCA100223 PBO 10.9
6  SCA30924 PBO 11.4
7  SCA40910 PBO 11.6
8  SCAB2001 PBO 10.4
```

14.3.2.2   Calculate ES: MD

We then calculate the ES using the simple MD with the following R code chunk:

```
> # Calculate the effect size
> esMADRS = escalc(measure="MD",
          n1i= nMADRS$x[nMADRS$TRT=="LTG"],
          n2i= nMADRS$x[nMADRS$TRT=="PBO"],
          m1i= mMADRS$x[mMADRS$TRT=="LTG"],
          m2i= mMADRS$x[mMADRS$TRT=="PBO"],
          sd1i= sdMADRS$x[sdMADRS$TRT=="LTG"],
          sd2i= sdMADRS$x[sdMADRS$TRT=="PBO"], append=T)
> # Use the study name as row name
> rownames(esMADRS) = nMADRS$Study[nMADRS$TRT=="LTG"]
> # Print the data
> esMADRS

                yi      vi
SCA100223  -0.8872  2.2421
SCA30924   -0.9503  1.9929
SCA40910   -1.1401  2.2278
SCAB2001   -5.4852  3.7504
```

Based on these ESs, we calculate the *p*-values associated with each study as follows:

```
> # Calculate the z-values
> z = esMADRS$yi/sqrt(esMADRS$vi)
> # Calculate the p-values
> pval = 2*(1-pnorm(abs(z)))
> # Print the p-values
> pval

[1] 0.55350 0.50084 0.44494 0.00462
attr(,"ni")
[1] 215 248 246 128
attr(,"measure")
[1] "MD"
```

Again from these *p*-values, the treatment effect is not statistically significant for first three studies.

14.3.2.3 Fixed-Effects and Random-Effects Meta-Analyses

For the meta-analysis, we fit the fixed-effects meta-model and the series of random-effects meta-model to compare the results, which can be easily implemented in R as follows:

```
> # The fixed-effects meta-analysis
> metaMADRS.MD.FE = rma(yi,vi,measure="MD",
                        method="FE", data=esMADRS)
> metaMADRS.MD.FE
```

```
Fixed-Effects Model (k = 4)

I^2 (total heterogeneity / total variability):   33.88%
H^2 (total variability / sampling variability):  1.51


Test for Heterogeneity:
Q(df = 3) = 4.5375, p-val = 0.2090


Model Results:
estimate      se     zval     pval    ci.lb     ci.ub
 -1.7116  0.7754  -2.2074   0.0273  -3.2313   -0.1919  *



> # The random-effects meta-analysis with "DL"
> metaMADRS.MD.DL = rma(yi,vi,measure="MD",
                         method="DL", data=esMADRS)
> metaMADRS.MD.DL

Random-Effects Model (k = 4; tau^2 estimator: DL)

tau^2 (estimated amount of total heterogeneity):1.2516
                                                (SE=3.0225)
tau (square root of estimated tau^2 value):      1.1187
I^2 (total heterogeneity / total variability):  33.88%
H^2 (total variability / sampling variability): 1.51


Test for Heterogeneity:
Q(df = 3) = 4.5375, p-val = 0.2090


Model Results:
estimate      se     zval     pval    ci.lb     ci.ub
 -1.8221  0.9615  -1.8952   0.0581  -3.7066   0.0623  .

> # The random-effects meta-analysis with "HS"
> metaMADRS.MD.HS = rma(yi,vi,measure="MD",
                         method="HS", data=esMADRS)
> metaMADRS.MD.HS

Random-Effects Model (k = 4; tau^2 estimator: HS)

tau^2 (estimated amount of total heterogeneity):0.3231
                                                (SE=1.6680)
tau (square root of estimated tau^2 value):      0.5685
I^2 (total heterogeneity / total variability):  11.69%
H^2 (total variability / sampling variability): 1.13
```

```
Test for Heterogeneity: Q(df = 3) = 4.5375, p-val = 0.2090

Model Results:
estimate      se      zval     pval     ci.lb    ci.ub
 -1.7474   0.8279  -2.1108   0.0348   -3.3700  -0.1248   *
```

```
> # The random-effects meta-analysis with "HE"
> metaMADRS.MD.HE = rma(yi,vi,measure="MD",
                        method="HE", data=esMADRS)
> metaMADRS.MD.HE
```

```
Random-Effects Model (k = 4; tau^2 estimator: HE)

tau^2 (estimated amount of total heterogeneity):2.5043(SE=4.1556)
tau (square root of estimated tau^2 value):      1.5825
I^2 (total heterogeneity / total variability):  50.63%
H^2 (total variability / sampling variability): 2.03

Test for Heterogeneity: Q(df = 3) = 4.5375, p-val = 0.2090

Model Results:
estimate       se      zval     pval     ci.lb    ci.ub
 -1.8852   1.1151  -1.6906   0.0909   -4.0707   0.3003   .
```

```
> # The random-effects meta-analysis with "SJ"
> metaMADRS.MD.SJ = rma(yi,vi,measure="MD",
                        method="SJ", data=esMADRS)
> metaMADRS.MD.SJ
```

```
Random-Effects Model (k = 4; tau^2 estimator: SJ)

tau^2 (estimated amount of total heterogeneity):2.6871(SE=2.5536)
tau (square root of estimated tau^2 value):      1.6392
I^2 (total heterogeneity / total variability):  52.39%
H^2 (total variability / sampling variability): 2.10

Test for Heterogeneity: Q(df = 3) = 4.5375, p-val = 0.2090

Model Results:
estimate       se      zval     pval     ci.lb    ci.ub
 -1.8922   1.1357  -1.6661   0.0957   -4.1180   0.3337   .
```

```
> # The random-effects meta-analysis with "ML"
> metaMADRS.MD.ML = rma(yi,vi,measure="MD",
                        method="ML", data=esMADRS)
 > metaMADRS.MD.ML
```

```
Random-Effects Model (k = 4; tau^2 estimator: ML)

tau^2 (estimated amount of total heterogeneity):0.0000
                                           (SE=1.6629)
tau (square root of estimated tau^2 value):    0.0010
I^2 (total heterogeneity / total variability):  0.00%
H^2 (total variability / sampling variability): 1.00

Test for Heterogeneity: Q(df = 3) = 4.5375, p-val = 0.2090

Model Results:
estimate     se     zval     pval     ci.lb     ci.ub
 -1.7116  0.7754  -2.2074  0.0273  -3.2313  -0.1919  *


> # The random-effects meta-analysis with "REML"
> metaMADRS.MD.REML = rma(yi,vi,measure="MD",
                          method="REML", data=esMADRS)
> metaMADRS.MD.REML

Random-Effects Model (k = 4; tau^2 estimator: REML)

tau^2 (estimated amount of total heterogeneity):0.5768
                                           (SE=2.4476)
tau (square root of estimated tau^2 value):    0.7595
I^2 (total heterogeneity / total variability):  19.11%
H^2 (total variability / sampling variability): 1.24

Test for Heterogeneity: Q(df = 3) = 4.5375, p-val = 0.2090

Model Results:
estimate     se     zval     pval     ci.lb     ci.ub
 -1.7714  0.8666  -2.0440  0.0409  -3.4699  -0.0729  *

> # The random-effects meta-analysis with "EB"
> metaMADRS.MD.EB = rma(yi,vi,measure="MD",
                        method="EB", data=esMADRS)
> metaMADRS.MD.EB

Random-Effects Model (k = 4; tau^2 estimator: EB)

tau^2 (estimated amount of total heterogeneity):1.7121(SE=3.4032)
tau (square root of estimated tau^2 value):    1.3085
I^2 (total heterogeneity / total variability):  41.21%
H^2 (total variability / sampling variability): 1.70
```

```
Test for Heterogeneity: Q(df = 3) = 4.5375, p-val = 0.2090

Model Results:
estimate     se     zval    pval    ci.lb   ci.ub
 -1.8490  1.0208  -1.8113  0.0701  -3.8497  0.1518  .
```

The same conclusion can be made that no `Test of Heterogeneity` is statistically significant, but the treatment effect is statistically significant which yields the same conclusion as the IPD pooled analysis.

14.4 Summary of Lamotrigine Analysis

In the above analysis, we used the simple MD by specifying `measure="MD"`. We also analyzed this data using *standardized MD* which can be specified easily by using `measure="SMD"`, and we reached the same conclusions.

In summary, when data from each study are analyzed separately, lamotrigine is not statistically more effective than the placebo in `HAMD`. For `MADRS`, there is a statistically significant treatment effect in study `SCAB2001`, but not in the other three studies of `SCA100223`, `SCA30924`, and `SCA40910`. However, when data from all four studies are pooled using the IPD pooled analysis and the meta-analysis, lamotrigine is statistically more effective than the placebo. Furthermore, there is no statistically significant difference among the studies indicating that there is no statistically significant heterogeneity among the four studies.

From the analysis, we can see that both the IPD pooled analysis and meta-analysis from the aggregated data yielded similar conclusions. In fact, this is true in general as demonstrated in Lin and Zeng (2010) in the setting of fixed-effects model. In this paper, the authors showed theoretically that for all commonly used parametric and semiparametric models, there is no asymptotic efficiency gain to analyze the original data when the parameter of main interest has a common value across studies and the SS are based on maximum likelihood theory regardless of different nuisance parameters among studies when the nuisance parameters have distinct values. The authors also demonstrated their results with simulations from the logistic regression setting. The R code for this simulation can be found from http://www.bios.unc.edu/ dzeng/Meta.html. Note that this conclusion generally fails to hold when the nuisance parameters have common values as discussed in Lin and Zeng (2010) and Simmonds and Higgins (2007).

In the next section, we follow this paper to design a simulation study following the continuous data structure reported from the lamotrigine clinical studies.

14.5   Simulation Study on Continuous Outcomes

We do not reproduce the theoretical work from Lin and Zeng (2010) because it is available from the literature for interested readers. This paper demonstrated both theoretically and numerically that there is little or no efficiency gain of IPD over meta-analysis. This provides assurance in performing a meta-analysis using SS. The practical implications from this work regarding whether to use IPD or meta-analysis are noted and emphasized. Usually patient-level data are not available for analysis and may be difficult and costly to obtain if available. In this section, we further illustrate this conclusion from a simulation based on the lamotrigine clinical studies.

14.5.1   Simulation Data Generator

We simulate data from K studies. Each study includes two interventions which are named treatment (TRT) and placebo (PBO) with n_i study participants in each study randomly assigned to the two treatments with binomial probability distribution of $p = 0.5$. The *nvec* denotes the vector of sample size from these K studies, i.e., $nvec = (n_1, \ldots, n_K)$. Similarly, we denote *meanvec* and *sdvec* as the vectors of means and standard deviations from these K studies.

For simplicity, we simulate data from a fixed-effects model setting where the model is

$$y_{ij} = \mu + \epsilon_{ij} \tag{14.1}$$

where i indexes the ith study ($i = 1, \ldots, K$) and j for observations within study ($j = 1, \ldots, n_i$), μ is the same for all K studies in the fixed-effects model, but different for each treatment. This setting can be easily modified for a random-effects model by adding an extra term μ_i to μ to simulate variation and heterogeneity among studies; we leave this to interested readers.

In this case, we build a data simulator (called **data.generator**) to generate data from K studies with two treatments as follows:

```
> # The function for data generation
> data.generator =  function(K, nvec, meanvec, sdvec){
  # Initialize data generation
  trt = study = mu = epsilon = NULL;
  # Loop to generate data for each study
  for(i in 1:K){
            # study identifier
            study = append(study,rep(i, nvec[i]))
            # indicator for treatment assignment
            trt0 = mu0 = which.trt = rbinom(nvec[i],1,0.5)
            # assign 1 to TRT and get its mean value
            trt0[mu0==1] = 1; mu0[mu0==1] = meanvec[i]
```

```
        # assign 0 for Placebo and get its mean value
        trt0[mu0==0] = 0; mu0[mu0==0] = meanvec[i+K]
        # epsilion
        epsilon0 = rnorm(nvec[i], 0, sdvec)
        # put together
        trt   = append(trt,trt0)
        mu    = append(mu, mu0)
        epsilon = append(epsilon, epsilon0)
              } # end of i-loop for data generation
# Put the data into a dataframe
trt[trt==1] = "TRT"
trt[trt==0] = "PBO"
y    = mu + epsilon
dat = data.frame(Study=as.factor(study), TRT = trt,mu=mu,y=y)
# Output the dataframe
dat
} # end of function "data.generator"
```

As an example, let us follow the Lamotrigine clinical studies to generate data with inputs as follows:

```
> # Set the seed for reproducibility
> set.seed(123)
> # The number of studies
> K    = 4
> # The number of observations for each study
> n    = 200
> nvec = rep(n, K); nvec

[1] 200 200 200 200

> # Treatment means from HAMD in Lamotrigine clinical study
> mTRT    = -10; mPBO = -8
> meanvec = c(rep(mTRT,K), rep(mPBO,K))
> # SDs for each study
> sdvec   = 8 + runif(K) ; sdvec

[1] 8.29 8.79 8.41 8.88
```

The SD for HAMD is close to 8 in the real data and we add values from a random uniform distribution to simulate study-level heterogeneity in this simulation. With these inputs, we call `data.generator` to generate IPD as follows:

```
> # Call `data.generator'
> dat =   data.generator(K,nvec,meanvec,sdvec)
> # Print the first few rows of data
> head(dat)
```

```
  Study TRT  mu     y
1     1 TRT -10 -12.0
2     1 PBO  -8 -11.1
3     1 TRT -10 -18.0
4     1 TRT -10 -10.4
5     1 TRT -10 -16.5
6     1 PBO  -8 -22.7
```

This dataframe "**dat**" has $4 \times 200 = 800$ observations with 4 columns as Study to denote the $K = 4$ studies, TRT to denote the treatment assignments, mu to denote the simulated true means, and y denotes the individual-level data from equation 14.1. We use R function **head** to see the *head* six data lines. The distribution of the generated data is graphically illustrated in Figure 14.3 using following R code chunk:

```
> # Call bwplot to make the figure
> print(bwplot(y~Study|TRT, data=dat,xlab="Study",
  ylab="Simulated Data",lwd=3,cex=1.3,pch=20,
  strip=strip.custom(bg="white"), type=c("p", "r")))
```

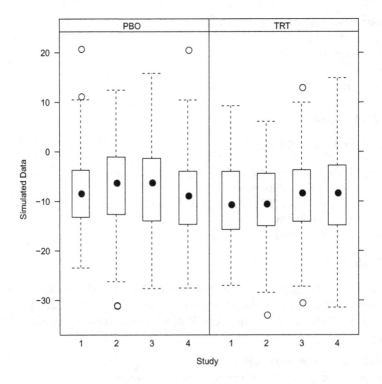

FIGURE 14.3
Simulated data from four studies.

14.5.2   Simulation Data Estimator

With the data generated from Section 14.5.1, we now estimate the relevant parameters from both IPD and SS models and design an estimator which is named as `data.estimator`. For this estimator, we design and contrast three analysis models. The first model is the analysis of variance model for each study which is in fact the t-test in this simulation since there are only two treatment groups. This analysis should be compared with the study-wise z-test in meta-analysis. The second model is an analysis model to pool the data from the K studies with model formulation of $y = \mu + TRT + Study + \epsilon$. The third model is the fixed-effects meta-analysis model which is used to compare results with the analysis model with pooled data. For the purpose of this simulation and estimation, we mainly keep track of the estimation results of treatment effect, standard errors, and the associated p-values from both IPD and SS models.

The input for this `data.estimator` is the `dat` from `data.simulator` from Section 14.5.1. The R implementation is as follows:

```
> # The function of `estimator'
> data.estimator = function(dat){
# 1. Get the study ID from the dataframe
idStudy = unique(dat$Study)
nStudy  = length(idStudy)
# 2. loop to get p-values for each study
eachIPD.pval = rep(0, nStudy)
for(i in 1:nStudy){
m4Study = lm(y~TRT, data=dat[dat$Study==idStudy[i],])
eachIPD.pval[i] = summary(m4Study)$coef[2,4]
            } # end of i-loop
# 3. The IPD with pooled data using linear model
mIPD        = lm(y~TRT+Study,dat)
# Extract parms from IPD model
poolIPD.trt.p   = anova(mIPD)["TRT","Pr(>F)"]
poolIPD.study.p = anova(mIPD)["Study","Pr(>F)"]
poolIPD.trt.est = summary(mIPD)$coef["TRTTRT","Estimate"]
poolIPD.trt.se  = summary(mIPD)$coef["TRTTRT","Std. Error"]
# 4. Meta-analysis
# 4.1. Aggregate the individual level data into study-level
ndat  = aggregate(dat$y, list(Study=dat$Study,TRT = dat$TRT),
          length)
mdat  = aggregate(dat$y, list(Study=dat$Study,TRT = dat$TRT),
          mean)
sddat = aggregate(dat$y, list(Study=dat$Study,TRT = dat$TRT),
          sd)
# 4.2. Call the library
library(metafor)
```

```
# 4.3 Calculate the ESs
esdat = escalc(measure="MD",
        n1i = ndat$x[ndat$TRT=="TRT"],
        n2i = ndat$x[ndat$TRT=="PBO"],
        m1i = mdat$x[mdat$TRT=="TRT"],
        m2i = mdat$x[mdat$TRT=="PBO"],
        sd1i= sddat$x[sddat$TRT=="TRT"],
        sd2i= sddat$x[sddat$TRT=="PBO"], append=T)
rownames(esdat) = ndat$Study[ndat$TRT=="TRT"]
# 4.4. z- and p-values for IPD in each study
z               = esdat$yi/sqrt(esdat$vi)
pval.studywise = 2*(1-pnorm(abs(z)))
# 4.5. Fixed-effects meta-analysis
meta.MD.FE = rma(yi,vi,measure="MD",method="FE", data=esdat)
# 4.6. Extract the estimate, p-values for ES and heterogeneity
MA.muhat.FE   = meta.MD.FE$b
MA.muhatse.FE = meta.MD.FE$se
MA.p.FE       = meta.MD.FE$pval
MA.pQ.FE      = meta.MD.FE$QEp
# 5. output from the estimator
out = list(
eachIPD.pval   = eachIPD.pval,
pval.studywise = pval.studywise,
IPD.trt.est    = poolIPD.trt.est,
IPD.trt.se     = poolIPD.trt.se,
IPD.trt.p      = poolIPD.trt.p,
IPD.study.p    = poolIPD.study.p,
MA.muhat.FE    = MA.muhat.FE,
MA.muhatse.FE  = MA.muhatse.FE,
MA.p.FE        = MA.p.FE,
MA.pQ.FE       = MA.pQ.FE)
# 6. Return the output
out
} # end of "data.estimator"
```

With this estimator, we call the function for the data we generated in Section 14.5.1 as follows:

```
> data.estimator(dat)

$eachIPD.pval
[1] 0.18036 0.00179 0.15436 0.98132

$pval.studywise
[1] 0.17821 0.00151 0.15149 0.98131
attr(,"ni")
```

```
[1]  200 200 200 200
attr(,"measure")
[1]  "MD"

$IPD.trt.est
[1] -1.76

$IPD.trt.se
[1]  0.604

$IPD.trt.p
[1]  0.00348

$IPD.study.p
[1]  0.764

$MA.muhat.FE
intrcpt -1.81

$MA.muhatse.FE
[1]  0.601

$MA.p.FE
[1]  0.00259

$MA.pQ.FE
[1]  0.183
```

As can be seen from the output for the individual studies, only the second study is statistically significant. But when the four studies are pooled in the IPD model, the estimated treatment difference is IPD.trt.est = -1.76 with standard error of IPD.trt.se $= 0.604$ and associated p-value IPD.trt.p $= 0.00348$. In addition, the associated p-value for study-effect is IPD.study.p $= 0.764$. Comparatively from the meta-analysis, the estimated treatment difference is MA.muhat.FE $= -1.81$ with standard error MA.muhatse.FE $= 0.601$ and associated p-value MA.p.FE $= 0.00259$. The associated p-value for study heterogeneity is MA.pQ.FE $= 0.183$.

14.5.3   Simulation

With the data generator in Section 14.5.1 and estimator in Section 14.5.2, we now run a large number of simulations to compare treatment effects as well as efficiency for both the IPD and SS models.

In order to effectively run the simulation, we develop another R function which is named IPD2MA, run the extensive simulations, and save the results for further graphical illustration and model comparison. This function has inputs from the `data.generator` with an additional input for the number of simulations which is denoted by `nsim`. This function is as follows with detailed annotations:

```
> # Main function for the simulation
> IPD2MA = function(nsim,K,nvec,meanvec,sdvec){
 # Put program checkers
 if(length(nvec)!= K)
   cat("Wrong for the number of obs in each study","\n")
 if(length(meanvec)!= 2*K)
   cat("Wrong for the study mean setup","\n")
 if(length(sdvec)!= K) cat("Wrong for the study SD setup","\n")

 # Output initialization
 IPD.trt.est=IPD.trt.se= IPD.trt.p=IPD.study.p =
 MA.muhat.FE=MA.muhatse.FE=MA.p.FE=MA.pQ.FE=rep(0, nsim)
 # Now loop-over for "nsim" simulation and extract the measures
 for(s in 1:nsim){
 cat("Simulating iteration =",s,sep=" ", "\n\n")
          # call "data.generator" to generate data
          dat = data.generator(K, nvec, meanvec, sdvec)
          # call estimator to get estimates from IPD and SS
          est = data.estimator(dat)
          # Extract the measures from the IPD and SS analyses
          IPD.trt.est[s]   = est$IPD.trt.est
          IPD.trt.se[s]    = est$IPD.trt.se
          IPD.trt.p[s]     = est$IPD.trt.p
          IPD.study.p[s]   = est$IPD.study.p
          MA.muhat.FE[s]   = est$MA.muhat.FE
          MA.muhatse.FE[s]= est$MA.muhatse.FE
          MA.p.FE[s]       = est$MA.p.FE
          MA.pQ.FE[s]      = est$MA.pQ.FE
          } #end of s-loop
 # Summary statistics
 out = data.frame(
 IPD.trt.est   = IPD.trt.est,    IPD.trt.se   = IPD.trt.se,
 IPD.trt.p     = IPD.trt.p,      IPD.study.p  = IPD.study.p,
 MA.muhat.FE   = MA.muhat.FE,    MA.muhatse.FE = MA.muhatse.FE,
 MA.p.FE       = MA.p.FE,        MA.pQ.FE      = MA.pQ.FE)
 # Return the dataframe "out"
 out
 } # end of "IPD2meta"
```

With the same inputs from Section 14.5.1, we run a simulation with 100,000 replications (note that if your computer is slower, you can reduce the number of simulations to 10,000) as follows:

```
> # The number of simulations
> nsim =100000
> # Call "IPD2MA" to run simulations
> IPD2MA.simu = IPD2MA(nsim,K,nvec,meanvec,sdvec)
```

This produces a dataframe named `IPD2MA.simu` to hold the 100,000 simulation results which includes 8 columns from both IPD and SS models. We now compare the performance between IPD and SS models with this dataframe. We first investigate the efficiency as noted in Lin and Zeng (2010) along with the estimates for treatment effect. The efficiency is defined as the ratio of estimated variance for the treatment effect between IPD and SS models – which is the squared value of the estimated standard errors and denoted by `relEff`. We also consider the relative estimates of treatment effect which is defined as the ratio of the estimates between IPD and SS models and denoted by `relEst`. We output the mean and mode along with the 95% CI from these 100,000 simulations using the following R code chunk:

```
> # The relative efficiency
> relEff = IPD2MA.simu$IPD.trt.se^2/IPD2MA.simu$MA.muhatse.FE^2
> # The mean
> mean(relEff)

[1] 1.01

> # The mode and 95% CI
> quantile(relEff, c(0.025, 0.5,0.975))

 2.5%    50% 97.5%
 0.99   1.01  1.03

> # The relative estimate
> relEst= IPD2MA.simu$IPD.trt.est/IPD2MA.simu$MA.muhat.FE
> # The mean
> mean(relEst)

[1] 1

> # The mode and 95% CI
> quantile(relEst, c(0.025, 0.5,0.975))

 2.5%    50% 97.5%
0.936  1.000 1.072
```

It can be seen that the mean and mode for the relative efficiency are both 1.01 with 95% CI of (0.99, 1.03) which indicates that both IPD and SS models have comparable efficiency and consistent with the finding from Lin and Zeng (2010). Further, the mean and mode for the relative estimates

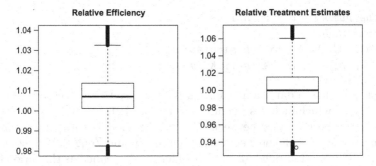

FIGURE 14.4
Distributions for the relative efficiency and relative estimates.

for treatment effect are both 1 with 95% CI of (0.936, 1.072) which again indicates the comparability between IPD and SS models. The distributions for both the relative efficiency and relative estimates for treatment effect can be graphically illustrated using `boxplot` as seen in Figure 14.4, which can be produced using following R code chunk:

```
> # Call boxplot to plot the relative efficiency and estimates
> par(mfrow=c(1,2))
> boxplot(relEff, main="Relative Efficiency",
         las=1,ylim=c(0.98,1.04))
> boxplot(relEst, main="Relative Treatment Estimates",
         las=1,ylim=c(0.93,1.07))
```

Separate from the above comparable relative measures, we also compare the number of simulations among these 100,000 simulations that report a statistically significant treatment effect which can be calculated as follows:

```
> # For IPD
> n4TRT.IPD = sum(IPD2MA.simu$IPD.trt.p<0.05)
> n4TRT.IPD
```

```
[1] 90606
```

```
> # For SS
> n4TRT.MA = sum(IPD2MA.simu$MA.p.FE<0.05)
> n4TRT.MA
```

```
[1] 90643
```

We see that the number of simulations among these 100,000 simulations that report significant treatment effect is 90606 from the IPD pooled model and 90,643 from the meta-analysis. Therefore, both models give similar results for testing treatment effect. The same can be done for testing heterogeneity among studies with the following R code chunk:

```
> # for IPD
> n4Study.IPD = sum(IPD2MA.simu$IPD.study.p<0.05)
> n4Study.IPD
```

[1] 5027

```
> # For SS
> n4Study.MA = sum(IPD2MA.simu$MA.pQ.FE<0.05)
> n4Study.MA
```

[1] 5158

Again, compatible results are obtained for both models.

14.6 Discussions

In this chapter, we started with real IPD on lamotrigine to treat bioploar depression in comparison to a placebo to illustrate the pros and cons of IPD and SS. A series of models were used to analyze this data and we concluded that both models yielded similar conclusions that lamotrigine is more effective than placebo in treating bioploar depression.

This analysis served as another real example for the conclusions reported in Lin and Zeng (2010). We further designed a simulation study using the data structure from the lamotrigine clinical studies and simulated 100,000 replications to compare the relative efficiency and the relative parameter estimates on treatment effects as well as the number of simulations that yielded statistically significant treatment effects. All demonstrated that both models yielded very comparable results.

This chapter thus serves to further promote meta-analysis using study-level SS. Without much loss in relative efficiency for testing treatment effect, SS is recommended since it is usually difficult to obtain original individual-level data and is costlier and more time-consuming.

Comparing the performance of IPD and SS models has received considerable debate in the meta-analysis literature. Olkin and Sampson (1998) and Mathew and Nordstrom (1999) showed their equivalence in comparing multiple treatments and a control. The theoretical results in Lin and Zeng (2010) are more general in this area as discussed in the paper.

A novel *confidence distributions* approach was proposed in Singh et al. (2005), Xie et al. (2011) and Xie and Singh (2013) to unify the framework for meta-analysis. This approach uses a (data-dependent) distribution function, instead of the point or interval estimates, to estimate the parameter of interest. This led to new developments in meta-analysis. An associated R package gmeta is created by Guang Yang, Jerry Q. Cheng, Minge Xie and Wei Qian which is available at http://stat.rutgers.edu/home/gmeta/. In his PH.D. dissertation (http://mss3.libraries.rutgers.edu/dlr/showfed.php?pid=rutgerslib:37435), Dr. Dungang Liu utilized this *confidence distributions* and developed an effective and efficient approach to combine heterogeneous studies. He showed that the new method can combine studies different in populations, designs or outcomes, including the cases pointed out in Sutton and Higgins (2008) and Whitehead et al. (1999). He showed theoretically and numerically that his approach was asymptotically as efficient as the maximum likelihood approach using individual-level data from all the studies. However different from the IPD analysis, his approach only requires SS from relevant studies and does not require the individual-level data. Several examples and cases were considered in this dissertation along with his theoretical theorems. We recommend this method to interested readers.

Other reviews on this topic can be found in Simmonds et al. (2005) and Lyman and Kuderer (2005) as well as the most recent study in Chen et al. (2020) on random-effects meta-analysis models.

15

Other R/Stata Packages for Meta-Analysis

To conclude this book, we give a summary of the three main R packages of meta, rmeta, and metafor used in this book. We additionally introduce and illustrate some extra R functions and packages designed for specific meta-analysis and provide discussion for listing more R packages for further reference. Readers can search the R homepage for packages for their own research and applications.

Specifically, we give a brief summary of the three R packages in Section 15.1. We further present methods to combine p-values from studies in Section 15.2. In Section 15.3, we introduce several R packages for meta-analysis of correlation coefficients and illustrate their applications to a real data set on land use intensity across 18 gradients from nine countries. We complete this book with Section 15.4 in which we discuss additional R packages and Section 15.5 to discuss additional Stata methods for meta-analysis for Stata users.

15.1   R Packages of meta, rmeta, and metafor

There are many R packages for meta-analysis and we have so far illustrated three commonly used ones: rmeta by Lumley (2009), meta by Schwarzer (2010), and metafor by Viechtbauer (2010), in previous chapters.

As seen from the illustrations in previous chapters in this book, all three packages can serve as "general purpose" packages for arbitrary effect-size and different outcome measures to fit fixed-effects or random-effects meta-analysis models. From our experience, all three packages are easy to use for meta-analysis with metafor having more methods implemented. For example, in random-effects meta-analysis, rmeta only implemented the DerSimonian-Laird estimator to estimate the between-study variance of τ^2, whereas metafor and meta include several other methods, such as the restricted maximum-likelihood estimator, the maximum-likelihood estimator, the Hunter-Schmidt estimator, the Sidik-Jonkman estimator, the Hedges estimator, and the Empirical Bayes estimator. In addition, `metafor` has a great feature for meta-regression as illustrated in Chapter 7 and can be used to include multiple continuous or categorical regression covariates as well as mixed-effects models, whereas `meta` can only include a single categorical regression covariate in fixed-effects, and meta-regression is not included in `rmeta`.

A comprehensive comparison and discussion of three packages can be found in Viechtbauer (2010). In this paper, he summarized all these three packages in his Table 2, which is reproduced here as Table 15.1 for readers' reference and easy access.

Note in Table 15.1, (1) in *Moderator Analyses* for `meta` is for only fixed-effects with moderators model, and (2) in *Other Analyses* for `meta` indicates that this is true when used together with the `copas` package as Carpenter and Schwarzer (2009).

TABLE 15.1
Comparison Among `metafor`, `meta`, and `rmeta` Packages

	metafor	meta	metafor
Model fitting			
Fixed-effects models	Yes	Yes	Yes
Random-effects models	Yes	Yes	Yes
Heterogeneity estimators	Various	DL	DL
Mantel-Haenszel method	Yes	Yes	Yes
Peto's method	Yes	Yes	No
Plotting			
Forest plots	Yes	Yes	Yes
Funnel plots	Yes	Yes	Yes
Radial plots	Yes	Yes	No
L'Abbe plots	No	Yes	No
QQ normal plots	Yes	No	No
Moderator analysis			
Categorical moderators	Multiple	Single[1]	No
Continuous moderators	Multiple	No	No
Mixed-effects models	Yes	No	No
Testing/Confidence intervals			
Knapp & Hartung adjustment	Yes	No	No
Likelihood ratio-test	Yes	No	No
Permutation tests	Yes	No	No
Other analyses			
Leave-one-out analysis	Yes	Yes	No
Influence diagnostics	Yes	No	No
Cumulative meta-analysis	Yes	Yes	Yes
Tests for funnel plot asymmetry	Yes	Yes	No
Trim and fill methods	Yes	Yes	No
Selection models	No	Yes[2]	No

15.2 Combining *p*-Values in Meta-Analysis

When summarizing a study for statistical purposes, a *p*-value is usually reported. In meta-analysis to combine several independent studies with reported *p*-values, we can combine the *p*-values to obtain an overall *p*-value.

There are several methods for combining *p*-values, see for example Hartung et al. (2008) and Peace (1991). The most commonly used one is Fisher's method. There is no need for a R package for this calculation since it is straightforward to write a simple R code for this purpose.

Fisher's method is known as Fisher's combined probability test which was developed to combine statistical *p*-values from several independent tests of the same hypothesis (H_0) using a χ^2-distribution. Specifically, suppose p_i is the *p*-value reported from *i*th study, then the statistic

$$X^2 = -2 \sum_{i=1}^{K} ln(p_i) \tag{15.1}$$

is distributed as χ^2-distribution with $2K$-degrees of freedom – since under the null hypothesis for test *i*, its *p*-value p_i follows a uniform distribution on the interval [0,1], i.e., $p_i \sim U[0,1]$. By taking the negative natural logarithm of a uniformly distributed value, $-ln(p_i)$ follows an exponential distribution. Multiplying this exponentially distributed statistic by a factor of two produces a χ^2-distributed quantity of $-2ln(p_i)$ with two degrees of freedom. The sum of K independent χ^2, each with two degrees of freedom , follows a χ^2 distribution with $2K$ degrees of freedom. Intuitively we can see that if the p_i are small, the test statistic X^2 would be large suggesting that the null hypothesis is not true for the combined test.

Based on this formulation, we can write a R function for Fisher's method as follows:

```
> # Create a function for Fisher's method
> fishers.pvalue = function(x){
 # Call chisq prob function for calculation
 pchisq(-2 * sum(log(x)),df=2*length(x),lower=FALSE)
 }
```

In this R function, *x* is the vector of *p*-values from all independent studies.

As an example, we make use of the data in Table 4.1 for coronary death or myocardial infarction (MI) among patients taking statins. In Section 4.2.1.2, we calculated the *p*-values for the 4 studies to compare the experimental to standard groups and the values are 0.106, 0.0957, 0.00166, and 0.0694, respectively. The following R code chunk illustrates the application of Fisher's method:

```
> # The reported p-values
> x = c(0.106, 0.0957, 0.00166, 0.0694)
```

```
> # Call function of fishers.pvalue
> combined.pval = fishers.pvalue(x)
> print(combined.pval)
```

[1] 0.000623

This gives a combined p-value of 0.00062 indicating strong statistical significance overall. A proper interpretation of this result is when the 4 studies are taken as an aggregate, Fisher's method for combining p-values provides evidence that intensive statin therapy is more effective than standard statin therapy in reducing the risk of MI or cardiac death.

15.3   Combining Correlation Coefficients in Meta-Analysis

There are several packages for meta-analysis of correlation coefficients. The R package of `meta` and `metafor` introduced above can be used to combine correlation coefficients from studies. We illustrate another package of `metacor` in this section for this purpose along with discussion for an additional R package `MAc`.

15.3.1   R Package `metacor`

Package `metafor` is designed for meta-analysis of correlation coefficients and is maintained by Etienne Laliberte (etiennelaliberte@gmail.com). The comprehensive information about this package can be seen from the website at http://cran.r-project.org/web/packages/metacor/index.html with package download and reference manual.

Readers can download the package from this webpage and load this package to the R console using:

```
> library(metacor)
```

For `help` about this package, simply use the general "help" function as follows:

```
> library(help=metafor)
```

It can be seen from this "help" function that two approaches are implemented to meta-analyze correlation coefficients as effect sizes reported from studies. These two approaches are the DerSimonian-Laird (DSL) and Olkin-Pratt (OP) methods as discussed in Schulze (2004). Based on these two methods, two functions are implemented in this package as:

1. `metacor.DSL` for DSL approach with correlation coefficients as effect sizes,

2. `metacor.OP` for OP approach with correlation coefficients as effect sizes.

15.3.2 Data on Land-Use Intensity

To illustrate the application of the approaches in this package, we make use of the data given in the package which is named as `lui`. This `lui` includes two correlation coefficients between *land use intensity* and response diversity (variable named as `r.FDis`) or functional redundancy (variable named as `r.nbsp`) along with the total observations (variable named as `n`) across 18 land use intensity gradients from nine countries and five biomes. We load the data into R as follows:

```
> # Load the data into R
> data(lui)
> # Print the data
> lui
```

	label	r.FDis	r.nbsp	n
15	New Zealand (TG)	-4.30e-01	-0.3790	72
1	Australia / NSW (STR)	-4.24e-01	-0.6042	176
4	Australia / Mungalli (TR)	-3.78e-01	-0.8438	36
12	Nicaragua / Rivas (TR)	-3.70e-01	-0.5482	42
5	Australia / Atherton (TR)	-3.29e-01	-0.4882	315
11	Nicaragua / Matiguas (TR)	-1.37e-01	-0.6163	42
2	Australia / QLD (STR)	-1.16e-01	-0.3791	117
14	Australia / NSW (TW)	-1.08e-01	-0.0841	332
16	Portugal (TF)	-4.58e-02	-0.0513	120
3	Australia / Tully (TR)	2.29e-17	0.1010	80
6	Costa Rica / Las Cruces (TR)	1.54e-02	-0.0400	297
17	Canada / Quebec (TF)	2.46e-02	0.0160	240
8	Costa Rica / La Palma (TR)	4.06e-02	0.0161	290
18	USA / North Carolina (TF)	1.11e-01	-0.4326	26
13	Laos (TR)	1.35e-01	0.0239	96
10	China / Hainan montane (TR)	1.39e-01	-0.1453	36
9	China / Hainan lowland (TR)	1.71e-01	-0.3880	48
7	Costa Rica / Puerto Jimenez (TR)	2.01e-01	0.1213	290

15.3.3 Meta-Analysis Using `metacor` Package

Meta-analysis for `r.FDis` is performed in the package as an example and we illustrate these two approaches for `r.nbsp`. The DSL approach meta-analysis can be performed with R code chunk as follows:

```
> # Call metacor.DSL for DerSimonian-Laird (DSL) approach
> nbsp.DSL.metacor = metacor.DSL(lui$r.nbsp, lui$n, lui$label)
> # Print the result
> nbsp.DSL.metacor
```

$z
```
 [1] -0.3988 -0.6997 -1.2343 -0.6158 -0.5337 -0.7190
 [7] -0.3990 -0.0843 -0.0513  0.1013 -0.0400  0.0160
[13]  0.0161 -0.4631  0.0239 -0.1463 -0.4094  0.1219
```

$z.var
```
 [1] 0.01449 0.00578 0.03030 0.02564 0.00321 0.02564
 [7] 0.00877 0.00304 0.00855 0.01299 0.00340 0.00422
[13] 0.00348 0.04348 0.01075 0.03030 0.02222 0.00348
```

$z.lower
```
 [1] -0.1629 -0.5506 -0.8932 -0.3020 -0.4227 -0.4051
 [7] -0.2155  0.0238  0.1299  0.3247  0.0743  0.1433
[13]  0.1318 -0.0545  0.2272  0.1949 -0.1172  0.2376
```

$r.lower
```
 [1] -0.1615 -0.5010 -0.7129 -0.2931 -0.3992 -0.3843
 [7] -0.2122  0.0238  0.1292  0.3137  0.0742  0.1423
[13]  0.1310 -0.0544  0.2233  0.1925 -0.1167  0.2332
```

$z.upper
```
 [1] -0.63479 -0.84867 -1.57553 -0.92967 -0.64462 -1.03281
 [7] -0.58261 -0.19236 -0.23252 -0.12203 -0.15431 -0.11134
[13] -0.09961 -0.87181 -0.17932 -0.48749 -0.70156  0.00617
```

$r.upper
```
 [1] -0.56134 -0.69038 -0.91790 -0.73044 -0.56804 -0.77503
 [7] -0.52456 -0.19002 -0.22842 -0.12143 -0.15310 -0.11089
[13] -0.09928 -0.70229 -0.17742 -0.45222 -0.60536  0.00617
```

$z.mean
```
[1] -0.286
```

$r.mean
```
[1] -0.278
```

$z.mean.se
```
[1] 0.0742
```

$z.mean.lower
```
[1] -0.14
```

```
$r.mean.lower
[1] -0.14

$z.mean.upper
[1] -0.431

$r.mean.upper
[1] -0.407

$p
[1] 5.85e-05
```

The first part of the results reports the study-specific z-values, the variances of each z, the lower/upper limits of the confidence intervals for each z, and the lower/upper limits of the confidence intervals for each r. The second part of the results reflects the combined results from the meta-analysis. From the study-specific confidence intervals, we can see that some studies have significant correlation coefficients and some do not. However, when combined, the correlation coefficient is -0.278 with lower CI bound of -0.14 and upper bound of -0.407. The p-value from the z-test is 0 which indicates significant correlation for the studies combined. The default setting in `metacor.DSL` provides the forest plot which is given by Figure 15.1.

Similar analysis can be performed for the OP approach. But we do not make the forest plot here rather we specify the `plot=F` (note that the `plot=T` is the default setting to generate the forest plot). Instead of printing all the results, we only print the p-value for the meta-analysis result to save space. The R code chunk is as follows:

```
> # Call metacor.OP for Olkin-Pratt (OP) approach
> nbsp.OP.metacor = metacor.OP(lui$r.nbsp, lui$n,
                    lui$label, plot=F)
> # Print the p-value only
> nbsp.OP.metacor$p

[1] 1.11e-18
```

15.3.4 Meta-Analysis Using `meta` Package

The same type of meta-analysis can be done by using the `metacor` function from R package `meta` with the following R code chunk; we print only the summary results without the individual-study data:

```
> # Load the library
> library(meta)
> # Call metacor for meta-analysis
```

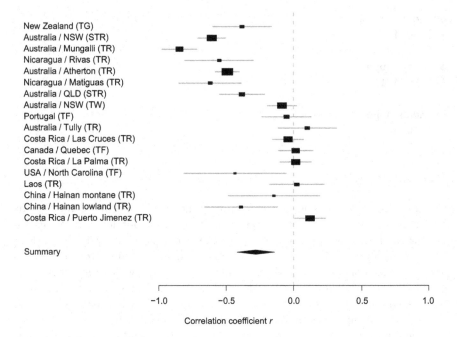

FIGURE 15.1
Meta-analysis for correlation coefficients of *nbsp*.

```
> nbsp.DSLfromMeta = metacor(cor=r.nbsp, n=n,
                        studlab=label, data=lui)
> # Print the summary result
> summary(nbsp.DSLfromMeta)

Number of studies combined: k = 18

                         COR            95%-CI       z
Fixed effect model    -0.1822 [-0.2191; -0.1448] -9.40
Random effects model  -0.2784 [-0.4066; -0.1396] -3.85
                        p-value
Fixed effect model    < 0.0001
Random effects model    0.0001

Quantifying heterogeneity:
 tau^2 = 0.0861 [0.0514; 0.2527]; tau = 0.2934 [0.2266; 0.5027];
 I^2 = 92.3% [89.3%; 94.5%]; H = 3.61 [3.06; 4.25]

Test of heterogeneity:
     Q d.f.  p-value
 221.10    17 < 0.0001
```

```
Details on meta-analytical method:
- Inverse variance method
- DSL estimator for tau^2
- Jackson method for confidence interval of tau^2 and tau
- Fisher's z transformation of correlations
```

Comparing these summary results (just the part of the random-effects model) with those from nbsp.DSL.metacort, we note that they are the same. Readers can call functions escalc and rma from R package metafor to reproduce the results. Notice that meta and metafor have more options to perform meta-analysis for correlation coefficients.

15.3.5 Further Discussions on Meta-Analysis for Correlations

R package MAc (Meta-Analysis for Correlations) can also be used to combine correlation coefficients. This package can be obtained from http://rwiki.sciviews.org/doku.php?id=packages:cran:ma_meta-analysis. The authors implemented the recommended procedures as described in Cooper and Valentine (2009). Including package MAc, there are in fact five related packages from this site which are MAc GUI, MAd (Meta-Analysis for Differences), MAd GUI, and compute.es. Note that compute.es is a package to convert and standardize various within-study effect-sizes and calculate the associated variances for further meta-analysis. The packages MAc and MAc GUI are the packages for meta-analysis of correlation coefficients with MAc GUI as the graphical user interface (GUI) version of MAc.

Because of this GUI, this package suite can integrate the meta-analytical approaches to achieve a user-friendly GUI so that meta-analysis can be performed in a menu-driven (i.e., "point and click") fashion for readers who are not versed in coding. Examples and illustrations can be found from the webpage.

15.4 Other R Packages for Meta-Analysis

There are many more R packages available from the R website. Searching "R Site Search" for "meta-analysis" produces several additional packages. We list a few more R packages for further reference and to promote the use of these packages.

1. metaMA is a package developed by Guillemette Marot for "Meta-Analysis for Microarray" (Marot et al., 2009) and is available at http://cran.r-project.org/web/packages/metaMA/. This package combines either p-values or modified effect-sizes from different microarray studies to find differentially expressed genes.

2. `MAMA`, developed by Ivana Ihnatova, is a similar package for "Meta-Analysis for Microarray" and is available at http://cran.r-project.org/web/packages/MAMA/. A detailed description of this package can be found at http://cran.r-project.org/web/packages/MAMA/vignettes/MAMA.pdf where nine different methods are described and implemented for meta-analysis of microarray studies.

3. `MetaDE`, developed by Xingbin Wang, Jia Li and George C Tseng, is another R package for microarray meta-analysis for differentially expressed gene detection and is available at http://cran.r-project.org/web/packages/MetaDE/. The reference manual can be found from http://cran.r-project.org/web/packages/MetaDE/MetaDE.pdf and describes the implementation of 12 major meta-analysis methods for differential gene expression analysis.

4. `mada`, developed by Philipp Doebler, is a package for meta-analysis of diagnostic accuracy and receiver operating characteristic curves and is available at http://cran.r-project.org/web/packages/mada/. A detailed description of this package can be found at http://cran.r-project.org/web/packages/mada/vignettes/mada.pdf. As described in the file, this package "provides some established and some current approaches to diagnostic meta-analysis, as well as functions to produce descriptive statistics and graphics. It is hopefully complete enough to be the only tool needed for a diagnostic meta-analysis."

5. `HSROC`, created by Ian Schiller and Nandini Dendukuri, is a package for joint meta-analysis of diagnostic test sensitivity and specificity with or without a gold standard reference test. This package is available at http://cran.r-project.org/web/packages/HSROC/ and "implements a model for joint meta-analysis of sensitivity and specificity of the diagnostic test under evaluation, while taking into account the possibly imperfect sensitivity and specificity of the reference test. This hierarchical model accounts for both within and between study variability. Estimation is carried out using a Bayesian approach, implemented via a Gibbs sampler. The model can be applied in situations where more than one reference test is used in the selected studies."

6. `bamdit`, created by Pablo Emilio Verde and Arnold Sykosch, is a package for Bayesian meta-analysis of diagnostic test data based on a scale mixtures bivariate random-effects model. This package is available at http://cran.r-project.org/web/packages/bamdit/.

7. `gemtc`, developed by Gert van Valkenhoef and Joel Kuiper, is a package for network meta-analysis and is available at http://cran.r-project.org/web/packages/gemtc/ or http://drugis.org/gemtc. As described in this package, network meta-analysis, known as mixed treatment comparison, "is a technique to

meta-analyze networks of trials comparing two or more treatments at the same time. Using a Bayesian hierarchical model, all direct and indirect comparisons are taken into account to arrive at a single, integrated, estimate of the effect of all included treatments based on all included studies."

8. `ipdmeta`, developed by S. Kovalchik, is a package for subgroup analyses with multiple trial data using aggregate statistics and is available at http://cran.r-project.org/web/packages/ipdmeta/. This package provides functions for an individual participant data (IPD) linear mixed effects model for continuous outcomes and any categorical covariate from study summary statistics. Other functions are also provided to estimate the power of a treatment-covariate interaction test.

9. `psychometric` is a package for psychometric applications and contains functions for meta-analysis besides the typical contents for correlation theory, reliability, item analysis, inter-rater reliability, and classical utility. This package is developed by Thomas D. Fletcher and is available at http://cran.r-project.org/web/packages/psychometric/.

10. `epiR`, created by Mark Stevenson with contributions from Telmo Nunes, Javier Sanchez, Ron Thornton, Jeno Reiczigel, Jim Robison-Cox, and Paola Sebastiani, is a package for the analysis of epidemiological data. It contains functions for meta-analysis besides the typical usage for analysis of epidemiological data, such as directly and indirectly adjusting measures of disease frequency, quantifying measures of association on the basis of single or multiple strata of count data presented in a contingency table, and computing confidence intervals around incidence risk and incidence rate estimates. This package is available at http://cran.r-project.org/web/packages/epiR/ or http://epicentre.massey.ac.nz.

11. `metamisc`, created by Thomas Debray, is a package for diagnostic and prognostic meta-analysis and is available at http://cran.r-project.org/web/packages/metamisc/. This package contains functions to estimate univariate, bivariate, and multivariate models as well as allowing the aggregation of previously published prediction models with new data. A further description given in the package is "The package provides tools for the meta-analysis of IPD and/or aggregate data. Currently, it is possible to pool univariate summary (with `uvmeta`) and diagnostic accuracy (with `riley`) data. Whereas the former applies a univariate meta-analysis using DerSimonian and Laird's method (method-of-moment estimator), the latter implements a bivariate meta-analysis (Restricted Maximum Likelihood) using the alternative model for bivariate random-effects meta-analysis by Riley et al. (2008). For this the

number of true positives, false negatives, true negatives, and false positives for each study must be known."

12. `metaLik`, created by Annamaria Guolo and Cristiano Varin, is a package for likelihood inference in meta-analysis and meta-regression models and is available at http://cran.r-project.org/web/packages/metaLik/.

Finally,

13. `MADAM`, created by Karl Kugler, Laurin Mueller, and Matthias Wieser, is a package that provides some basic methods for meta-analysis and is available at http://cran.r-project.org/web/packages/MADAM/. This package is aimed at implementing and improving meta-analysis methods used in biomedical research applications.

We recommend interested readers to search for packages for their own applications since more and more new packages are being developed.

15.5   Other Stata Methods for Meta-Analysis

As introduced in Section 1.2, we have used the suite of `metan` in this book for meta-analysis for `Stata` users. All corresponding `Stata` programs are included as appendix in each chapter. In this suite, we mainly used the commands/functions of `metan` and `meta` to illustrate the meta-analyses aligning with the meta-analysis performed in R.

There are many more `Stata` packages/features/commands available from the `Stata`. A more comprehensive compilation of functions can be found in https://www.stata.com/support/faqs/statistics/meta-analysis/. As seen from this link, There are 50 more meta-analysis commands listed besides the `metan` (as the first command). A full list of official meta-analysis features can be found from https://www.stata.com/features/meta-analysis/. We do not intend to repeat the entire lists in the book again and interested readers are recommended to read these links and study these functions for their meta-analysis.

With all these discussions and illustrations, we conclude this book!

Thank You and We Hope That You Have Enjoyed Your Reading!

Bibliography

Adler, J. (2012). *R In a Nutshell, 2nd Edition*. Sebastopol, CA: O'Reilly Media, Inc.

Begg, C. B. and M. Mazumdar (1994). Operating characteristics of a rank correlation test for publication bias. *Biometrics 50*, 1088–1101.

Berkey, C. S., D. C. Hoaglin, A. Antezak-Bouckoms, F. Mosteller, and G. A. Colditz (1998). Meta-analysis of multiple outcomes by regression with random effects. *Statistics in Medicine 17*, 2537–2550.

Berkey, C. S., D. C. Hoaglin, F. Mosteller, and G. A. Colditz (1995). A random-effects regression model for meta-analysis. *Statistics in Medicine 14(4)*, 395–411.

Berman, N. G. and R. A. Parker (2002). Meta-analysis: Neither quick nor easy. *BMC Medical Research Methodology 2(10)*, 1–9.

Bhaumik, D. K., A. Amatya, S. T. Normand, J. Greenhouse, E. Kaizar, B. Neelon, and R. D. Gibbons (2012). Meta-analysis of rare binary adverse event data. *Journal of the American Statistical Association 107(498)*, 555–567.

Bohning, D., E. Dietz, P. Schlattmann, C. Viwatwonkasem, A. Biggeri, and J. Bock (2002). Some general points in estimating heterogeneity variance with the dersimonian–laird estimator. *Biostatistics 3*, 445–457.

Borenstein, M., L. V. Hedges, J. P. T. Higgins, and H. R. Rothstein (2009). *Introduction to Meta-Analysis*. West Sussex, United Kingdom: Wiley.

Bujkiewicz, S., J. R. Thompson, A. J. Sutton, N. J. Cooper, M. J. Harrison, D. P. Symmons, and K. R. Abrams (2013). Multivariate meta-analysis of mixed outcomes: a bayesian approach. *Statistics in Medicine 32(22)*, 3926–3943.

Cai, T., L. Parast, and L. Ryan (2010). Meta-analysis for rare events. *Statistics in Medicine 29(20)*, 2078–2089.

Calabrese, J. R., R. F. Huffman, R. L. White, S. Edwards, T. R. Thompson, and J. A. Ascher (2008). Lamotrigine in the acute treatment of bipolar depression: results of five double-blind, placebo-controlled clinical trials. *Bipolar Disorder 10*, 323–333.

Cannon, C. P., B. A. Steinberg, S. A. Murphy, J. L. Mega, and E. Braunwald (2006). Meta-analysis of cardiovascular outcomes trials comparing intensive versus moderate statin therapy. *Journal of the American College of Cardiology 48*, 438–445.

Carpenter, J. and G. Schwarzer (2009). **copas**: Statistical methods to model and adjust for bias in meta-analysis. *R package version 0.6-3*.

Chambers, J. M. (1998). *Programming with Data*. New York: Springer.

Chambers, J. M. (2008). *Software for Data Analysis: Programming with R*. New York: Springer.

Chen, D. G., D. Liu, X. Min, and H. Zhang (2020). Relative efficiency of using summary versus individual data in random-effects meta-analysis. *Biometrics.*, 1–15.

Chen, D. G. and K. E. Peace (2010). *Clinical Trial Data Analysis Using R*. Boca Raton, FL: Chapman & Hall/CRC.

Chen, D. G. and K. E. Peace (2013). *Applied Meta-Analysis Using R*. Chapman & Hall/CRC: Boca Raton, FL, USA.

Chen, D. G., K. E. Peace, and P. G. Zhang (2017). *Clinical Trial Data Analysis Using R and SAS*. Boca Raton, FL: Chapman & Hall/CRC.

Chen, H., A. K. Manning, and J. Dupuis (2012). A method of moments estimator for random effect multivariate meta-analysis. *Biometrics*, (Epub May 2, 2012).

Clarke, M. and T. Clarke, T (2000). A study of the references used in Cochrane protocols and reviews. Three bibles, three dictionaries and nearly 25,000 other things. *International Journal of Technology Assessment in Health care, 16*, 907–909.

Cochran, W. G. (1952). The chi-squared test of goodness of fit. *Annals of Mathematical Statistics 23*, 315–345.

Cochran, W. G. (1954). The combination of estimates from different experiments. *Biometrics*, 101–129.

Cohen, J. (1988). *Statistical power analysis for the behavioral sciences (2nd ed.)*. Hillsdale, NJ: Lawrence Erlbaum.

Colditz, G. A., T. F. Brewer, C. S. Berkey, M. E. Wilson, E. Burdick, H. V. Fineberg, and F. Mosteller (1994). Efficacy of bcg vaccine in the prevention of tuberculosis: Meta-analysis of the published literature. *Journal of the American Medical Association 271*, 698–702.

Cooper, H., H. L. V. and J. C. Valentine (2009). *The Handbook of Research Synthesis and Meta-Analysis (2nd edition)*. New York: Russell Sage Foundation.

Dahabreh, I. J. (2008). Meta-analysis of rare events: an update and sensitivity analysis of cardiovascular events in randomized trials of rosiglitazone. *Clinical Trials 5*, 116–120.

DerSimonian, R. and N. Laird (1986). Meta-analysis in clinical trials. *Controlled Clinical Trials 7*, 177–188.

Dickersin, K. and Y. I. Min (1993). NIH clinical trials and publication bias. Online Journal of Current Clinical Trials, Doc No 50.

Dickersin, K., Y. I. Min, and C. L. Meinert (1992). Factors influencing publication of research results: Follow-up of applications submitted to two institutional review boards. *Journal of the American Medical Association*, 263, 374–378.

Duval, S. and R. Tweedie (2000a). A nonparametric 'trim and fill' method of accounting for publication bias in meta-analysis. *Journal of the American Statistical Association*, 95, 89–98.

Duval, S. and R. Tweedie (2000b). Trim and fill: A simple funnel-plot-based method of testing and adjusting for publication bias in meta-analysis. *Biometrics*, 56, 455–463.

Easterbrook, P. J., J. A. Berlin, R. Gopalan, and D. R. Matthews (1991). Publication bias in clinical research. *Lancet*, 337, 867–872.

Emerson, J. D. (1994). Combining estimates of the odds ratios: the state of the art. *Statistical Methods in Medical Research 3*, 157–178.

Egger, M., G. Davey Smith, M. Schneider, and C. Minder (1997). Bias in meta-analysis detected by a simple, graphical test. *British Medical Journal*, 315, 629–634.

Everitt, B. and T. Hothorn (2006). *A Handbook of Statistical Analyses Using R*. Boca Raton, FL: Chapman & Hall/CRC.

Faraway, J. J. (2004). *Linear Models with R*. Boca Raton, FL: Chapman & Hall/CRC.

Faraway, J. J. (2006). *Extending Linear Models with R: Generalized Linear, Mixed Effects and Nonparametric Regression Models*. Boca Raton, FL: Chapman & Hall/CRC.

Field, A. P. (2003). The problems in using fixed-effects models of meta-analysis on real-world data. *Understanding Statistics 2*, 77–96.

Gardener, M. (2012). *Beginning R: The Statistical Programming Language*. Indianapolis, IN: John Wiley & Sons, Inc.

Gasparrini, A. Armstrong, B. and M. G. Kenward (2012). Multivariate meta-analysis for non-linear and other multi-parameter associations. *Statistics in Medicine Epub ahead of print*(doi: 10.1002/sim.5471).

Geddes, J. R., J. R. Calabrese, and G. M. Goodwin (2009). Lamotrigine for treatment of bipolar depression: independent meta-analysis and meta-regression of individual patient data from five randomized trials. *The British Journal of Psychiatry. 194*, 4–9.

Götzsche P. C. (1987). Reference bias in reports of drug trials. *BMJ*, 295, 654–656.

Hardy, R. J. and S. G. Thompson (1998). Detecting and describing heterogeneity in meta-analysis. *Statistics in Medicine 17*, 841–856.

Hartung, J., G. Knapp, and B. K. Sinha (2008). *Statistical Meta-Analysis with Applications*. Hoboken, New Jersey: John Wiley & Sons, Inc.

Harwell, M. (1997). An empirical study of hedge's homogeneity test. *Psychological Methods 2*, 219–231.

Hedges, L. V. (1981). Distribution theory for glass's estimator of effect size and related estimators. *Journal of Educational Statistics 6*, 107–128.

Hedges, L. V. (1982). Estimating effect size from a series of independent experiments. *Psychological Bulletin 92*, 490–499.

Hedges, L. V. (1984). Estimation of effect size under nonrandom sampling: The effects of censoring studies yielding statistically insignificant mean differences. *Journal of Educational Statistics*, 9, 61–85.

Hedges, L. V. (1989). Estimating the normal mean and variance under a selection model. In L., Gieser, M. D. Perlman, S. J. Press, A. R. Sampson. *Contributions to Probability and Statistics: Essays in Honor of Ingram Olkin* (pp. 447–458). New York, NY: Springer Verlag.

Hedges, L. V. and I. Olkin (1985). *Statistical Methods for Meta-Analysis*. Orlando, FL: Academic Press, Inc.

Hedges, L. V. and J. L. Vevea (1998). Fixed- and random-effects models in meta-analysis. *Psychological Methods 3*, 486–504.

Higgins, J. P. T. and S. G. Thompson (2002). Quantifying heterogeneity in a meta-analysis. *Statistics in Medicine 21*, 1539–1558.

Higgins, J. P. T., S. G. Thompson, J. J. Deeks, and D. G. Altman (2003). Measuring inconsistency in meta-analyses. *British Medical Journal 327*, 557–560.

Huizenga, H. M., B. M. van Bers, J. Plat, W. P. van den Wildenberg, and M. W. van der Molen (2009). Task complexity enhances response inhibition deficits in childhood and adolescent attention-deficit/hyperactivity disorder: a meta-regression analysis. *Biological Psychiatry 65,* 39–45.

Hunter, J. E. and F. L. Schmidt (2004). *Methods of Meta-Analysis: Correcting Error and Bias in Research Findings. 2nd Edition.* Newbury Park, CA: Sage.

Ihaka, R. and R. Gentleman (1996). R: A language for data analysis and graphics. *Journal of Computational and Graphical Statistics 5(3),* 299–314.

Ishak, K. J., R. W. Platt, L. Joseph, J. A. Hanley, and J. J. Caro (2007). Meta-analysis of longitudinal studies. *Clinical Trials 4*(5), 525–539.

Jackson, D., R. Riley, and I. R. White (2011). Multivariate meta-analysis: potential and promise. *Statistics in medicine 30*(20), 2481–2498.

Jiini, P., F. Holenstein, J., Sterne, J., C. Bartlett, and M. Egger (2002). Direction and impact of language bias in meta-analyses of controlled trials: empirical study. *International Journal of Epidemiology,* 31, 115–123.

Kabacoff, R. I. (2011). *R In Action: Data Analysis and Graphics with R.* New York: Manning Publications Co.

Katcher, B. S. (2006). *MEDLINE: A Guide to Effective Searching in PubMed and Other Interfaces.* San Francisco, CA: Ashbury Press.

Lane, P. W. (2012). Meta-analysis of incidence of rare events. *Statistical Methods in Medical Research,* 2012 Jan 4 Epub.

Law, M. R., N. J. Wald, and S. G. Thompson (1994). By how much and how quickly does reduction in serum cholesterol concentration lower risk of ischaemic heart disease? *British Medical Journal 308,* 367–373.

Lau, J., E. M. Antman, J. Jimenez-Silva, B. Kupelnick, F. Mosteller and, T. C. Chalmers (1992). Cumulative meta-analysis of therapeutic trials for myocardial infarction. *New England Journal of Medicine,* 327, 248–254.

Li, Y., L. Shi, and H. D. Roth (1994). The bias of the commonly-used estimate of variance in meta-analysis. *Communications in Statistics-Theory and Methods 23,* 1063–1085.

Light, R. J. and D. B. Pillemer (1984). *Summing up: The Science of Reviewing Research.* Cambridge, MA: Harvard University Press.

Light, R. J., J. D. Singer, and J. B. Willett (1994). *The visual presentation and interpretation of meta-analyses.* In M. Cooper & L. V. Hedges (eds), The Handbook of Research Synthesis. New York, NY: Russell Sage Foundation.

Lin, D. Y. and D. Zeng (2010). On the relative efficiency of the using summary statistics versus individual-level data in meta-analysis. *Biometrika 97(2),* 321–332.

Linares, O. (2014). https://www.amazon.com/Applied-Meta-Analysis-Chapman-Hall-Biostatistics/dp/1466505990/ref=cm_cr_arp_d_product_top?ie=UTF8.

Liu, D., R. Y. Liu, and M. Xie (2015). Multivariate meta-analysis of heterogeneous studies using only summary statistics: efficiency and robustness. *Journal of the American Statistical Association 110*(509), 326–340.

Lumley, T. (2009). rmeta: Meta-Analysis. R package version 2.16. URL http://CRAN.R-project.org/package=rmeta.

Lyman, G. H. and N. M. Kuderer (2005). The strengths and limitations of meta-analyses based on aggregate data. *BMC Medical Research Methodology 5*, 1–7.

Mallet, S., S. Hopewell, and M. Clarke (2002). The use of grey literature in the first 1000 Cochrane reviews. *Paper presented at the Fourth Symposium on Systematic Reviews: Pushing the Boundaries;* 2002 Jul 2–4; Oxford, UK.

Mantel, N. and W. Haenszel (1959). Statistical aspects of the analysis of data from retrospective studies of disease. *Journal of the National Cancer Institute 22(4)*, 719–748.

Marot, G., J.-L. Foulley, C.-D. Mayer, and F. Jaffrezic (2009). Moderated effect size and p-value combinations for microarray meta-analyses. *Bioinformatics 25(20)*, 2692–2699.

Mathew, T. and K. Nordstrom (1999). On the equivalence of meta-analysis using literature and using individual patient data. *Biometrics 55*, 1221–1223.

Morris, C. N. (1983). Parametric empirical bayes inference: Theory and applications (with discussion). *Journal of the American Statistical Association 78*, 47–65.

Murrell, P. (2005). *R Graphics*. Boca Raton, FL: Chapman & Hall/CRC.

Nissen, S. E. and K. Wolski (2007). Effect of rosiglitazone on the risk of myocardial infarction and death from cardiovascular causes. *The New England Journal of Medicine 356*, 2457–2471.

Normand, S. L. (1999). Meta-analysis: Formulating, evaluating, combining and reporting. *Statistics in Medicine 18*, 321–358.

Olkin, I. and A. Sampson (1998). Comparison of meta-analysis versus analysis of variance of individual patient data. *Biometrics 54*, 317–322.

Orwin, R.G. and R. F. Boruch (1983). RRT meets RDD: statistical strategies for assuring response privacy in telephone surveys. *Public Opinion Quarterly, 46*, 560–571.

Peace, K. E. (1991). Meta-analysis in ulcer disease. In *Swabb and Szabo (Eds.), Ulcer Disease: Investigation and basis for Therapy*, pp. 407–430. Marcel Dekker, Inc.

Peace, K. E. and D. G. Chen (2010). *Clinical Trial Methodology*. Boca Raton, FL: Chapman & Hall/CRC.

Petitti, D. B. (2000). *Meta-Analysis, Decision Analysis, and Cost-Effectiveness Analysis: Methods for Quantitative Synthesis in Medicine. 2nd Edition*. Oxford: Oxford University Press.

Pigott, T. D. (2012). *Advances in Meta-Analysis*. New York: Springer.

Ravnskov, U. (1992). Frequency of citation and outcome of cholesterol lowering trials. *BMJ*, 305–717.

Reed, J. G. and P. M. Baxter (2009). *Using reference databases*. In H. Cooper, L.V. Hedges & J. Valentine (eds), The Handbook of Research Synthesis (2nd edn). New York, NY: Sage Publications.

Riley, R. D. (2009). Multivariate meta-analysis: the effect of ignoring within-study correlation. *Journal of the Royal Statistical Society: Series A (Statistics in Society) 172*(4), 789–811.

Riley, R. D., J. R. Thompson, and K. R. Abrams (2008). An alternative model for bivariate random-effects meta-analysis when the within-study correlations are unknown. *Biostatistics 9*, 172–186.

Rizzo, M. L. (2008). *Statistical Computing with R*. Boca Raton, FL: Chapman & Hall/CRC.

Roberts, C. and T. D. Stanley (2005). *Meta-Regression Analysis: Issues of Publication Bias in Economics*. Blackwell:Wiley.

Robins, J., N. Breslow, and S. Greenland (1986). Estimators of the mantel-haenszel variance consistent in both sparse data and large strata models. *Biometrics 42*, 311–323.

Rothstein, H. R. (2006). Use of unpublished data in systematic reviews in the *Psychological Bulletin* 1995–2005. Unpublished manuscript.

Rosenthal, R. (1979). The 'file drawer problem' and tolerance for null results. *Psychological Bulletin*, 86, 638–641.

Rothstein, H. R. and S. Hopewell (2009). *The Grey literature*. In H. Cooper, L. V. Hedges & J. Valentine (eds), The Handbook of Research Synthesis (2nd edn). New York, NY: Sage Publications.

Rothstein, H. R., A. J. Sutton, and M. Borenstein (2005). *Publication Bias in Meta-analysis: Prevention, Assessment and Adjustments*. Chichester, UK, John Wiley & Sons, Ltd.

Rucker, G., G. Schwarzer, J. Carpenter, and I. Olkin (2009). Why add anything to nothing? the arcsine difference as a measure of treatment effect in meta-analysis with zero cells. *Statistics in Medicine 28(5)*, 721–738.

Sarkar, D. (2008). *Lattice: Multivariate Data Visualization with R.* New York: Springer.

Schulze, R. (2004). *Meta-analysis: a comparison of approaches.* Gottingen, Germany:Hogrefe & Huber.

Schwarzer, G. (2010). meta: Meta-Analysis with R. R package version 1.6-0, URL http://CRAN.R-project.org/package=meta.

Schwarzer, G., J. R. Carpenter, and G. Rucker (2015). *Meta-Analysis with R.* Springer.

Shuster, J. J., L. S. Jones, and D. A. Salmon (2007). Fixed vs random effects meta-analysis in rare event studies: the rosiglitazone link with myocardial infarction and cardiac death. *Statistics in Medicine 26(24)*, 4375–4385.

Shuster, J. J. and D. A. Schatz (2008). The rosigliazone meta-analysis: Lessons for the future. *Diabetes Care 31(3), March 2008*, 10.

Sidik, K. and J. N. Jonkman (2005a). A note on variance estimation in random effects meta-regression. *Journal of Biopharmaceutical Statistics 15*, 823–838.

Sidik, K. and J. N. Jonkman (2005b). Simple heterogeneity variance estimation for meta-analysis. *Journal of the Royal Statistical Society, Series C, 54*, 367–384.

Simmonds, M. C. and J. P. T. Higgins (2007). Covariate heterogeneity in meta-analysis: Criteria for deciding between meta-regression and individual patient data. *Statistics in Medicine 26*, 2982–2999.

Simmonds, M. C., J. P. T. Higgins, L. A. Stewartb, J. F. Tierneyb, M. J. Clarke, and S. G. Thompson (2005). Meta-analysis of individual patient data from randomized trials: a review of methods used in practice. *Clinical Trials 2*, 209–217.

Singh, K., M. Xie, and W. E. Strawderman (2005). Combining information from independent sources through confidence distribution. *Annals of Statistics 33*, 159–183.

Stata 16 manual (2019). *Stata meta-analysis reference manual release 16.* A Stata Press Publication, StataCorp LLC, College Station, Texas.

Sterne, J. A. C., D. Gavaghan, and M. Egger (2000). Publication and related bias in meta analysis: Power of statistical tests and prevalence in the literature. *Journal of Clinical Epidemiology, 53*, 1119–1129.

Sutton, A. J., N. J. Cooper, P. C. Lambert, D. R. Jones, K. R. Abrams, and M. J. Sweeting (2002). Meta-analysis of rare and adverse event data. *Expert Review of Pharmacoeconomics and Outcomes Research 2(4)*, 367–379.

Sutton, A. J. and J. P. T. Higgins (2008). Recent developments in meta-analysis. *Statistics in Medicine 27*, 625–650.

Sweeting, M. J., A. J. Sutton, and P. C. Lambert (2004). What to add to nothing? use and avoidance of continuity corrections in meta-analysis of sparse data. *Statistics in Medicine 23*, 1351–1375.

Thompson, S. G. and J. P. T. Higgins (2002). How should meta-regression analyses be undertaken and interpreted? *Statistics in Medicine 21(11)*, 1559–1573.

Thompson, S. G. and S. Sharp (1999). Explaining heterogeneity in meta-analysis: a comparison of methods. *Statistics in Medicine 18*, 2693–2708.

Tian, L., T. Cai, M. Pfeffer, N. Piankov, P. Cremieux, and L. Wei (2009). Exact and efficient inference procedure for meta-analysis and its application to the analysis of independent 2 by 2 tables with all available data but without artificial continuity correction. *Biostatistics 10(2)*, 275–281.

Tramer, M. R., D. J. Reynolds, R. A. Moore, and H. J. McQuay (1997). Impact of covert duplicate publication on meta-analysis: a case study. *BMJ, 315*, 635–640.

van Houwelingen, H. C., L. R. Arends, and T. Stijnen (2002). Tutorial in biostatistics: Advanced methods in meta-analysis: Multivariate approach and meta-regression. *Statistics in Medicine 21*, 589–624.

Viechtbauer, W. (2005). Bias and efficiency of meta-analytic variance estimators in the random-effects model. *Journal of Educational and Behavioral Statistics 30*, 261–293.

Viechtbauer, W. (2010). Conducting meta-analyses in R with the *metafor* package. *Journal of Statistical Software 36(1)*, 1–48.

Wang, J., C. Zhao, Z. C., X. Fan, Y. Lin, and Q. Jiang (2011). Tubeless vs standard percutaneous nephrolithotomy: a meta-analysis. *British Journal of Urology International 109*, 918–924.

Weisz, J. R., B. Weiss, S. S. Han, D. A. Granger, and T. Morton (1995). Effects of psychotherapy with children and adolescents revisited: a meta-analysis of treatment outcome studies. *Psychological Bulletin, 117*, 450–468.

West, S., V. King, T. S. Carey, K. N. Lohr, N. McKoy, S. F. Sutton, and L. Lux (2002). Systems to Rate the Strength of Scientific Evidence. Evidence Report/Technology Assessment No. 47 (Prepared by the Research Triangle

Institute-University of North Carolina Evidence-based Practice Center under Contract No. 290-97-0011). *In AHRQ Publication No. 02-E016. Rockville, MD: Agency for Healthcare Research and Quality*, 64–88.

Whitehead, A. (2003). *Meta-Analysis of Controlled Clinical Trials.* New York, NY:John Wiley & Sons, Inc.

Whitehead, A., A. J. Bailey, and D. Elbourne (1999). Combining summaries of binary outcomes with those of continuous outcomes in a meta-analysis. *Journal of Biopharmaceutical Statistics 9*(1), 1–16.

Xie, M. and K. Singh (2013). Confidence distribution, the frequentist distribution estimator of a parameter – a review. *International Statistical Review.*, In Press.

Xie, M., K. Singh, and W. E. Strawderman (2011). Confidence distributions and a unifying framework for meta-analysis. *Journal of the American Statistical Association 106*, 320–333.

Yusuf, S., R. Peto, J. Lewis, R. Collins, and P. Sleight (1985). Beta blockade during and after myocardial infarction: an overview of the randomized trials. *Progress in Cardiovascular Diseases 27*, 335–371.

Zeng, D. and D. Lin (2015). On random-effects meta-analysis. *Biometrika 102*(2), 281–294.

Index

Note: **Bold** page numbers refer to tables, *Italic* page numbers refer to figures.

Printed in the United States
by Baker & Taylor Publisher Services